Healthy Dining
in Orange County

Fifth Edition

Restaurant Nutrition Guide

Featuring Healthy Entrees from
Popular Orange County Restaurants

Including:

- ✓ **Calories**
- ✓ **Fat**
- ✓ **Cholesterol**
- ✓ **Sodium**

Diabetic Food Exchanges, Fruit & Vegetable Servings,
Protein, Carbohydrate & Fiber Information

by

Accents On Health, Inc.

Authors and Contributors:
Anita Jones-Mueller, M.P.H.
Esther Hill, Ph.D.
Susan Goldstein
Erica Bohm, M.S.
Nicole Quartuccio

Healthy Dining in Orange County

Fifth Edition

Restaurant Nutrition Guide

by

Accents On Health, Inc.

Authors and Contributors:

Anita Jones-Mueller, M.P.H., Esther Hill, Ph.D., Susan Goldstein, Erica Bohm, M.S., and Nicole Quartuccio

Published by:

Healthy Dining Publications
Accents On Health, Inc.
8305 Vickers Street, Suite 106
San Diego, CA 92111
(858) 541-2049
FAX (858) 541-0508
www.healthy-dining.com

Cover graphics by Andrew Curl, logo by Ramon Hutson, staff photos by Michael Ross, clip art by Microsoft.

 Published in U.S.A.

Library of Congress Cataloging in Publication Data
Jones, Anita
Healthy Dining in Orange County
1, Nutrition.
2, Diet.
3, Restaurant Food
91-71724
ISBN 1-879754-14-2

Table of Contents

About **Healthy Dining** and Accents On Health iv
Forward by The American Cancer Society vi
Preface by Dr. Donald Lyman, California Department of Health Services vii
A Message from Marilu Henner, author and actress viii
Healthy Dining Extravaganzas ix
People are Talking about **Healthy Dining** x
Disclaimer xii
Healthy Dining's Distinguished Advisory Board xiii
A Message from the **Healthy Dining** Team xviii

Part I Healthy Dining Tips: Realistic Guidelines and Practical Information 1
Introduction How to Use This Book 3
Chapter 1 Health, Lifestyle, Diet, Misconceptions & ... Dining Out 7
Chapter 2 Is Restaurant Food Fattening and Unhealthy? 12
Chapter 3 Do Your Calories Have a Purpose? 18
Chapter 4 Fat - How Much and What Type? 22
Chapter 5 Cholesterol - A Hot Topic 27
Chapter 6 Sodium - To Salt or Not to Salt? 31
Chapter 7 Protein, Carbohydrates & Diabetic Exchanges 34
Chapter 8 Fruits & Vegetables - Nutrition Heavyweights 37
Chapter 9 Additional Tips for Healthy Dining 42
Appendix Analysis Methods and Accuracy 44

Part II Healthy Dining Menus (arranged alphabetically) 45

Part III Chefs' Recipes 113

Part IV Health Resource Guide 171

Part V Other Editions of **Healthy Dining, Questionnaire & Order Form** 185
Healthy Dining in Los Angeles Participating Restaurants 186
Healthy Dining in San Diego Participating Restaurants 187
"Thank You" Notes to Restaurants 189
Questionnaire 191
Book Order Form with $5.00 Discount 192

Part VI Restaurant Coupons 193

Part VII Restaurant Indexes 215
Cuisine 216
Location 218
Alphabetical 222

About **Healthy Dining** and Accents On Health

Healthy Dining's team of highly qualified nutrition and health professionals is committed to an ambitious and exciting vision: to foster an ever-expanding trend toward healthier menu selections in restaurants. The **Healthy Dining** project began in San Diego in 1990 and expanded to Orange County and Los Angeles. The team has worked with hundreds of restaurants throughout Southern California and has analyzed over 10,000 menu items for nutrition content. No other company in the country matches Accents On Health's expertise in restaurant nutrition analysis.

Healthy Dining is earning respect from all corners -- health professionals, the media, the restaurant industry, and tens of thousands of consumers, many of whom write and call, expressing appreciation for the impact that **Healthy Dining** continues to make in Southern California. Accents On Health completed a 3-year landmark study/campaign called **TrEAT Yourself Well** which was funded by the California Department of Health Services, and has been honored by the California Dietetic Association with a Meritorious Service Award.

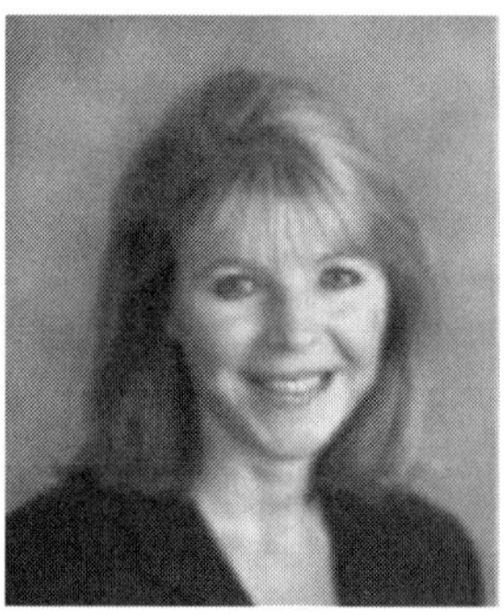

Anita Jones-Mueller, M.P.H. – Director

Anita earned her Master's Degree in Public Health from San Diego State University. Her background includes extensive work in the health and nutrition fields, both with individuals and with community group education and support sessions. Anita is one of the founders of the **Healthy Dining** program and the lead author of the book series. She has directed the **Healthy Dining** project from its inception into a growing community program, and was director of the **TrEAT Yourself Well** research study. Anita oversees the nutrition analysis, directs marketing and public relations, and speaks frequently to health professionals and community groups.

Esther Hill, Ph.D. – Editor/Publisher

Esther Hill, a physiologist with a Ph.D. in Biomathematics, worked for over 15 years in medical research at the University of California at San Diego. Dr. Hill's motivation for being involved in this project comes largely from dealing with her son's unstable diabetes. Her family found traveling and restaurant dining difficult and understands why nutrition information is so important to those with dietary restrictions. She is one of the founders of the **Healthy Dining** program and was Principal Investigator of the **TrEAT Yourself Well** research study. Currently she edits and publishes the **Healthy Dining** books.

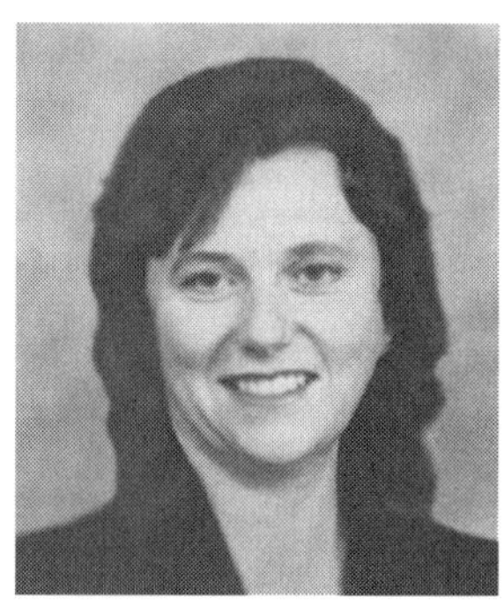

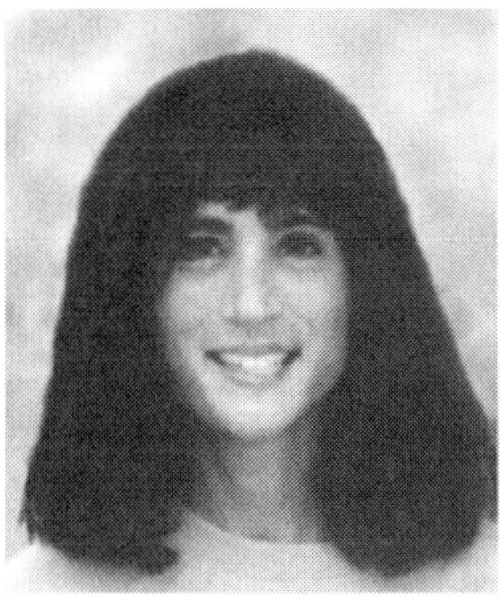

Susan Goldstein – Orange County Regional Director

Susan Goldstein earned her Bachelor of Science Degree with distinction in Human Development from Cornell University. Her background and knowledge in nutrition, health promotion, and fundraising combine over 15 years' professional and volunteer experience. She is also a Board Member of the Juvenile Diabetes Research Foundation, Orange County chapter. Susan works closely with the restaurants to develop the **Healthy Dining** books and expand participation in the community. She is involved in program promotion and projects with health professionals, local businesses, education and marketing, the media, and community events.

Erica Bohm, M.S. – San Diego Regional Director

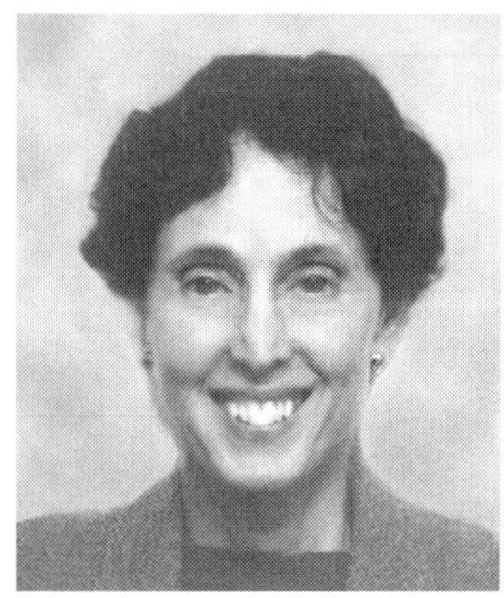

Erica Bohm earned her Master's Degree in Community Health Sciences from New York City's Hunter College. Her experience includes nutrition education, cholesterol reduction, weight control and smoking cessation. During her 20+ years in the health field, Erica has worked for the American Red Cross, the American Health Foundation, and other health organizations, research projects and businesses. Her roles in **Healthy Dining** include seminars, program promotion, and networking with restaurants, health professionals and organizations, community groups, businesses and the media. Erica was also Campaign Manager for the **TrEAT Yourself Well** study.

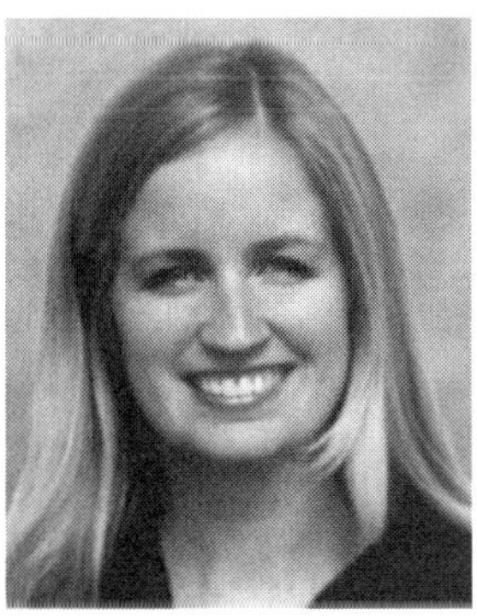

Nicole Quartuccio – Nutrition & Communications Manager

Nicole Quartuccio earned her Bachelor of Science Degree in Foods and Nutrition from San Diego State University and is currently a dietetic intern with Sodexho. She coordinates the nutrition analysis for the books, which includes working with the restaurant chefs and managers. Nicole also provides nutrition education for restaurant staff, assists with community events, publishing and book distribution, and manages **Healthy Dining's** e-mail newsletter and website, www.healthy-dining.com.

Acknowledgments

Healthy Dining wishes to thank Alia Tanous for volunteering her assistance. We also especially thank the participating restaurants and all health-conscious diners who support **Healthy Dining**. Thanks for your enthusiasm and best wishes for many years of healthy dining out!

For a majority of Americans who do not smoke, dietary choices and physical activity are the most important modifiable determinants of cancer risk. Evidence suggests that one third of all cancers deaths that occur in the United States each year can be attributed to poor diet and lack of physical activity.

The American Cancer Society publishes nutrition and physical activity guidelines to advise health care professionals and the general public about dietary and other lifestyle practices that can reduce cancer risk. Although no diet can guarantee full protection against any disease, these guidelines offer the best information currently available about how diet and physical activity can reduce the risk of cancer.

Studies have shown that populations whose diets are high in vegetables and fruits and low in animal fat, meat and/or calories have a reduced risk of some of the most common types of cancer. In addition to these individual actions, a recommendation for community action is also included in the guidelines. This recommendation underscores the importance of community measures to support healthy behaviors by increasing access to healthful food choices and opportunities to be physically active.

The Healthy Dining program educates people on how to make healthful choices and creates an environment that supports healthy food choices which is consistent with the American Cancer Society's Nutrition and Physical Activity Cancer Prevention Guidelines. Thank you to the restaurants participating in the program for providing healthy dining options.

Sincerely,

Georjean Stoodt, MD, MPH
President Elect & Chair
Mission Delivery Group
American Cancer Society

Diane J. Fink, MD
Chief Mission Delivery Officer
American Cancer Society
California Division, Inc.

The American Cancer Society Guidelines on Nutrition and Physical Activity for Cancer Prevention

1. Eat a variety of healthful foods with an emphasis on plant sources
2. Adopt a physically active lifestyle
3. Maintain a healthful weight throughout life
4. If you drink alcoholic beverages, limit consumption
5. Public, private and community organizations should work to create social and physical environments that support the adoption and maintenance of healthful nutrition and physical activity behaviors

California
Department of
Health Services

State of California—Health and Human Services Agency

Department of Health Services

ARNOLD SCHWARZENEGGER
Governor

January 29, 2004

Dear Fellow Californians,

We live in a great State! At the California Department of Health Services (CDHS), it is our mission to enhance the health of all Californians. In the past fifteen years, our State has realized a 66 percent decrease in the consumption of tobacco, translating into an impressive 10 percent decrease in cancer incidence, compared to a 1 percent decrease nationally. *That is a significant success for California.*

With this accomplishment, we are now transitioning the CDHS priorities and efforts to improving the nutritional status of Californians. An estimated 35,000 premature deaths and $24.6 billion in health care and related costs every year can be linked to poor diet and physical inactivity in our state. We are challenged to turn this situation around as we have with tobacco use.

With nutrition a priority, it is of utmost importance that Californians have access to healthy choices, whether at home, at work, or when eating out. I applaud the restaurants participating in ***Healthy Dining***. These restaurants are leading the nation in providing healthier cuisine. Whenever I am in Southern California, I look forward to using this ***Healthy Dining*** book to guide me to restaurants that offer healthy menu choices. This book makes it easy to enjoy great-tasting meals at popular restaurants.

Congratulations and best wishes in your efforts to lead a healthier lifestyle!

Sincerely,

Donald O. Lyman, MD, Chief
Chronic Disease and Injury Control

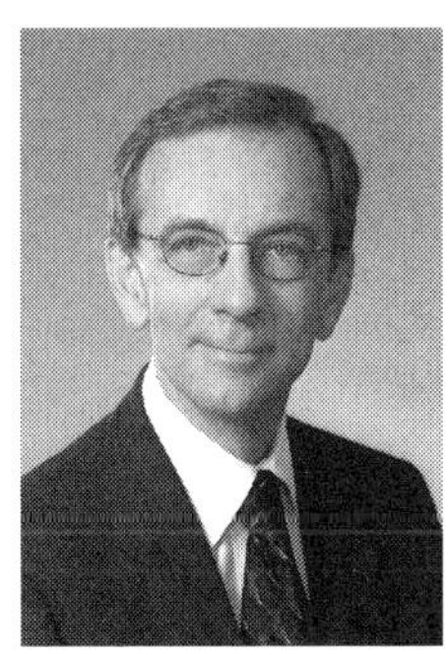

Division of Chronic Disease and Injury Control, MS 7200, P.O. Box 997413, Sacramento, CA 95899-7413
(916) 449-5700
Internet Address: www.dhs.ca.gov/cdic

A Message from Marilu Henner

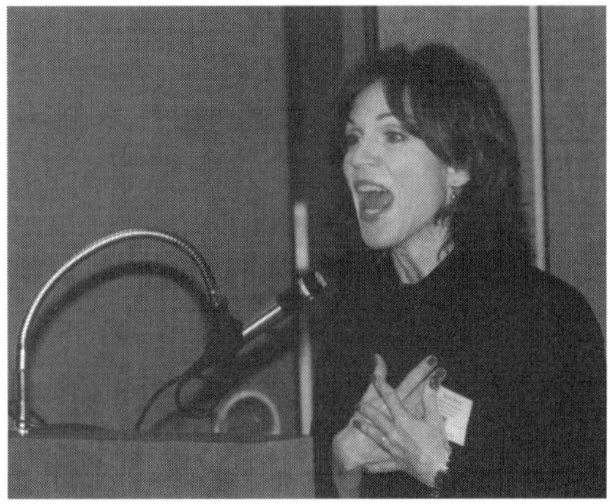

Marilu at the March 1, 2000 media launch of **Healthy Dining's TrEAT Yourself Well** *campaign.*

With good health, you can do it all. And without health, what do you really have? Health is the single most important factor in your life. It's the basis from which every aspect of your life stems. You can have all the money in the world, you can have all the power in the world, but if you do not have your health, you have nothing. You have been dealt a certain hand in life, and you have been given all the opportunity to play that hand the best you can. Disease doesn't discriminate.

Everything you need to live a longer, happier, healthier life is literally at your fingertips. And, **what you eat makes all the difference**! Whole, natural, high-quality foods will get -- and keep -- you in top form. Lots of fresh fruits and vegetables, whole grains and lean proteins will bring you health and vitality and add years to your life.

Congratulations to the chefs and restaurants participating in the ***Healthy Dining*** program. They truly have your health and tastebuds in mind. Enjoy the delicious dishes featured in this book. And, best wishes for a very happy, healthy and balanced life!

Sincerely,

Marilu Henner

"With good health you can do it all." And "do it all," she does. Marilu Henner is a celebrated television and film actress, best known for her role as Elaine Nardo on *Taxi* and her role opposite Burt Reynolds in *Evening Shade*. She recently starred in the smash Broadway musical *Chicago*. Marilu is the author of two *New York Times* best-selling nutrition books: *Total Health Makeover* and *30-Day Total Health Makeover*. She has just released a new recipe book called *The Total Health Kitchen*. Marilu is the mother of two young boys and is also the author of a parenting book, *I Refuse to Raise a Brat*.

Looking for a fun & delicious event for your company, organization, or conference?

The **Healthy Dining** Extravaganza

Combines 5 "ingredients:"

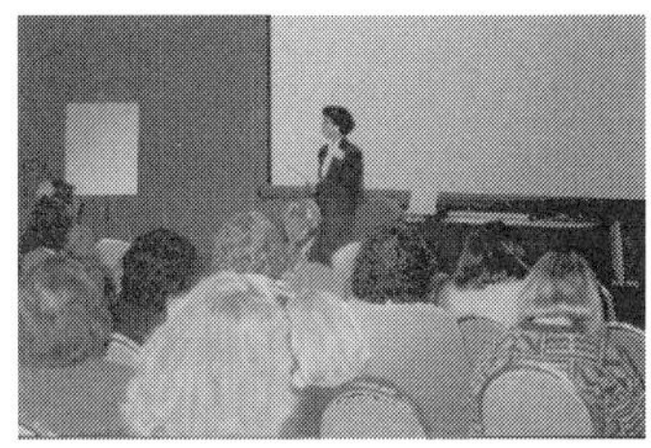

1. An illuminating, interactive seminar about restaurant dining and health;
2. Lunch or dinner featuring a tasting of **Healthy Dining** dishes from popular restaurants;

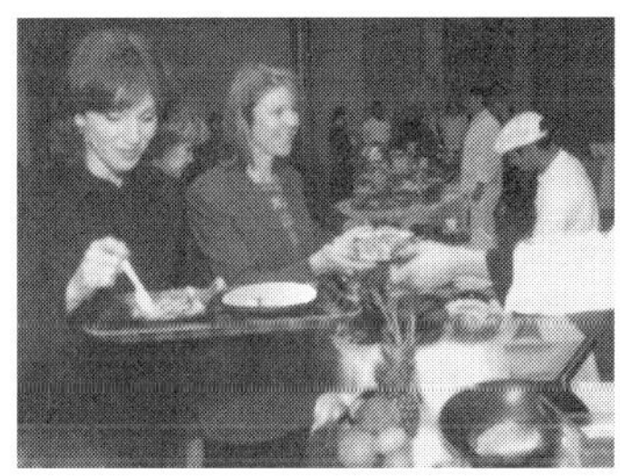

3. The book **Healthy Dining in Orange County** for each guest to keep (which can be labeled with your organization's name/logo);
4. A cooking demonstration by a professional chef featuring tips on preparing beautiful, healthy dishes;

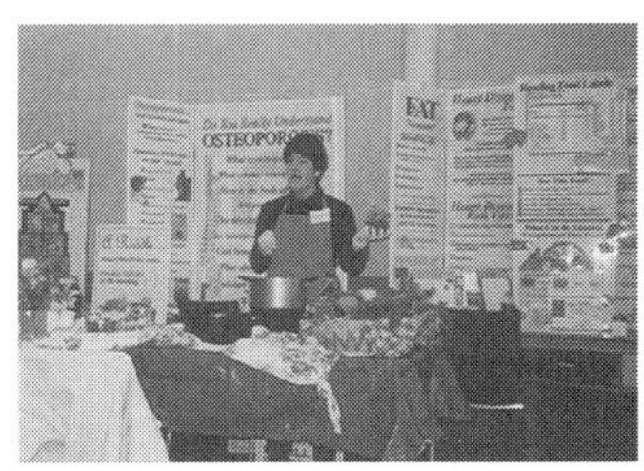

5. A drawing for a gift certificate to a **Healthy Dining** restaurant.

For more information or to schedule a program,
please call **Healthy Dining** at (800) 953- DINE (3463).

People Are Talking About Healthy Dining...

"All restaurants should offer consumers a real choice–one that also includes healthful selections– as part of every menu. This book is an invaluable resource for customers who want that choice."
– Marion Nestle, Ph.D., M.P.H., nutrition professor, author, speaker, researcher & policy advisor

"A road map gets you where you want to go when you travel. *Healthy Dining* does the same thing when you dine out and do not want to do yourself in."
– Annette Globits, R.D., nutrition education and counseling

"*Healthy Dining* has been a wonderful addition to the American Cancer Society's worksite wellness program, Active for Life. It is an excellent resource and we are delighted to be working with you."
– Florence L. Dann, Worksite Wellness Programs, American Cancer Society

"This is something very near and dear to my heart. I think every restaurant should have a *Healthy Dining* section on its menu."
– Tom Feltenstein, C.E.O., Feltenstein Partners; Chairman & Founder, Neighborhood Marketing Institute

"Thank you for the *Healthy Dining* book. My husband is very conscious about his diet, and I haven't been able to pry the book out of his hands yet. All I have to do now is convince him that it's healthier to eat at these restaurants than it is for me to cook!"
– Kathleen C. Peleti, C.P.A. and Healthy Dining customer

"Wonderful book! Wish I had several to showcase to other individuals...as mine is very dog-eared."
– County of Orange Commuter Club Member

"Patients love the coupons...keeps eating out enjoyable and fun. Also encourages patients to try new entrees and new restaurants."
– Paula Partch, M.S., R.D., C.D.E., St. Joseph Heritage Healthcare

"*Healthy Dining* makes it possible for us to find restaurants serving a variety of styles, including our favorite ethnic foods, staying within the guidelines my diabetes requires. This is the best book on healthy dining I've read. Without it, I'd never eat out!"
– Joan W. Derrick, Healthy Dining customer

"I love this book! In the perpetual battle of the bulge, it arms me with the knowledge to finally win the war."
– Rieva Lesonsky, Senior Vice President/Editorial Director, Entrepreneur Magazine

People Are Talking About Healthy Dining...

"I've discovered new favorite restaurants because of your book."
– Marilyn Biggica, Community College Foods & Nutrition Instructor

"I'm proud and honored to be a part of *Healthy Dining* which has been a terrific organization... [it] has made a difference in getting the word out to our guests, as well as educating the rest of the industry about better dining choices. Thank you for filling such a huge void."
– Steve Karfaridis, Director of Operations, Wahoo's Fish Taco

"The American Heart Association applauds the participating restaurants for accommodating today's customer, the customer that cares about good health."
– Patricia Lozada-Santone, M.P.H., American Heart Association volunteer

"It's so exciting that *Healthy Dining* is available! It helps people realize that they can enjoy eating out and being healthy. Having a good time while doing what's good for them is doubly reinforcing! I love recommending it to my clients!"
– Ali Chambers, M.A., lifestyle educator, Kaiser Permanente

"I encourage patients to use the book whenever they dine out. It's great that there is finally a 'nutrition label' for restaurant dining. That's exactly what Healthy Dining provides for health-conscious Americans."
- Mary Felando, M.S., R.D., Cardiac Rehab Nutritionist

"What a great book. Will buy one for my sister's birthday today! Thank you for being there. This is great inspiration."
– American Cancer Society "Active for Life" participant

"What you eat makes all the difference! Lots of fresh fruits and vegetables, whole grains and lean proteins will bring you health and vitality and add years to your life. Congratulations to the chefs and restaurants participating in the *Healthy Dining* program. They truly have your health and tastebuds in mind."
– Marilu Henner, nutrition author and television, film & stage actress

"The restaurants are fabulous! We're so delighted to be partnering with *Healthy Dining* and a very, very informative book. You shouldn't leave home without it."
– Babette Hubert, R.N., Manager of Heart Center Program Development, St. Joseph Hospital

Disclaimer:

The purpose of this book is to provide nutrition information for selected menu items from restaurants that have chosen to participate in the **Healthy Dining** program. Please note that the items listed in this book are not necessarily appropriate or healthful for all individuals. Some people need to be more careful about certain items such as salt or sugar, or have food allergies which put additional restrictions on their food choices. Each individual is responsible, in cooperation with his or her physician, dietitian or other health consultant, for making personal dietary decisions. We have not included all the restaurants that serve healthy food, nor are we recommending all entrees from restaurants that are included in this book.

It is also important to note that the numerical values for the nutrition information included in this book are approximations only, and that the categories "Good Choice" and "Excellent Choice" give a better overall indication of the nutrition content of the menu items.

The nutrition information provided is based on the United States Department of Agriculture (USDA) nutrition information database, the source most commonly used for estimating nutritional content of foods. Generally participating restaurants supplied their recipes for the computerized analysis (a few provided the nutrition analysis which had been performed elsewhere). Analyses by **Healthy Dining** were completed using the Nutritionist IV and ESHA Food Processor computer programs. If values for recipe ingredients were not available from the USDA database, the manufacturer was contacted for the nutrition information. If the manufacturer did not have nutrition information, ingredients were closely matched to a similar product's nutrition information. Data were rounded as follows: for calories, cholesterol and sodium, to the nearest 5 mg; for fat, protein, carbohydrates and fiber, to the nearest whole number; and for diabetic exchanges to the nearest ¼ exchange.

All information contained in this book has been carefully compiled and reviewed by qualified health professionals. Nutrition information is based on recipes supplied by the restaurants. Participating restaurants have agreed to prepare food according to the recipes submitted for a period of one year, or to clearly notify customers otherwise.

The authors are not responsible for maintaining quality control over the food that is prepared by the restaurants. The restaurants are ultimately responsible for the quality of the food they serve.

Healthy Dining's Distinguished Advisory Board

The following individuals serve on **Healthy Dining**'s Advisory Board. Each advisor completes a review of one of our publications – the San Diego, Orange County, or Los Angeles edition – and provides feedback and suggestions. The **Healthy Dining** team is proud, honored, and fortunate to gain the input of such a distinguished group. We thank every Advisory Board member for his or her commitment to this important community health program.

Margot J. Aiken, MD, FRCPC, FACE. Dr. Aiken is a board certified internist and endocrinologist in clinical practice with Scripps Health and XIMED Medical Group. Dr. Aiken is involved in education programs and professional societies related to infertility, menopause and endocrinology. She is a member of numerous professional organizations including The Am. Assoc. of Clinical Endocrinology, The Am. Soc. of Reproductive Medicine, The Pacific Coast Reproductive and Endocrine Society and The International. Menopause Society.

Robert Ashley, Host, Fox News Radio Talk Show, "Eat This! America's Radio Kitchen with Chef Robert Ashley." Chef Robert was formerly Director of Nutrition Services and Executive Chef at the exclusive University of California San Diego Medical Center's Thornton Hospital in La Jolla, California. He has cooked for numerous heads of state, royalty and celebrities throughout the world. With travels to 102 different countries, Chef Robert has won national and international acclaim by using ingredients indigenous to regional food creations with an emphasis on improving the nutritional profile of these international cuisines. He has hosted television programs, radio programs and lectured around the world on the benefits of his internationally acclaimed, tasty and nutritious world cuisine.

Marilyn Biggica, Instructor of Foods & Nutrition, San Diego Community College. Marilyn teaches low-fat cooking at San Diego Community College and is active in the Community College District, where she serves on the Curriculum Council and Advisory Committee. Marilyn is an active member of the International Association of Cooking Professionals. She also advises restaurants about healthier alternatives on their menus, and teaches that healthy food can taste good, as reflected in her cookbook *"101 Ways to Eat for Health and Pleasure."*

Mary Donkersloot, RD, Nutrition Therapist. Mary is a Beverly Hills-based consulting nutritionist who treats clients dealing with diabetes, weight control, eating disorders, and fitness and nutrition issues. She is the author of *The Simply Gourmet Diabetes Cookbook* and *Fast-Food Diet, Quick and Healthy Eating.* Mary is also the nutrition consultant for numerous national food corporations.

Lisa Dougherty, Owner of Whole Body Fitness in Costa Mesa and Past President, Nutrition and Fitness Council of Orange County Inc. Lisa has an extensive background in nutrition and fitness. She graduated from the Fitness Instructor Program at UC Irvine, and is a certified ACE personal trainer and Lifestyle and Weight Management Consultant. She has designed a unique 6-week lifestyle weight management program with a focus on daily physical activity and weekly goal setting. You can learn more about all of Lisa's services or sign up for her newsletter at www.wholebodyfitness.biz.

Karen C. Duester, MS, RD, President, Food Consulting Company. Karen has been providing nutrition analysis, food nutrition facts labels, food labeling content, and foods labels regulatory expertise to food companies and restaurant owners since she founded Food Consulting Company in 1993. The company has grown substantially since its beginning and has now served over 1,000 clients across America and around the globe.

Judith Ewing, Adult Education Instructor, San Diego Community College District. With a Bachelor's degree in Home Economics, Judith is involved in a variety of projects and programs related to health. For the past 27 years, she has been an Instructor at the San Diego Community College, where she teaches cooking classes. Judy is an adjunct faculty member of Pt. Loma Nazarene University, and also does appliance demonstrations.

Mary Felando, MS, RD, Cardiac Rehab Dietitian, Cedars-Sinai Medical Center, Los Angeles. With a Master's degree in Human Nutrition from Cornell University, Mary has worked in the nutrition field for 25 years. Currently employed as a cardiovascular nutrition specialist at Cedars-Sinai Medical Center in Los Angeles, she is responsible for the development and implementation of the nutrition component of one of the largest cardiac rehabilitation programs in the country.

Gail C. Frank, DrPH, RD, CHES, Professor of Nutrition, Cal. State University Long Beach. Gail has been active in the fields of nutrition and health for over 30 years. Along with directing many programs at Cal State Univ. Long Beach, Gail is an Adjunct Professor of Primary Care and Internal Medicine at Univ. of Cal., Irvine, and Co-Principal Investigator for the Women's Health Initiative. She is active in several professional organizations, and has served as the Media Spokesperson for the American Dietetic Association for 17 years. Gail has had over 700 media interviews including the *LA Times, Orange County Register*, CNN, NPR, "Dateline NBC," KABC, *US News & World Report* and *USA Today*.

Linda Gigliotti, MS, RD, CDE, Program Director, University of California Irvine, Weight Management Program. Linda is a registered dietitian with a degree in education and extensive experience in outpatient and community education. Her expertise is in weight management and lifestyle modification, working with clients to make choices to manage their health. She is a certified diabetes educator and has received certification from the American Dietetic Association in both adult and childhood and adolescent weight management.

Robyn L. Goldberg, R.D., Private Practice. Robyn began her career at Cedars-Sinai Medical Center in Los Angeles as the inpatient dietitian in the Department of Cardiology. She currently has her own private practice in Beverly Hills, CA, where she specializes in medical conditions, disordered eating, preventative nutrition and athletes maximizing optimal nutrition. Robyn promotes opportunity to excel in personal health and fitness maintenance through a lecture series in association with several medical groups. She serves as a Nutrition Consultant for the Celiac Disease Foundation, and is the nutritionist for the Susan Krevoy Eating Disorders Program.

De'Anna Gullotta, Mrs. California, United States 2002-2003; Mrs. Southern California, America 2003-2004. De'Anna is the community spokesperson for the Ronald McDonald house and works with The Special Olympics. She does public speaking on healthy food choices, volunteerism and breast cancer awareness. De'Anna is also a part-time model and voiceover artist and was previously a stuntwoman and actress for a variety of television shows.

Michelle Heilpern, Managing Partner, The Center for Health Enhancement. Michelle has over 20 years of professional experience in marketing, strategic planning and fundraising in the health care field. She is currently co-owner and managing partner at The Center for Health Enhancement at Saint John's Health Center in Santa Monica, California, which offers a wide range of preventative, integrative and alternative medicine services.

Greg Hernandez, Executive Director, Lifestyles Health & Fitness Consulting. Greg is an ACE Gold Certified Clinical Exercise Specialist in practice for 7 years and has provided health, fitness and nutrition services for several Southern California hospitals, medical groups, companies, and individuals. He is also a former president and current board member of the Orange County Wellness Coalition and owner of Salsa Swing Connection Dance Studio in Costa Mesa, CA. With a commitment to motivating the "inactive" population to adopting a healthy lifestyle, he has worked to develop new programs for the American Cancer Society, American Diabetes Association, and the American Heart Association.

Steve Karfaridis, Director of Operations, Wahoo's Fish Taco. Steve was born and raised on the coast of Northern Greece and immigrated to the US, where he earned a Bachelor's Degree in Business Administration and Molecular Biology. He has been involved in the restaurant industry for the better part of the last 30 years as a line cook, server, chef, general manager and consultant. He has been with Wahoo's Fish Taco for over 12 years, where he was promoted to district manager and then partner and Director of Operations, helping the company to grow from two locations to 23 in two states. He enjoys being part of the drive to provide restaurant guests with healthier, fresher, better dining choices.

Kay Kimball, RN, MSN, OCN. Coordinator, Cancer Resource Centers/Patient Education & Support Services, Palomar Pomorado Health. Kay is an oncology certified nurse. She maintains the Cancer Resource Centers at Palomar Medical Center and Pomerado Hospital in North San Diego County. Through these centers she coordinates patient education classes addressing the prevention, detection, diagnosis and treatment of cancer. Information on nutrition is always offered as part of an 8-week I Can Cope program presented 3 times yearly and co-sponsored by Palomar Pomerado Health and the American Cancer Society.

Jeffrey Krebs, MD, FACP. Dr. Krebs has been practicing Internal Medicine in San Diego County since 1989. He is an Associate Clinical Professor of Medicine at the UCSD School of Medicine. Dr. Krebs has served on the Council of the San Diego County Medical Society and is past Chair of the California Medical Association's Young Physician Section. As a former competitive athlete, Dr. Krebs has always had an interest in nutrition.

Rieva Lesonsky, Senior Vice President/Editorial Director, Entrepreneur Media, Inc. Rieva has over 20 years experience at Entrepreneur Media, currently serving as SVP/Editorial Director of *Entrepreneur* and *Business Start-Ups* magazines. Rieva served on the Small Business Administration's (SBA) National Advisory Council from 1994 - 2000. The SBA has also honored her as a Small Business Media Advocate and a Woman in Business Advocate. For five years, Business News Reporter has named her one of the Top 100 Most Influential Journalists.

Phyllis Ann Marshall, FCSI, President, FoodPower, Inc. Phyllis is a foodservice industry consultant specializing in concept development and strategic plans to increase sales and profits of restaurants. She holds a B.A. degree from Cornell University and has extensive experience in the areas of market positioning, menu development, merchandising and four-walls marketing. Phyllis develops growth strategies with an eye to adding new profit centers and establishing brands. She assists shopping centers with the development of new food service and the retrofitting of existing properties in order to create destination restaurant locations.

April Morgan, VP of Sports and Fitness, The Sports Club Company. April has over 20 years experience in the fitness industry and holds a Bachelor's degree in Commercial Recreation. In her current position, she oversees all member programs such as private training, group exercise, nutrition, sports and children's programs for The Sports Club Company which operates upscale health and fitness clubs throughout the country under The Sports Club/LA name.

Marion Nestle, PhD, MPH, Professor and Chair, Dept. Nutrition, Food Studies & Public Health, NY University. Dr. Nestle received her Ph.D. in molecular biology and M.P.H. in public health nutrition from UC Berkeley, and has since been on the faculty at Brandeis University, UC San Francisco School of Medicine, and NY University. She has served as advisor in the Department of Health and Human Services and as a member of the FDA Food Advisory Committee and Science Board, the USDA/DHHS 1995 Dietary Guidelines Advisory Committee, and American Cancer Society committees that issue dietary guidelines for cancer prevention. Her research focuses on analysis of the scientific, social, cultural, and economic factors that influence dietary recommendations and practices. She is the author of *Food Politics: How the Food Industry Influences Nutrition and Health* (2002).

Paula Partch, MS, RD, CDE, Health Educator, St. Joseph Heritage Healthcare. Paula received a BS degree in Dietetics from UC Davis and a Masters degree in Nutrition from the University of Arizona. She has worked in the field of dietetics for over 25 years. Her health educator role focuses on nutrition counseling in the areas of diabetes, gestational diabetes, weight management, and cardiovascular health. She values the behavior changes her clients need to incorporate to support healthy eating and finds the *Healthy Dining* publication a valuable tool to be used.

Victoria Pepper, MS, RD, Marketing & Promotions Coordinator, Kaiser Permanente Preventive Medicine. Victoria has worked for Kaiser Permanente's Positive Choice Wellness Center since 1987. She teaches nutrition and weight management for the wellness center. In addition, she coordinates the marketing and promotion for the Department of Preventive Medicine, which includes the Positive Choice Wellness Center and Health Appraisal.

Diane Powers, Owner, Bazaar del Mundo. Diane is the founder, owner and operator of Bazaar del Mundo, the landmark San Diego tourist destination which includes 5 restaurants and helps attract over 7 million visitors to Old Town State Historic Park each year. She received the "Entrepreneur of the Year" Award from the California Travel Industry Association and the "San Diego Woman of Achievement" Award from the League of Women Voters, along with numerous honors for her achievements in design, recycling/environment, marketing and management.

Elyse Resch, MS, RD, FADA, Nutrition Therapist. Elyse is a Fellow of the American Dietetic Association and has been in private practice in Beverly Hills for over 21 years, specializing in eating disorders, intuitive eating and preventative nutrition. She is the co-author of "Intuitive Eating" (St. Martin's Press 1995, 2003) and does regular speaking engagements. She is a certified child and adolescent obesity expert and was the treatment team nutritionist on the Eating Disorder Unit at Beverly Hills Medical Center. She participates in a variety of organizations and activities including the Sports, Cardiovascular and Wellness Nutrition Practice Group of the American Dietetic Association, The International Association of Eating Disorder Professionals, and National Association of Anorexia Nervosa and Associated Disorders.

Joan W. Rupp, MS, RD, Director, Project LEAN (Leaders Encouraging Activity & Nutrition) and Assistant Clinical Professor, University of California San Diego. Joan is an Assistant Clinical Professor in the Department of Family and Preventative Medicine at the University of California San Diego and a Lecturer in the Department of Exercise and Nutritional Sciences at San Diego State University. She is also the Director of the Southern Coast Region of Project LEAN, a state-wide nutrition education program involving restaurants, chefs, grocery stores, schools and the media promoting the healthy eating message. Ms. Rupp also directs the San Diego Nutrition Network, a partnership of over 60 agencies working to improve the health of San Diego residents.

John Ryan, General Manager, Walt's Wharf Restaurant. John has been in the food industry business for over 20 years. He is a firm believer in healthy dining and its counterpart, physical fitness. His position at Walt's Wharf has been a perfect fit, with a menu emphasizing freshness and healthy choices. John, wife Dana and two sons have many fitness accomplishments that currently include swimming and triathlon competition.

Mary Ryzner, MS, RD, Clinical Dietitian, Palomar Medical Center. Since receiving her Master's Degree in Nutrition in 1988 from California State University, Northridge, Mary has worked as a Clinical Dietitian for various hospitals and care centers. Mary is active in the San Diego Dietetic Association and is the event coordinator for the Nutrition Fuels Fitness 5K/10K Run/Walk. She has her own business specializing in weight regulation, and is also the team coordinator for the San Diego Track Club Masters Women's team.

Jamie Steele, President & Fitness Director, Steele Bodies. Jamie has been in the health and fitness industry for over 20 years. His company, Steele Bodies, a personalized fitness, wellness and nutrition program, specializes in high-intensity training principles. Jamie has owned and operated 10 health and fitness facilities in California and Arizona and worked in upper level management and business development for a large California health and fitness chain.

Michel Stroot, Executive Chef, The Golden Door Spa. As Executive Chef of the renowned Golden Door spa, Michel Stroot is expert at making cuisine both healthy and delicious. His book, *The Golden Door Cookbook*, received special praise from *Vogue Magazine*, CNN, CBS and The Today Show. It also received a James Beard Foundation Award nomination, making him the first spa chef to be so honored. His third and latest cookbook, published in 2003, is *The Golden Door Cooks Light and Easy*. Chef Stroot combines fresh ingredients from The Golden Door's on-site organic gardens with French style cooking to achieve "tantalizing and singularly inspiring creations," according to the *New York Times*. *InStyle* magazine says, "If The Golden Door is the mother of American luxury spas, its Chef, Michel Stroot, must be spa cuisine's favorite son."

Steve Sweeney, Director of Marketing, The Old Spaghetti Factory Restaurants. Steve has a BA degree from the University of San Francisco and a Master of Business Administration from the University of Oregon. He joined The Old Spaghetti Factory in 1980 as a waiter and bartender, and then worked through management positions to eventually become the Director of Marketing for the entire corporation in 1996. His current responsibilities include menu development and printing, beverage purchasing, marketing, managing advertising agencies and printing vendors, creating advertising and promotions, and planning of advertising.

Christopher Trela, Journalist, OC Metro Magazine/"Metro Menus". Christopher is the restaurant writer for Metro Menus and the theatre critic for the OC Metro Magazine. He also writes a Health & Fitness column for the OC Metro Magazine, and is a freelance writer and photographer for many local magazines, a public relations consultant, and the President and owner of Paradise West Creative Services.

Evelyn Tribole, MS, RD, Nutritionist for LifetimeTV.com. Evelyn is an award-winning registered dietitian, with a nutrition counseling practice in Irvine, CA. She has written six books including the million-copy bestseller *Healthy Homestyle Cooking* and *Intuitive Eating* (co-author). She is currently the nutritionist for LifetimeTV.com and was contributing editor for *Shape* magazine where her monthly column, *Recipe Makeovers*, appeared for 11 years. Tribole was the nutrition expert for Good Morning America and was a national spokesperson for the American Dietetic Association for 6 years.

Bruce Vancil, Director, American Cancer Society's Orange County Region. Bruce has worked for ACS since 1982 in social work, patient counseling, ethnic outreach, legislative advocacy, research promotion, and related activities. He serves on many community-based coalitions, including the Orange County Breast Cancer Coalition (currently president), the Breast Cancer Detection Partnership, Cancer Genetics Research Advisory Board, Tobacco Use Prevention Coalition, Nutrition Alert Coalition, and a committee advising use of tobacco settlement funds. He is also the So. Calif. Chapter President of the Steamship Historical Society of America, a member of the group's National Board of Directors, and an avid fan of the Queen Mary and other old steamships.

Terry Zierenberg, BS, RN, CDE, Education Manager, Marketing Dept. at Medtronic MiniMed. Terry has spent many years educating health care professionals, patients and the community about diabetes. Previously, she was a Diabetes Nurse Clinician for the Diabetes Treatment Centers of America, Tarzana, Ca. and the Program Coordinator for the Diabetes Care Center at Encino-Tarzana Regional Medical Center. Her affiliations include the American Association of Diabetes Educators, the American Diabetes Association and the Juvenile Diabetes Research Foundation.

A Message from the Healthy Dining Team

Welcome to the **Healthy Dining** "family." This program has grown from San Diego to Orange County to Los Angeles. More than 2000 individuals have participated in this effort, including restaurant chefs and management, health professionals, and members of community organizations. You, the **Healthy Dining** reader and restaurant diner, are also an essential "ingredient."

Why? Because restaurants are responsive to their customers. They need to hear from you that health-conscious menu items and nutrition information are important to you.

Here's how you can help **Healthy Dining** grow in your community:

1. Dine at the restaurants listed in the book and tell the restaurant staff and owners that you appreciate and value their participation in **Healthy Dining**.
2. Request the **Healthy Dining** menus at participating restaurants and use the discount coupons.
3. Tell friends, family and business associates about **Healthy Dining**.
4. Tell other restaurants about **Healthy Dining** and recommend that they participate next year.
5. Give **Healthy Dining** books as gifts for birthdays, holidays, incentives, client or staff appreciation, etc.
6. Use **Healthy Dining** as a fund-raiser or for health education/fairs/events (call for information).
7. Use **Healthy Dining** restaurants for your catering and party needs.
8. Invite **Healthy Dining** authors to speak for your organization or conference (see page ix).
9. Visit our website (www.healthy-dining.com) to stay up-to-date on health and restaurant news and events and to register for your free e-newsletter, "Cuisine Connection."
10. Please call or e-mail us with suggestions and feedback: (800) 953-DINE (3463), or books@healthy-dining.com.

Thanks! Together we can make Southern California a healthier place to live and dine.

Part I

Healthy Dining Tips

Realistic Guidelines and Practical Information

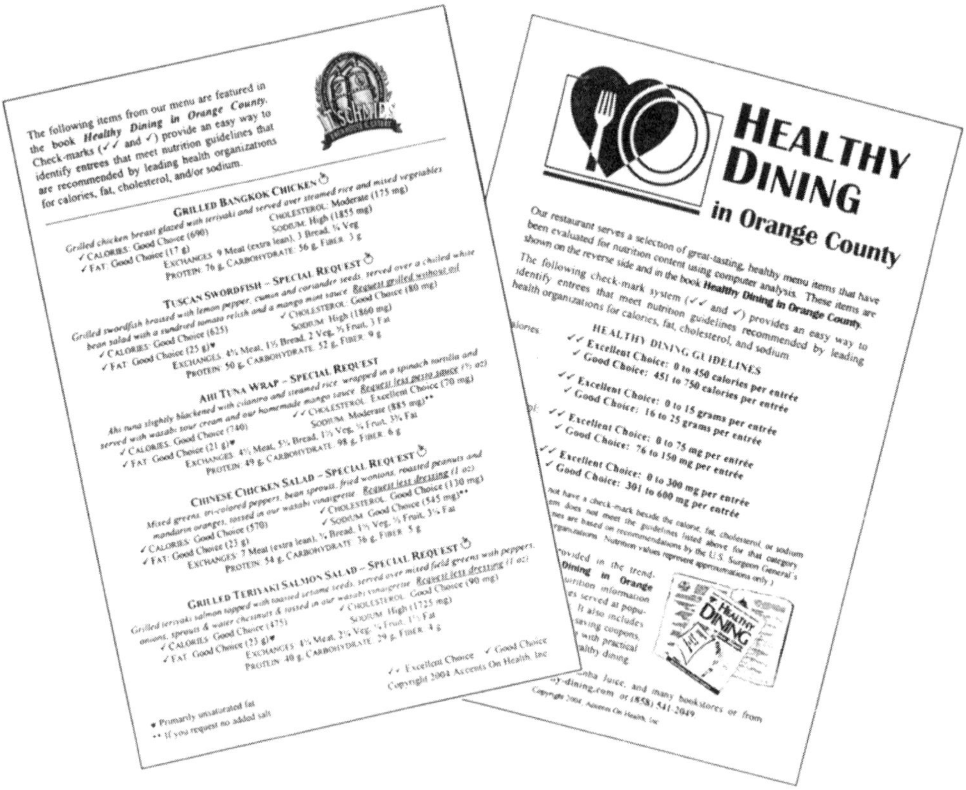

Healthy Dining menus available at participating restaurants for customer convenience.

The **Healthy Dining** menus illustrated above are condensed versions of the menu pages in your book. We encourage all the restaurants to pass out their **Healthy Dining** menus along with their regular menus. Some restaurants, however, don't automatically provide them - *you need to request these special menus*. And please do! The more that restaurants hear customers asking for specific nutrition information and ordering "Special Requests," the more they will recognize how important healthy dining is to many people.

If nutrition information is important to you, if you want to have the choice to "order healthy," please request **Healthy Dining** menus in the restaurants and let them know that you appreciate the healthy menu choices.

How to Use This Book

This introduction summarizes how to interpret the nutrition information for the restaurant menu items. Part I provides more in-depth information to help you become better informed about health and restaurant dining. Part II features nutrition profiles for specific entrees at participating restaurants at over 350 locations in Orange County. Part III presents a wonderful selection of Chefs' Recipes and Part IV includes a Health Resource Guide. Part V contains a list of other **Healthy Dining** books, Thank You Notes to give to restaurants, a Questionnaire, and a Book Order Form. Part VI contains over $350 in Restaurant Discount Coupons, and finally, Part VII contains three Restaurant Indexes for quick reference.

The Check Mark System – An easy way to find entrees to fit your goals

The nutrition profiles of restaurant meals vary widely. For this book, we strived to feature dishes that are low in fat, cholesterol, calories and sodium and contain fruits and/or vegetables. Not all of the dishes included in the book, however, meet <u>all</u> of these criteria. The check mark system described below will help you easily and quickly identify which entrees best fit your individual dietary goals. Also, be sure to look for the ♥ and 🍎 symbols, which identify items that contain primarily unsaturated fat and at least two servings of fruits and/or vegetables, respectively.

Nutritional guidelines are difficult to set because each individual has different nutritional needs. For example, caloric needs vary according to age, gender, activity level, body weight and health goals (e.g., reducing body fat, lowering cholesterol, etc.). Nevertheless, the following are general guidelines to make the menu information easy to interpret. These guidelines are based on recommendations by the U.S. Surgeon General's Office and the American Heart Association. Details about how the values were developed are included in Chapters 3 through 6, but here's a quick summary of the check mark meanings:

<u>ENTREE GUIDELINES</u>

Calories	✓✓	Excellent Choice = 0 to 450 calories/entree
	✓	Good Choice = 451 to 750 calories/entree
Fat	✓✓	Excellent Choice = 0 to 15 grams (g)/entree
	✓	Good Choice = 16 to 25 grams (g)/entree
Cholesterol	✓✓	Excellent Choice = 0 to 75 milligrams (mg)/entree
	✓	Good Choice = 76 to 150 milligrams (mg)/entree
Sodium	✓✓	Excellent Choice = 0 to 300 milligrams (mg)/entree
	✓	Good Choice = 301 to 600 milligrams (mg)/entree

It's important to note...

Although some individuals prefer stricter criteria for their meal guidelines (especially people on very low-fat or low-sodium diets), the **Healthy Dining** guidelines represent fairly high standards for restaurant entrees and are realistic goals for most diners, as discussed in Chapters 3 through 6.

We occasionally include a menu item that is described as "moderate" or "high" in one of the nutrient categories because it does not fit within our "Excellent Choice" or even "Good Choice" guidelines. "High" indicates that the nutrient contains more than double the amount of a "Good Choice" (or for sodium over 1,000 mg). For example, an item that is considered "high" in cholesterol would have to contain over 300 mg, of cholesterol since a "Good Choice" can contain 76 to 150 mg. Finally, "moderate" means the nutrient value falls somewhere between a "Good Choice" and "high."

The **Healthy Dining** guidelines are general guidelines developed for the general public. You, your physician and your dietitian are responsible for setting individual nutritional guidelines according to your particular health needs. **Please note also that the numerical values for the nutrition information are approximations only, based on recipes supplied by the restaurants**.

If you are health-conscious and looking for better ways to eat and enhance your overall health, this book will provide an easy way to choose entrees that don't have the hidden calories, fat, cholesterol and sodium you'd rather avoid.

- If you want to lose weight, select items listed as Excellent Choice (✓✓) or Good Choice (✓) in the calorie and fat categories. For more information, see Chapters 3 and 4.
- If you want to reduce your blood cholesterol level, choose from items that are listed as Excellent Choice (✓✓) or Good Choice (✓) for both cholesterol and fat (see Chapter 5).
- To reduce dietary sodium, select those menu items that are shown as Excellent Choice (✓✓) or Good Choice (✓) in sodium, and request no added salt (see Chapter 6).
- If you have diabetes, the "Exchanges" (i.e., Diabetic Exchanges used by the American Diabetes Association) are particularly useful, along with values for carbohydrate and protein. For more details, see Chapter 7.

If your physician or dietitian has given you daily limits in terms of sodium, cholesterol, etc., by all means note the numerical values as well as the check marks, and be sure they fit your restrictions. You may need to ask for additional modifications to your meal.

We've included brief entree descriptions, but they are not complete ingredient lists. Therefore, if you have food allergies or sensitivities, be sure to emphasize this to the restaurant personnel so they will understand how important it is to prepare your meal according to your specifications.

Comments about serving sizes, dressings and sauces, and side dishes

The nutrition information published in this book is based on the FULL SERVING (unless stated otherwise). Restaurant portions are frequently large, so you may not want to eat the full serving. If you eat only ⅔ of the entree, you're only consuming ⅔ of the calories, fat, cholesterol, sodium, etc.

In some cases the nutrition analysis includes dressings or sauces, and in other cases it does not. We generally recommend that you order sauces and dressings on the side and use them sparingly. Dressings and sauces usually contain 5 to 10 grams of fat (45 to 90 calories) per tablespoon.

Depending on your goals, you may choose to completely avoid them, or order them on the side and limit the amount you use. You will likely be served more than one tablespoon, so don't assume you can pour it all on your meal. You can measure out the amount you want using your teaspoon, keeping in mind that 3 teaspoons (tsp.) are equivalent to one tablespoon (Tbs.) or ½ ounce (oz).

The check mark system and guidelines listed on the previous page apply to main entrees only. The calorie, fat, cholesterol and sodium guidelines for side dishes, appetizers, and desserts are equal to ⅓ of the entree guidelines. Other items, such as breads, are not generally shown because the nutrition values are fairly standard.

GUIDELINES for SIDE DISHES, APPETIZERS & DESSERTS †

Calories	✓✓ Excellent Choice = 0 to 150 calories/serving
	✓ Good Choice = 151 to 250 calories/serving
Fat	✓✓ Excellent Choice = 0 to 5 grams (g)/serving
	✓ Good Choice = 6 to 8 grams (g)/serving
Cholesterol	✓✓ Excellent Choice = 0 to 25 milligrams (mg)/serving
	✓ Good Choice = 26 to 50 milligrams (mg)/serving
Sodium	✓✓ Excellent Choice = 0 to 100 milligrams (mg)/serving
	✓ Good Choice = 101 to 200 milligrams (mg)/serving

Footnotes and other symbols

† Side dish guidelines are ⅓ of Entree Guidelines
♥ Primarily unsaturated fat (see Chapter 4)
** If you request no added salt (see Chapter 6)
at least 2 fruit/vegetable servings (see Chapter 8)

At the end of each restaurant's introductory paragraph, a price range symbol appears:

$	Average entree under $10
$$	Average entree $10 to $20
$$$	Average entree over $20

How are restaurants selected to be included in **Healthy Dining?**

Our goal is to include a wide variety of restaurants. We do not specifically look for restaurants that specialize in serving "health food," but for a selection of popular restaurants that have a sincere interest in providing healthful options and nutrition information. If you want organic, natural foods and vegetarian dishes, we include restaurants that cater to these preferences as well. A good clue for identifying vegetarian dishes (at more conventional restaurants) is to look for items with no cholesterol (no animal products) or very low values, which may indicate small quantities of cheese or dairy products. You may, of course, double check with the restaurant personnel before ordering.

Restaurants participating in this book have a genuine interest in offering healthy choices. They pay a fee for the nutrition analysis, and they have signed an agreement with Accents On Health to prepare the selected entrees in accordance with the recipes they submitted or clearly notify customers otherwise. We highly respect the restaurants included in this book for their interest and commitment to serving healthy entrees. We purposely include many different types of cuisines with a wide range of prices and believe this will have the greatest impact in encouraging all restaurants to offer healthy, delicious choices.

How are entrees selected?

When a restaurant participates in the **Healthy Dining** Program, our staff of qualified health professionals works with the chef to select recipes that are low in fat, cholesterol, calories and sodium.

Our first choice is to find items already on the menu, without making any modifications to the original recipe. This would be the easiest for you as well as for the restaurant. However, in some cases the original recipe doesn't meet the **Healthy Dining** guidelines, so we work with the chef to develop a "Special Request" version that is lower in calories, fat, cholesterol and/or sodium than the original dish (see Chapter 2). The analyses listed in this book for the "Special Request" items correspond to the lower calorie, fat, etc., content that you will be served if and only if you make the "Special Request." Otherwise you will be served a meal with considerably higher fat and calorie values.

You can make a difference!

The restaurants in this book devote time, money and effort to participate in **Healthy Dining**. In many cases, the restaurants have modified recipes to meet your needs. Now they need to hear that this nutrition information is important to you and that you appreciate their participation in this unique program.

We encourage all the restaurants to pass out **Healthy Dining** menus along with their regular menus. These menus are condensed versions of the book pages. Some restaurants, however, do not automatically provide them – *you must request the* **Healthy Dining** *menus.* And please do! The more that restaurants hear customers asking for specific nutrition information and ordering "Special Requests," the more they will recognize how important healthy dining is to many people.

So, if this information is important to you, if you want to have the choice to "order healthy," **please tell the Healthy Dining restaurants**! Please tell other restaurants that you'd like them to participate. This will enable us to include more restaurants and an even greater variety of healthy choices in the next edition of **Healthy Dining in Orange County.**

Please ask for the **Healthy Dining** menus
at participating restaurants.

We welcome your ideas

This program is growing, and we welcome your ideas on how to enhance it. Please write or email us with your comments. We update this publication periodically and will continue to add more restaurants, more healthy entrees, and more nutrition information.

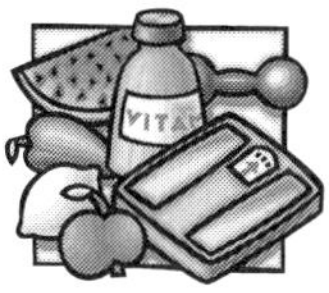

CHAPTER 1

Health, Lifestyle, Diet, Misconceptions & ... Dining Out

In 1988, the Surgeon General made a startling announcement to the American public:

> "If you don't smoke, what you eat may be
> the biggest factor influencing your health."

In December 2001, Surgeon General David Satcher said:

> "Overweight and obesity may soon cause as much
> preventable disease and death as cigarette smoking."

We've come a long way...

Diet has always strongly influenced health and disease. Until the early decades of this century, our country suffered from problems of *undernutrition*. Rickets, pellagra, scurvy, beriberi and goiter plagued our nation. Fortunately, in the United States, advances in medicine, fortification of foods, and successful cures virtually eliminated the vicious diseases caused by a lack of essential nutrients.

Currently, we've reached a whole new perspective on health and disease. A large body of medical research shows that lifestyle greatly influences health status. It is well recognized that daily health habits – what we eat and drink, whether or not we smoke, how much exercise we get and how effectively we manage stress – contribute to *how well and how long* we live.

The 1988 Surgeon General's Report on Nutrition and Health outlines the substantial impact of dietary practices on health. Today, the four leading causes of death by disease (heart disease, cancer, stroke, and diabetes), which together account for over ⅔ of all deaths in the U.S., are directly related to diet. The main conclusion of the 1988 report is:

> "*Overconsumption* of certain dietary components is now a major concern for Americans. While many food factors are involved, chief among them is the disproportionate consumption of foods high in fats, often at the expense of foods high in complex carbohydrates and fiber that may be more conducive to health."

-- 1988 Surgeon General's Report on Nutrition and Health --

Clearly, a priority for Americans is to reduce intake of calories, fat and especially saturated fat, because of the relationship between excess consumption of these nutrients and the development of many leading chronic diseases.

Dietary guidelines for Americans

The following guidelines are based on recommendations by leading health organizations.

1. Reduce overall consumption of fat, especially saturated fat. No more than 20 to 35% of total calories should come from fat (the average American diet contains approximately 35% fat). Saturated fat should comprise no more than 10% of the daily diet. Choose foods low in fat such as vegetables, fruits, whole grain foods, fish, lean meats and non-fat dairy products. Use food preparation methods that add little or no fat.

2. Reduce cholesterol consumption to less than 300 mg. per day. The average American consumes about 400 – 600 mg. of cholesterol daily.

3. Reduce intake of sodium by choosing foods relatively low in sodium and limiting the amount of salt in food preparation and at the table. No more than 2400 mg. sodium per day should be consumed. The average American consumes about 4,000 – 6,000 mg. daily.

4. Achieve and maintain a desirable body weight. To do so, choose a balanced diet in which energy (calorie) intake is consistent with energy expenditure. To reduce caloric intake, limit consumption of foods relatively high in calories, fat, and sugar, and minimize alcohol consumption. Increase energy expenditure through regular exercise.

5. Eat a variety of foods. Increase consumption of complex carbohydrates and fiber, such as whole grain foods, cereals, vegetables, fruits, dried beans, peas, and lentils.

6. Limit sugar in your diet, and if you drink alcoholic beverages, do so in moderation.

Americans are catching on!

More of us are watching what we eat. Learning more about what we eat. Making healthier choices. We're beginning to cherish our health for its influence on all other aspects of our lives. For top performance, we're eating more high-quality fuel – fruits, vegetables and whole grains – and less beef, butter, whole milk and other foods high in saturated fat.

Since the mid-1970s, consumption of saturated fats has decreased significantly. In addition, U.S. death rates from heart disease have fallen dramatically, close to 25 percent in the last decade. Leading health organizations attribute some of this decline to better medical care but give most of the credit to healthier diets and lifestyles.

Food manufacturers are catching on, but...

Marketing efforts toward our increasingly health-conscious society have intensified in the past several years. Close to 30% of food advertising includes some type of health message. Although this spiraling emphasis on healthy eating from food makers is encouraging, it can be very misleading. For example, lunchmeats frequently flaunt a "96% FAT FREE" label, yet this means that only 4% of the meat's weight is fat, not 4% of the calories (a high percentage of the weight is water, thus decreasing the percentage weight from fat). Cookies, crackers and chips leap out from shelves with bright "NO CHOLESTEROL" or "FAT FREE" labels, yet the product may be high in calories, sodium or sugar to make up for the lost flavor.

Reading between the lines

Until recently, deciphering food labels was a difficult task. Nutrition information on labels was often misleading, confusing and incomplete. Terms such as "low-fat," "light," "natural," and "healthy" had virtually no standardized meaning and could be added to any package, regardless of contents.

In 1994, the Food and Drug Administration (FDA) implemented guidelines requiring almost all food packages to display a universal nutrition information label. The revised labels help you to easily identify important nutrition information. The FDA has also developed strict guidelines for several nutritional claims commonly used by food manufacturers. For example, any food package stating the product is "low-fat" must have 3 grams of fat or less per serving. A "low-calorie" food must contain 40 calories or less per serving. A food package promoting the product as "light" (e.g., light mayonnaise) must contain 50% less fat or one-third fewer calories than the food with which it is being compared (e.g., regular mayonnaise).

The **Healthy Dining** guidelines differ from the guidelines set by the FDA for food packages in that the **Healthy Dining** guidelines usually represent a full meal, whereas the FDA guidelines are designed for a single product or serving (often as small as a ½ or one oz. serving).

A crusader for healthier fast foods

In April 1990, Phil Sokolof and his non-profit organization, The National Heart Savers Association, attacked American fast food restaurants with full-page ads in large newspapers accusing them of "poisoning" Americans with foods high in saturated fat. A Gallup poll showed that almost 40% of those who saw the ads immediately decreased their visits to fast food restaurants. Just three weeks later, McDonald's responded by removing beef tallow from their French fries. Other fast food chains quickly followed. Sokolof points out that his major goal was to stop fast food from being a *"fast track to a heart attack."*

With Sokolof paving the way, consumers demanded to know – just what are we getting in fast food meals? As a result, most fast food restaurants now provide nutrition information on menu items for customers who inquire. At last, the fast American favorites have exposed their "fat facts."

Some fat facts

A McDonald's Big Mac has 580 calories, 33 grams of fat and 1050 milligrams of sodium. If you add medium fries and a small shake, the meal adds up to 1460 calories, 67 grams of fat and 1550 mg of sodium. Even the Filet-O-Fish has 470 calories, 27 grams of fat and 730 milligrams of sodium. Add fries and a shake and you're drowning in calories, fat and sodium.

Three pieces of Original Recipe Kentucky Fried Chicken Breast contain a whopping 1140 calories, 57 grams of fat and 3450 milligrams of sodium. Add coleslaw, mashed potatoes with gravy and a biscuit, and you get a total of 1640 calories, 79 grams of fat and 4710 milligrams of sodium. That's over a full day's recommended allowance for both fat and sodium in just one meal, and 54% of the total calories come from fat!

Salads are usually considered a healthy choice. However, many salads have over 1000 calories, over 50 grams of fat, and over 1000 milligrams of sodium. Sometimes salads are higher in calories and fat than many other items on the menu.

Better alternatives

In response to their new "fat visibility," many fast food restaurants have added items that look much better on the nutritional charts. As a result of health-conscious consumers speaking out, we now have more choices to "order healthy" at fast food restaurants. "The public does not realize the dramatic power it wields," Sokolof emphasizes. "The consumer's wish is big business' command."

In place of traditional fast food, many people are finding healthier meals at the growing number of convenient *"quick-service"* restaurants. For example:

Pick Up Stix specializes in take-out and prepares its food in exhibition kitchens. Each order is freshly wok'd with minimal oil, including the Buddha's Feast with only one gram of fat and 370 calories, the Szechwan Chicken with 10 grams of fat and 590 calories, and the Chicken with Vegetables with 10 grams of fat and 650 calories (excluding the rice).

Baja Fresh offers a new "Lighten Up" menu, which features seven items that are healthy and delicious with 10 grams of fat or less. In addition to the Lighten Up items, Baja Fresh serves several delicious tacos and burritos using only fresh, quality ingredients and flavorful recipes.

Charo Chicken features a diverse menu, including their Smoky BBQ Ranch Chicken Salad, Veggie Bowl, Fiesta Ensalada, and various side dishes like corn on the cob. Items are prepared hourly at each locations for a delicious dining experience.

But what about dining out in other restaurants?

What's healthy and what's not?

If dining out were only for special occasions, the rich and creamy dishes could be wonderful treats. After all, an occasional splurge is not so bad. But because restaurant dining for business, pleasure and convenience has become so common, it is important to find healthier choices.

That's what **Healthy Dining** is all about. It's the first book of its kind. Never before has so much information been available for restaurant menu items. Each restaurant has its own unique recipes, prepared in its own special way. So nutrition information must be compiled restaurant-by-restaurant, recipe-by-recipe, and that's a lot of work!

There are books and other materials that give general information for dining out. They list common entrees to avoid and those that are probably best to order. However, as restaurants become more specialized and creative, "common" entrees are not so common, and so general guidelines are not always accurate or useful.

As you read on about what we've discovered in our research, you'll find that often you can't tell what you're getting by the menu description. It may portray a healthy item, but many times there are hidden ingredients, and the method of preparation is not specified. Without complete nutrition information, you don't know what you're getting, and over the long run, that can pose health risks! **Healthy Dining** makes the process of ordering healthy food much easier.

Goals of Healthy Dining in Orange County:

1. **To guide you in ordering healthier entrees served at popular restaurants.**

2. **To provide you with easy-to-read nutrition profiles for selected entrees.**

3. **To give you useful, practical guidelines and advice for healthier restaurant dining.**

4. **To encourage restaurants to prepare and serve a wide variety of healthy choices.**

CHAPTER 2

Is Restaurant Food Fattening and Unhealthy?

It can be if you're not careful! But it doesn't have to be.

Many restaurants smother meals with excess fat, sodium, cholesterol and calories. Butter, oil, cream, cheese and salt are frequently added to achieve the taste and texture that the average American expects. To make matters worse, many restaurant diners have the habit of adding "extras" such as salad dressing, sour cream, and butter (which push up the calorie and fat count even more). Let's take a shocking look at a popular restaurant dinner:

Chicken Breast
Topped with a Creamy Parmesan Sauce
Served with Dinner Salad, Baked Potato and Sautéed Vegetables

	Calories	Fat (g)	Cholest. (mg)	Sodium (mg)
Dinner Salad	32	0	0	53
Blue Cheese Dressing (4 Tbs.)	308	32	36	668
Chicken Breast with Sauce	1312	91	481	1517
Baked Potato	220	0	0	16
Butter (2 Tbs.)	200	23	61	232
Sour Cream (2 Tbs.)	62	6	13	15
Sautéed Vegetables	117	11	0	207
Meal Total	2251	163	591	2708

Now let's evaluate these numbers relative to daily recommendations:

Calories: Close to a FULL day's recommended calories in one meal.
Fat: Almost three times the recommended fat intake for a FULL Day.
Cholesterol: Almost twice the recommended cholesterol intake for a FULL Day.
Sodium: Almost the entire recommended sodium intake for a FULL Day.

Other fat-filled favorites:

	Calories	Fat (g)	Cholest. (mg)	Sodium (mg)
Salad bar - with potato & tuna salad, dressing, and muffins with butter	1715	89	310	2954
Ultimate cheeseburger with fries & shake	1625	96	165	1708
Lasagna with garlic bread & salad	1538	77	194	2805
Beef & cheese enchiladas, rice & refried beans	1510	88	210	3516
Italian manicotti with garlic bread	1393	79	411	2330
Pizza - sausage & mushroom	1290	48	84	1656
Chicken sandwich with onion rings & shake	1282	68	82	2290
Stir fry chicken with rice & egg rolls	1213	62	99	2907
Seafood platter - fried - with tarter sauce	1195	70	97	1780
Fried chicken - with potato salad & cole slaw	1124	71	239	2552
Chicken fried steak with fries	1119	77	205	1895
Salmon - smothered in a cream sauce	1024	76	283	1017
Chimichanga with sour cream & cheese	922	68	205	2125
Omelet with hashbrowns	850	53	892	852

Does dining out have to be so destructive to our health?

Some say, "Order grilled fish, salads or vegetarian dishes. By avoiding red meat, fried foods and creamy sauces, you can dine out and stay on your diet."

Be careful! We've analyzed hundreds of apparently "healthy" entrees and found that many were diet disasters. The menu descriptions portrayed healthy items, but when we looked into the preparation methods, we found the items contained excessive amounts of ingredients that should be consumed sparingly or avoided altogether.

Surprising nutrition information about seemingly "healthy" meals:

Grilled Swordfish - *Marinated in herbs and olive oil.*

884	Calories	
71	Fat (g)	Nearly a full day's recommended fat intake.
115	Cholesterol (mg)	Too much olive oil used in the preparation!
846	Sodium (mg)	

Vegetarian Pasta Primavera - *Fresh vegetables and garlic sautéed in a vegetable broth. Served over fettucini noodles and tossed with Parmesan cheese.*

816	Calories	The menu description doesn't mention that the pasta was
45	Fat (g)	heavily tossed with oil, and the vegetables were sautéed
139	Cholesterol (mg)	in both broth *and butter.* This brings the fat total to 75%
892	Sodium (mg)	of a FULL day's recommended fat intake.

The "Healthy" Sandwich - *Avocado, tomato & cheese on whole wheat bread.*

746	Calories	
50	Fat (g)	May be healthy ingredients, but too much
66	Cholesterol (mg)	avocado, cheese, and mayonnaise add
958	Sodium (mg)	up to too much fat and sodium for a healthy meal.

Cobb Salad - *Crispy greens topped with chicken, avocado, bacon, tomato, hard-boiled egg and blue cheese crumbles. Served with a generous portion of your favorite dressing.*

1296	Calories	Salads can be good sources of vegetables, but with several
102	Fat (g)	high fat ingredients, it is much too high in fat, cholesterol,
647	Cholesterol (mg)	sodium and calories.
2553	Sodium (mg)	

Shrimp Stirfry - *Shrimp and assorted vegetables with chow mein noodles.*

866	Calories	Too much fat, calories, cholesterol and sodium.
64	Fat (g)	1 oz. oil to sauté (27 g fat), butter/cream
392	Cholesterol (mg)	sauce (25 g fat), and the chow mein noodles
668	Sodium (mg)	(9 g fat) quickly add up.

Tostada - *Mexican beans, guacamole, lettuce, tomato and cheese.*

1416	Calories	
77	Fat (g)	The cheese alone contributes 519 calories,
288	Cholesterol (mg)	43 grams of fat, 137 mg cholesterol and
2010	Sodium (mg)	802 mg sodium.

We also found other items labeled "Light" or "Light-Fare" that included potato skins (deep fried), vegetables with cheese sauce, a hamburger patty and cottage cheese (too much saturated fat), cheese quesadillas (there's that saturated fat in the cheese again) and deep fried fish tacos.

Accents On Health also discovered that even many entrees with a ♥ next to them were too high in fat. Here are a few examples:

??? Heart Healthy Entrees ???

♥	Eggplant Salad	34 grams fat - 86% of calories from fat
♥	Pasta with Tomatoes & Garlic	42 grams fat - 50% of calories from fat
♥	Grilled Halibut	64 grams fat - 75% of calories from fat

How can these items be designated as "healthy" or "light" when, in fact, they aren't? A bit of history is in order. As we noted in Chapter 1 when discussing packaged foods, health sells; and so food manufacturers were quick to tout the health benefits of their products. Restaurants soon followed, with menus and banners promoting the healthfulness of certain dishes.

As demonstrated in the previous pages, however, many dishes described as "healthy" actually are not. A restaurant may designate a meal as healthy simply because it is vegetarian or contains no butter, but in most cases, dishes with health claims have never been analyzed for nutrition content. And until recently, there were no standards for what really constituted a healthy or low-fat restaurant meal. The hearts used on most restaurant menus have no standardized meaning, and often there is no explanation of the meaning that the restaurant is attributing to their heart designation. In this **Healthy Dining** book, we use the heart symbol to identify meals that contain primarily unsaturated fat (see Chapter 4), and the footnotes at the bottom of the restaurant menu pages clearly identify its meaning.

Restaurant regulations

In an attempt to protect consumers from vague, incorrect, or misleading information, the Food and Drug Administration (FDA) implemented regulations for restaurants that make health and nutrition claims about their food. The regulations require that dishes with descriptions such as "low fat" or "low calorie" meet specified criteria; and that restaurants provide nutrition information to substantiate any health claims made.

Unfortunately, however, the large majority of restaurants choose not to provide healthful menu items with credible nutrition information. This leaves diners, in most cases, at a loss for determining the nutritional content of restaurant meals.

The menu items featured in this book represent meals created with an eye on nutrition and taste, substantiated by credible nutrition data. These dishes are great for your health and your tastebuds.

Some scrumptious and healthy examples:

Susan's Healthy Gourmet (Home delivery or pick-up)

MOM'S POT ROAST

An old-fashioned supper served with garlic mashed potatoes, gravy, green beans and fresh corn.

✓✓ CALORIES: Excellent Choice (370) ✓✓ CHOLESTEROL: Excellent Choice (55 mg)
✓✓ FAT: Excellent Choice (6 g) ✓ SODIUM: Good Choice (370 mg)

Angie's Cuisine Italiano (Tustin)

CAPELLINI POMODORO

Angel hair sautéed with olive oil, garlic, sweet basil and diced tomatoes.

✓✓ CALORIES: Excellent Choice (430) ✓✓ CHOLESTEROL: Excellent Choice (0 mg)
✓✓ FAT: Excellent Choice (15 g)♥ ✓✓ SODIUM: Excellent Choice (10 mg)**

Walt's Wharf (Seal Beach)

OAK GRILLED VEGETABLE PLATTER

with artichoke, zucchini, crookneck squash, Bermuda onion, eggplant, and red & green peppers.

✓✓ CALORIES: Excellent Choice (275) ✓✓ CHOLESTEROL: Excellent Choice (35 mg)
✓✓ FAT: Excellent Choice (13 g) ✓✓ SODIUM: Excellent Choice (270 mg)**

McCormick & Schmick's (Irvine)

GRILLED HALIBUT WITH FRESH SALSA

Topped with the Chef's special salsa-of-the-day and served with seasonal vegetables.

✓✓ CALORIES: Excellent Choice (375) ✓✓ CHOLESTEROL: Excellent Choice (65 mg)
✓✓ FAT: Excellent Choice (13 g)♥ ✓✓ SODIUM: Excellent Choice (225 mg)**

♥ Primarily unsaturated fat

** If you request no added salt

Some scrumptious and healthy examples (continued):

The Taco Company (Orange)

CAMARON TACO

Charbroiled shrimp with a soft shell. Analysis is for two tacos.

✓✓ CALORIES: Excellent Choice (200)
✓ CHOLESTEROL: Good Choice (85 mg)
✓✓ FAT: Excellent Choice (2 g)♥
✓✓ SODIUM: Excellent Choice (190 mg)**

Whole Foods Market (Tustin)

LEMON CAPELLINI SALAD *(½ lb. serving)*

✓✓ CALORIES: Excellent Choice (285)
✓✓ CHOLESTEROL: Excellent Choice (0 mg)
✓✓ FAT: Excellent Choice (12 g)♥
✓✓ SODIUM: Excellent Choice (245 mg)

Santa Monica Seafood (Costa Mesa, Orange, Santa Monica)

SUSHI ROLL COMBINATION

Includes tuna roll, cucumber roll, salmon roll and California roll.

✓✓ CALORIES: Excellent Choice (405)
✓✓ CHOLESTEROL: Excellent Choice (55 mg)
✓✓ FAT: Excellent Choice (5 g)♥
✓✓ SODIUM: Excellent Choice (125 mg)**

Baja Fresh (many Orange County locations)

BAJA MAHI MAHI TACO

Fresh mahi mahi, sliced avocado, cabbage, fresh pico de gallo salsa, and zesty avocado salsa.

✓✓ CALORIES: Excellent Choice (260)
✓✓ CHOLESTEROL: Excellent Choice (20 mg)
✓✓ FAT: Excellent Choice (10 g)
✓ SODIUM: Good Choice (460 mg)

Red Rock Chili Co. (Newport Beach)

WHITE ROCK CHILI *(8 oz.)*

with chicken, white beans, peppers, onions, chilies, tomato sauce, and lots of spices!

✓✓ CALORIES: Excellent Choice (150)
✓✓ CHOLESTEROL: Excellent Choice (20 mg)
✓✓ FAT: Excellent Choice (2 g)
✓ SODIUM: Good Choice (445 mg)

The menu items on the previous pages and in the following chapters are just a taste of the wonderful entrees served at the restaurants participating in **Healthy Dining in Orange County.** We invite you to visit the restaurants featured in this book. You'll discover a whole new world of menu items that are marvelously delicious and so good for you!

"Special Requests"

In some cases, after analyzing the restaurant recipes, we found dishes that contained too many calories and/or too much fat, cholesterol or sodium. So we recommended that the chef modify the dishes to meet the **Healthy Dining** guidelines. We note these dishes as "Special Requests." "Special Requests" may be prepared with less oil or butter, salad dressing or sauce served on the side, less cheese, etc. When you order, you must ask for the "Special Request" for your meal to correspond to the published nutrition information. See the examples below to find out how many calories and grams of fat you save by ordering some of these "Special Requests."

♥ Primarily unsaturated fat

** If you request no added salt

Examples of "Special Requests:"

Old Spaghetti Factory (Newport Beach, Fullerton, Riverside, R. Cucamonga)
SPINACH TORTELLINI WITH MUSHROOM SAUCE – SPECIAL REQUEST
Hat shaped pasta, stuffed with a delicious blend of meat & cheese. Request Mushroom Sauce instead of Alfredo.
This request saves 155 calories and 14 grams of fat!

The Beach House (Dana Point, Laguna Beach)
BAKED GULF PRAWNS – SPECIAL REQUEST
Butterflied with parmesan cheese, sherry and garlic, served with wild rice pilaf.
Request less cheese (½ oz.) and less butter (1 Tbs.) in preparation.
This request saves 570 calories, 51 grams of fat and 130 mg cholesterol!

McKenna's (Long Beach)
WOOD GRILLED VEGETABLE SALAD – SPECIAL REQUEST
Fresh in-season grilled vegetables over greens with goat cheese.
Request dressing and avocado on the side (not included in analysis).
This request saves 515 calories and 56 grams of fat!

La Salsa (Multiple Locations)
CHILE-LIME SALAD – SPECIAL REQUEST
Chicken, Romaine, Cotija cheese, tomatoes & avocado, with our own Chile-lime dressing.
Request dressing on the side (not included in analysis) or use mango salsa as an excellent alternative.
This request saves 255 calories, 24 grams of fat and 585 mg cholesterol!

> Remember: Any dish marked "**Special Request**" means you must specifically order the "Special Request" for it to correspond to the published nutrition information.

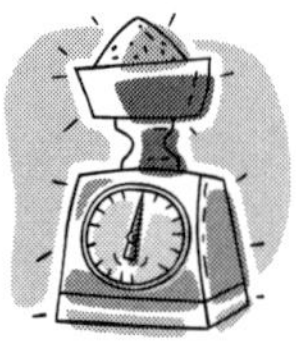

CHAPTER 3

Do Your Calories Have a Purpose?

Calories have a bad reputation in our society. We're counting calories and cutting calories, as though we've forgotten that calories are what keep us alive. Food and water fuel our bodies to do the miraculous tasks we perform each day. Instead of focusing on just cutting calories, we need to look at the *quality* of the calories we consume.

Just what are you getting from your calories?

Calories add up from the amounts of protein, carbohydrate and fat in foods. Each type of calorie has a very different function in the body. The following chapters explain the functions in more detail, but briefly:

Protein calories help the body to build and restore.

Carbohydrate calories are the body's main energy source; complex carbohydrates provide the most nutrients.

Fat of certain types is essential for healthy bodies, but too much fat supplies excess calories that can easily turn into body fat.

In general, protein and complex carbohydrate calories supply our bodies with nutrients necessary to function optimally. We need a small amount of what are called "essential" fats, but because fat is so prevalent in most meals, most Americans suffer from an excess of dietary fat, not a deficiency.

We should strive to eat foods with high-quality, nutritious calories. Recommendations vary according to individual needs, but generally 45% to 65% of total daily calories should come from carbohydrates, 10% to 35% from protein, and 20 to 35% from fat. Because most Americans get enough protein and too much fat, the best way to determine the quality of your calories is to determine the percentage of calories from fat, and keep it between 20-35%.

Percentage of calories from fat

The 20 to 35% fat recommendation is the suggested average for the whole day. Some foods will add little, if any, fat to your diet, while other foods may supply a big chunk of the fat for the day.

Of course, it's best to avoid (or use sparingly) foods which have a high percentage of fat (e.g., butter, margarine, oils, sour cream, cheese, cream cheese, etc.).

A fattening example:

Salmon - *Smothered in a cream sauce*

Total Calories:	1024
Protein:	77 grams
Carbohydrate:	8 grams
Fat:	76 grams

How to calculate the percentage of calories from fat:

Each gram of fat has nine calories. Using this information, you can calculate the percentage of calories from fat as shown in the following example. For the **Salmon with Cream Sauce**:

1. Multiply the number of grams of fat by 9 (number of calories per gram of fat):
   76 grams x 9 cals/gram = 684 calories from fat

2. Divide by total calories to get the fraction of calories from fat:
   684 calories ÷ 1024 calories = 0.67

3. Multiply by 100 to get the percentage:
   0.67 x 100 = 67%

67% of calories in this dish come from fat!

Carbohydrate and protein percentages can be calculated in the same way, except that the number of grams of each is multiplied by 4 rather than 9, because carbohydrates and proteins provide 4 calories per gram. The division step is the same. For this example, these calculations show that 3% of calories come from carbohydrate and 30% from protein. Cholesterol and sodium do not contribute to calories.

The amounts of carbohydrate and protein in this salmon dish are typical of and appropriate for meat, poultry and fish entrees. In terms of fat content, the salmon example above contains excessive amounts of cream and butter, which are not necessary to create a delicious tasting entrée.

Let's look at a healthier salmon dish:

Grilled Coho Salmon

Seven ounces of grilled, herb-seasoned salmon, served with veggies and baked potato.

Analysis for salmon alone:

Total Calories:	275
Protein:	38 grams
Carbohydrates:	0 grams
Fat:	12 grams

To calculate the percentage of calories from fat:

1. Multiply grams of fat by 9 calories per gram:
   12 grams x 9 cals/gram = 108 calories from fat

2. Divide by total calories and multiply by 100 to get a percentage:
   108 calories / 275 calories x 100 = 39%

39% of calories from this dish come from fat – much less than the example above, but still above the recommended maximum of 20% to 35% of calories from fat.

Remember, the guideline of 20 to 35% of calories from fat applies to the overall diet – an entire day or week, not just one entree. Restaurants differ greatly in the ways meals and side dishes are presented. If you order a lean meat or fish entree, it consists mainly of protein and fat, and the percentage of fat will generally appear to be high. By themselves, many lean meats and fish contain 30% to 50% fat. Even soybeans contain about 40% of their calories from fat. But generally these high-protein entrees are not eaten by themselves. If you choose quality carbohydrate side dishes such as vegetables, grains, breads, and fruits, the percentage of fat for the overall meal is significantly less. Entrees that are made up largely of carbohydrates (such as pasta or rice dishes) generally have a lower percentage of calories from fat.

As an example of how the side dishes change the overall percentage fat, let's include the side dishes that are served with this entree:

	Calories	Fat (g)
Salmon	275	12
Vegetables	32	1
Plain Baked Potato	375	1
Butter (1 tsp)	33	4
Totals	715	18

To calculate percentage of calories from fat:

18 grams of fat x 9 cals/gram = 162 calories from fat
162 calories from fat / 715 total calories x 100 = 23%

Only 23% of total calories from this meal come from fat, which is within the recommended guidelines and significantly less than the percentage of fat calculated for the salmon alone.

This example demonstrates how a meal can be a good choice even when the protein-rich part of the meal by itself (the salmon, in this case) exceeds 30% of calories from fat. Also, remember that a meal like this one will probably be the largest of your day, and your choices for the remainder of the day can also bring the overall percentage of fat down. Finally, note that salmon contains essential omega-3 oils and is primarily unsaturated fat (see Chapter 4 for more about types of fat).

Grams of fat vs. percentage of calories from fat

We list grams of fat for each of the dishes on the menu pages rather than percentage of calories from fat. The previous example illustrates how calculating the percentage of calories from fat for a single menu item does not adequately reflect values for the entire meal or the entire day. Chapter 4 discusses in more detail how to choose guidelines for fat intake that are appropriate for you.

How the check mark guidelines for calories are set

The **Healthy Dining** guidelines assume an average intake of 2,000 calories per day. Next, we assume that the restaurant meal accounts for the largest of the day's meals, up to 40% of the daily calorie allotment, or 800 calories. So 750 calories for the main entree would fit into the calorie budget. Thus, an upper limit of 750 calories is labeled as a "Good Choice" for calories. The "Excellent Choice" value of 450 calories represents a proportionately lower level, corresponding to about 1200 to 1500 calories per day:

✓✓ Excellent Choice = 0 to 450 calories/entree
✓ Good Choice = 451 to 750 calories/entree

> Glance through the restaurant pages and use the quick, easy check mark system to see the wide variety of entrees which contain high-quality, nutritious calories and are "Excellent Choice" (✓✓) or "Good Choice" (✓) for calories.

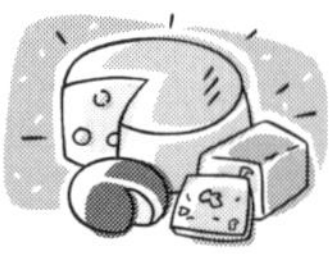

CHAPTER 4

Fat—How Much and What Type?

Fat – it clogs our arteries and builds up around the stomach, thighs and buttocks. Too much body fat, almost always caused by too much fat in our diet, too many calories and/or too little exercise in our day, increases the risks of high blood pressure, elevated blood fats (triglycerides and cholesterol), heart disease, stroke, diabetes, cancer and other health problems.

How much is too much?

The guidelines recommended by leading health organizations (see Chapter 1) suggest that fat should contribute no more than 20 to 35% of total calories. Chapter 3 shows examples of calculating percentage of calories from fat. This section deals with counting grams of fat. If we assume a daily intake of 2000 calories, then no more than 400 to 700 calories per day (20 to 35%) should come from fat. Since each gram of fat contributes 9 calories, then about 77 grams of fat (700 ÷ 9) is the suggested upper limit of fat intake per day. If you're not careful, it's easy to exceed that with just one meal!

How the check mark guidelines for fat are set

What is a reasonable limit per meal or per entree? If we assume the restaurant meal is the largest meal of the day and allow up to 40% of the upper limit of the daily fat allotment (77 grams) for that meal, that sets a limit of about 30 grams of fat for your entire restaurant meal. Main entrees usually contribute the largest amount of fat to the meal (assuming you're careful about side dishes), so we set entrée guidelines of:

✓✓ Excellent Choice = 0 to 15 grams of fat/entree
✓ Good Choice = 16 to 25 grams of fat/entree

If you're very active and take in more calories, then a higher limit would be appropriate. If you're on a weight loss diet or very low fat diet, then the "Excellent Choice" guideline of up to 15 grams of fat per entree is probably more appropriate.

Notice that these recommended guidelines represent an average intake for an average meal. Don't be overly concerned about the cutoff between our designations of "Good Choice" and "Excellent Choice." Unless you're on a very restricted diet, the difference between an entree with 16 grams of fat (which would receive one check mark) and one with 15 grams of fat (two check marks) is probably not worth worrying about. An occasional meal with somewhat more fat (but don't overdo it!) can be fairly easily compensated for by reducing fat intake during other meals.

Portion sizes

Be aware of portion sizes. Restaurant portions tend to be very large. The entrees listed in this book often represent 6 to 10 ounces of a very filling meal. In some cases, for a large serving, we may note that the nutrition information is based on only a part (e.g., ½ or ⅔) of a full serving. This means that only the recommended portion of the meal corresponds to the nutrition information. So, because it is a large serving, eat ½ or ⅔ and save the rest for the next day – or share with a friend.

Types of fat

Together with protein, fats form the structures in our bodies, including muscles, nerves, membranes and blood vessels. "Saturated" and "unsaturated" refer to the chemical structure of the fat molecules. We need very little fat to perform these functions, and only *unsaturated* sources of fat aid in these processes.

Unsaturated Fats - Monounsaturated, Polyunsaturated. You should include in your diet small to moderate amounts of these "good" types of fat. A low total fat intake, with the majority of fat from unsaturated sources, appears to lower blood cholesterol levels. The best sources for these "good" fats are natural grains, seeds and nuts, and fish. Many oils are primarily unsaturated, such as olive, canola, peanut, corn, safflower, sesame, cottonseed and soybean. Look for menu items with the ♥ alongside the fat content for dishes that contain primarily unsaturated fat. This ♥ indicates that at least 90% of the fat contained in the dish comes from foods containing the "good," unsaturated types of fat.

Omega-3 Fats. Fish and seafood contain unique polyunsaturated fats called omega-3 fatty acids. These fatty acids seem to make blood platelets less likely to clot, thus decreasing risk of artery blockage and heart attack. Fish with high amounts of omega-3 include salmon, albacore tuna, mackerel, herring and rainbow trout.

Saturated Fats. Saturated fats are the *very unhealthy* fats that raise blood cholesterol and triglyceride levels. Excess saturated fat is related to an increased risk of cardiovascular disease. Foods that contain saturated fats are usually hard at room temperature. Saturated fat is found mostly in animal products (beef, chicken, butter, ice cream, and cheese), processed and fast foods and some vegetable oils (palm oil, coconut oil, and partially hydrogenated oils).

Hydrogenated Oils and Trans-Fatty Acids. Also *very unhealthy*, vegetable oils found in most margarines and in many packaged and processed foods (such as cookies, pastries, crackers, chips, pudding, fish sticks, etc.) are "hydrogenated." During the hydrogenation process, hydrogen is added to liquid oil, thereby changing its chemical structure. The result is a harder, more saturated fat product, which many people find appealing for spreads and in cooking. Manufacturers use the hydrogenation process because it increases product stability and shelf life, saving them money. Unfortunately, consumption of hydrogenated products contributes to elevated blood cholesterol levels and an increase in heart disease risk, partly because the hydrogenation produces more saturated fat.

In addition to making the fat more saturated, hydrogenation also produces unnatural compounds called *trans-fatty acids* that have a more rigid molecular structure than natural fats do. Many scientists now believe that these trans-fats are harmful because they block the important functions of the "good" types of fat and because the trans-fats cannot be metabolized properly by the body.

Fortunately, recent legislation will require manufacturers to list the amount of trans-fat in their products as of 2006. Regardless, it is probably wise to opt for unprocessed foods rather than foods that contain "hydrogenated" or "partially hydrogenated" oils.

A summary of fat

When assessing the fat content of food, it is important to look at:

1. The number of grams of fat
2. The percentage of calories from fat
3. The type of fat - minimize or avoid saturated and hydrogenated fats

One Last Word on Fat: Although unsaturated fats do not raise blood cholesterol levels, they are a very concentrated source of calories. Too much fat – saturated or unsaturated – may make *you* fat, and excess body fat is a risk factor for many chronic diseases.

> On the restaurant menu pages, the heart symbol (♥) next to the grams of fat indicates that the fat is primarily unsaturated (the "good" type). Look for it!

Some delicious examples of "Excellent" and "Good" choices for fat:

Notice that many contain primarily unsaturated fat (designated with the ♥).

El Pollo Loco (many locations in Orange County)

POLLO BOWL

Flame-broiled boneless skinless breast with pinto beans, Spanish rice, tomato, onion and cilantro.

✓✓ FAT: Excellent Choice (10 g)

Fitness Grill & Fitness Pizza (Brea & Yorba Linda)

SEAFOOD BROCHETTE

Variety of marinated and grilled halibut, shrimp & scallops served over basmati wild rice & steamed spinach.

✓✓ FAT: Excellent Choice (10 g)♥

Ho Sum Bistro (Newport Beach)

QUENELLES

Five dumplings stuffed with a light blend of chicken, vegetables and its own sauce.

✓✓ FAT: Excellent Choice (3 g)

Wahoo's Fish Taco (many Orange County locations)

CHARBROILED FISH BURRITO

✓✓ FAT: Excellent Choice (12 g)

Examples of "Excellent" and "Good" choices for fat (continued):

Finbars (Costa Mesa and Seal Beach)
CHICKEN GIARDINA
Bite size pieces of chicken breast sautéed with olive oil, garlic, onion, diced tomatoes, carrots, celery, oregano and fresh basil, served over rice.
✓✓ FAT: Excellent Choice (11 g)

Pick Up Stix (many Orange County locations)
SZECHWAN CHICKEN
Chicken in a blend of seared red chili peppers mixed with green and white onions, carrots and celery. (Analysis does not include rice.)
✓✓ FAT: Excellent Choice (10 g)

Café Chin Chin (Lakewood Mall and Tustin Market Place)
LITE GINGER WINE SHRIMP – SPECIAL REQUEST
Classic light sauce with shrimp, ginger, snow peas, water chestnuts, carrots & Chinese wine. Request LITE preparation.
✓✓ FAT: Excellent Choice (2 g)♥

Vie de France (Costa Mesa)
SEARED AHI TUNA NICOISE – SPECIAL REQUEST
Ahi tuna on a mound of green beans, tomato wedges, red bliss potatoes, hard cooked egg, black olives and red onions over mixed greens, splashed with fat-free dressing. Request fat-free vinaigrette.
✓✓ FAT: Excellent Choice (9 g)

Pascal (Newport Beach)
FREE RANGE CHICKEN BREAST PROVENCAL
Roasted breast of chicken served with olives, sweet garlic and tomatoes. Garnished with steamed asparagus.
✓ FAT: Good Choice (19 g)

J T Schmid's Brewhouse & Eatery (Anaheim)
GRILLED BANGKOK CHICKEN
Grilled chicken breast glazed with teriyaki and served over steamed rice and mixed vegetables.
✓ FAT: Good Choice (17 g)

Sammy's Woodfired Pizza (Fountain Valley)
HEALTHY DINING VEGETARIAN PIZZA (½ PIZZA)
Grilled eggplant, onions, bell peppers, fontina, garlic, zucchini and Roma tomatoes with fat-free mozzarella. Analysis is for ½ of a pizza.
✓ FAT: Good Choice (21 g)♥

The Beach House (Laguna Beach and Dana Point)
SAUTÉED BLUENOSE BASS
Served with fresh steamed vegetables.
✓✓ FAT: Excellent Choice (11 g)♥

♥ Primarily unsaturated fat

Now – how well are YOU doing?

If you're not careful, all the "extras" in your meal can add too much fat to your diet very quickly. Consider the following high-fat culprits:

	Calories	Fat (g)	Cholest.(mg)	Sodium (mg)
Salad Dressings: (3 Tbs.)				
Blue Cheese	231	24	27	501
Oil & Vinegar	215	24	0	0
Italian	206	21	0	348
French	201	19	6	642
Thousand Island	176	17	15	327
Ranch	162	17	12	291
Toppings: (2 Tbs.)				
Margarine	202	23	0	264
Butter	200	23	61	232
Mayonnaise	198	22	16	157
Tarter Sauce	150	16	18	196
Cream Cheese	100	10	31	85
Cheese (1 oz. cheddar)	114	9	30	176
Sour Cream	67	6	13	15
Desserts:				
Cheesecake	386	24	82	284
Ice Cream (1 cup)	349	24	88	108
Chocolate Cake	407	17	5	300
Apple Pie	323	14	28	207

Instead try:

- Fat-free or low-fat salad dressings
- Salsa, low-fat cottage cheese, or plain yogurt as salad dressing or topping for potatoes
- Only very small amounts of regular or high-fat salad dressings
- Frozen yogurt, sorbet, sherbet or fruit for dessert

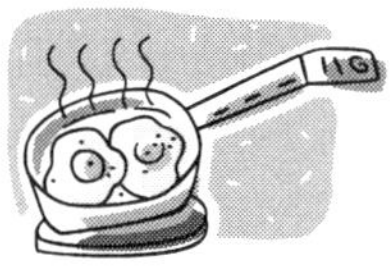

CHAPTER 5

Cholesterol—A Hot Topic

Cholesterol continues to be a hot topic enmeshed in controversy. Medical research is progressing on this subject, and we hope to clear up some misconceptions concerning cholesterol.

Where does cholesterol come from?

Most of the cholesterol in your blood is manufactured by your liver. Our bodies use cholesterol to form hormones and cell membranes, producing about 1,000 milligrams (mg) of cholesterol each day. In addition, the average American consumes 400 to 600 mg daily from food. Dietary cholesterol is found only in animal products. The cholesterol we derive from our diets is essentially the same as the cholesterol our bodies manufacture

However, the average high-fat/high-cholesterol diet tends to add too much cholesterol to the bloodstream. The excess cholesterol and other substances accumulate in the walls of the blood vessels. Over time the arteries become narrowed, and eventually the flow of blood is cut off, leading to a heart attack or stroke.

What determines blood cholesterol levels?

1. **Genetics**. Some individuals, no matter how prudent their diet or how regularly they exercise, can't achieve a low cholesterol level without the help of a physician and cholesterol-lowering medications.

2. **Lipoproteins**. Cholesterol is carried through the blood in protein packages called lipoproteins. The amounts and types of lipoproteins are an important indicator of your heart disease risk. The two major lipoproteins include LDL and HDL.

LDLs (low-density lipoproteins) are commonly termed "bad" cholesterol. LDLs increase heart disease risk because they keep cholesterol in blood circulation and carry it to the arteries to be deposited. Excess body fat and a diet high in saturated fat tend to increase LDL levels.

HDLs (high-density lipoproteins) are the "good" cholesterol that protect against heart disease. They actually carry cholesterol AWAY from the arteries to the liver to be excreted from the body. Individuals with high HDL levels have a lower risk of heart disease. Regular exercise, maintaining appropriate body weight, and not smoking help to increase HDL levels.

3. **Diet**. Foods high in saturated fat increase cholesterol levels. These include butter, whole milk products, palm and coconut oils, cheese, beef, pork, and egg yolks. In addition, many packaged and processed foods are high in saturated fat or (partially) hydrogenated oils, which also have a cholesterol-raising effect.

A diet *low in total fat*, with fat intake primarily from unsaturated fat sources, reduces cholesterol levels. Unsaturated fats include olive, corn, safflower, sesame, canola, soybean, and sunflower oils. *High fiber foods*, especially oat bran, apples, carrots, oranges, and legumes (beans, peas and lentils) decrease cholesterol levels by inhibiting the absorption of cholesterol into the bloodstream. *Fish and fish oils*, which contain omega-3 fatty acids, also decrease cholesterol levels.

4. **Smoking, stress and some medications** also raise cholesterol levels.

How should blood cholesterol be measured?

For an accurate and complete cholesterol measure, a tube of blood should be drawn from the arm by a qualified health professional. You should not eat or drink anything (except water) for 12 hours before the blood draw. The laboratory which analyzes the blood sample should follow the reference methods set by the U. S. Centers for Disease Control. The fingertip method found in shopping malls and health fairs may not provide results that are as accurate or thorough (many do not measure HDL levels).

Important facts on dietary cholesterol and fat

Too much of any fat (even unsaturated oils!) can increase body weight, which may increase blood cholesterol levels. Oils, margarine, and butter all have approximately the same number of calories and fat grams per ounce, and so all have the same potential to make you fat. Therefore it's important to limit your total intake of all types of fat.

Even though oils, margarine, and butter have about the same calorie and fat counts, there is a big difference in the chemical make-up of these fats. Butter is high in saturated fat, and saturated fats increase blood cholesterol levels. Saturated fats stimulate the production of LDLs ("bad cholesterol"), resulting in increased blood cholesterol levels. Therefore, if you avoid only dietary cholesterol in the food you eat, without reducing the amount of saturated fat, you may not decrease your blood cholesterol level at all.

Avoid hydrogenated fats too, because they are also saturated. Margarine, although cholesterol-free, is partially hydrogenated and contains trans-fatty acids, which have been shown to have a cholesterol-raising effect.

Vegetable oils are generally unsaturated fats. Liquid oils (such as olive, corn, canola, etc.) in small amounts may help to decrease cholesterol levels. Remember though, that all oils are 100% fat and high in calories, so use only small amounts.

The amount of cholesterol found in foods is not as important as the amount of saturated fat. But you should minimize intake of very concentrated sources of cholesterol such as egg yolks and liver. Shellfish is very low in saturated fat, but moderately high in cholesterol. Most medical experts agree that shellfish, in moderate quantities, is a healthy choice.

Cholesterol is found only in animal products. Don't be misled, though – just because foods don't contain cholesterol doesn't mean they are also low in fat! In fact, many "no-cholesterol" foods are loaded with fat. Be sure to check the number of fat grams on nutrition labels.

How the check mark guidelines for cholesterol are set

The Surgeon General's Office and the American Heart Association recommend that cholesterol consumption be limited to 300 mg per day. If the day's total were evenly divided in thirds, this would suggest a limit of 100 mg per meal. We set our guidelines for cholesterol as follows:

✓✓ Excellent Choice = 0 to 75 mg cholesterol/entree
✓ Good Choice = 76 to 150 mg cholesterol/entree

If every meal in your day were at the "Good Choice" limit of 150 mg, you would exceed the recommended amount. But since a restaurant meal usually contains a larger portion of meat or other cholesterol-containing foods than side dishes or other meals of the day, we assumed that this cholesterol intake can easily be compensated for by choosing foods with little or no cholesterol for the remaining selections.

If you are watching your blood cholesterol level, select items that are:

1. "Excellent Choice" or "Good Choice" for fat
2. Primarily unsaturated (designated with the ♥)
3. "Excellent Choice" or "Good Choice" for cholesterol

Flavorful examples of "Excellent" and "Good" choices for cholesterol:

Old Spaghetti Factory (Newport Beach, Fullerton, Riverside, Rancho Cucamonga)
SPAGHETTI WITH MUSHROOM SAUCE
Fresh tender mushrooms, swimming in authentic Italian tomato sauce.
✓✓ FAT: Excellent Choice (7 g)♥ ✓✓ CHOLESTEROL: Excellent Choice (0 mg)

Blackboard Bistro (Seal Beach)
ROSEMARY CHICKEN
A fresh double breast of chicken marinated in rosemary, herbs, and extra virgin olive oil, served with brown rice and veggies.
✓✓ FAT: Excellent Choice (12 g) ✓ CHOLESTEROL: Good Choice (145 mg)

The Flame Broiler (Costa Mesa, Fullerton, Orange, Stanton)
BEEF VEGGIE BOWL
Teriyaki beef with broccoli, cabbage and carrots served over steamed rice and topped with teriyaki sauce.
✓✓ FAT: Excellent Choice (10 g) ✓✓ CHOLESTEROL: Excellent Choice (70 mg)

Examples of "Good" & "Excellent" choices for cholesterol (continued):

Luigi's D'Italia (Anaheim)

VEGETARIAN CHEESELESS PIZZA (⅓ MEDIUM PIZZA) 🍎

✓ FAT: Good Choice (22 g)♥ ✓✓ CHOLESTEROL: Excellent Choice (0 mg)

La Salsa (multiple Orange County locations)

SONORA MAHI MAHI TACO

Flour tortilla taco filled with grilled Mahi Mahi, lettuce, tomatoes, Jack and Cheddar cheeses and topped with our Sonora sauce and a squeeze of lime.

✓✓ FAT: Excellent Choice (8 g) ✓✓ CHOLESTEROL: Excellent Choice (30 mg)

The Culinary Wrap (Brea, Costa Mesa, and Cal State Long Beach campus)

GREEK WRAP 🍎

Roasted red peppers and eggplant, tomatoes, red onion, cucumbers, lettuce and feta tossed in a balsamic vinaigrette.

✓ FAT: Good Choice (21 g)♥ ✓✓ CHOLESTEROL: Excellent Choice (25 mg)

Z Pizza (multiple Orange County locations)

Z TUNA SALAD 🍎

Tuna over romaine and looseleaf lettuce, with cucumber, tomato, basil, and Oriental non-fat dressing.

✓✓ FAT: Excellent Choice (2 g) ♥ ✓✓ CHOLESTEROL: Excellent Choice (25 mg)

Baja Fresh (multiple locations in Orange County area)

BAJA STYLE CHARBROILED CHICKEN TACO

✓✓ FAT: Excellent Choice (5 g) ✓✓ CHOLESTEROL: Excellent Choice (25 mg)

Mother's Market & Kitchen (Costa Mesa, Huntington Beach, Irvine, Laguna Woods)

SPRINGTIME SALAD 🍎

A colorful selection of broccoli, cauliflower, grated beets and carrots, tomato, cucumber, mushrooms and avocado slices atop organic mixed greens.

✓ FAT: Good Choice (16 g)♥ ✓✓ CHOLESTEROL: Excellent Choice (0 mg)

Newport Beach Brewing Co. (Newport Beach)

BREWERY LETTUCE WRAPS 🍎

Broiled chicken, sesame seeds, lettuce leaves, carrots, bean sprouts and sides of Thai, plum and curry sauces (sauce analyses separate).

✓✓ FAT: Excellent Choice (7 g) ✓ CHOLESTEROL: Good Choice (150 mg)

Pat & Oscar's (Buena Park, Irvine, Lake Forest, and Orange)

BARBEQUE CHICKEN PIZZA (2 SLICES)

BBQ chicken, red onions, cilantro & BBQ sauce. Analysis is for 2 slices (⅓ pizza).

✓✓ FAT: Excellent Choice (14 g) ✓✓ CHOLESTEROL: Excellent Choice (50 mg)

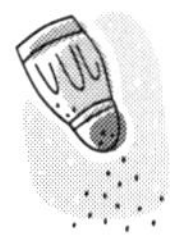

CHAPTER 6

Sodium — To Salt or Not to Salt?

That is the question. Sodium is an essential nutrient. It helps to maintain blood volume, regulate the balance of water in the cells, and transmit nerve impulses. The kidneys control sodium balance by increasing or decreasing sodium in the urine.

In general, Americans consume more sodium than needed. Many foods contain sodium naturally, and it is commonly added to foods during preparation or processing in the form of salt. Sodium is also found in drinking water, prescription drugs and over-the-counter medications.

The American Heart Association recommends a maximum intake of 2,400 mg of sodium per day. That's the amount in about 1 tsp. of salt. Other condiments contain significant amounts of sodium, such as seasoning salts (1620 - 1850 mg per teaspoon), monosodium glutamate (MSG, 492 mg per teaspoon), soy sauce (343 mg per teaspoon), and meat tenderizer (1750 mg per teaspoon). Packaged and processed foods also tend to be very high in sodium.

In the United States, nearly one in three adults has elevated blood pressure. Sodium intake is only one of the factors known to affect blood pressure, and not everyone is equally susceptible. The sensitivity to sodium seems to be very individualized. At present, there is not a good method to predict who is salt-sensitive or who will develop high blood pressure. Low-sodium diets may help some people avoid high blood pressure. Low-sodium diets may help some people with high blood pressure to control their blood pressure. And in some individuals, a low-sodium diet will not affect blood pressure at all.

Since most Americans consume more sodium than needed, consider reducing your sodium intake. Use less table salt, read labels carefully, and eat sparingly those foods which have large amounts of sodium. Remember that a substantial amount of the sodium you eat may be "hidden" - either occurring naturally in foods or as part of a preservative or flavoring agent that has been added.

To avoid too much sodium:

- Learn to enjoy the flavors of unsalted foods.
- Cook without salt or with only small amounts of added salt.
- Flavor foods with herbs, spices, and lemon juice.
- Add little or no salt to food at the table.
- Limit your intake of salty foods such as potato chips, pretzels, salted nuts and popcorn, condiments (soy sauce, steak sauce, garlic salt), pickled foods, cured meats, cheeses, and canned foods.
- Read food labels carefully to determine the amounts of sodium.
- Use lower sodium products, when available, to replace those with higher sodium content.

To avoid too much sodium when dining out:

1. Order entrees listed as "Excellent Choice" or "Good Choice" for sodium levels, and
2. Request no added salt whenever possible.

The sodium content for dishes featured in this book reflects three sources: (1) the sodium that occurs naturally in foods that are part of the recipe, (2) sodium in the form of salt that is included in a prepared sauce, marinade or other recipe in which the salt cannot be reduced for an individual portion (for example, soups, which are typically made in advance in large quantities), and (3) soy sauce, teriyaki sauce, and other ingredients that contain high concentrations of sodium, as discussed in more detail below.

There are two circumstances in which the amount of salt in your restaurant meal can be reduced: (1) Often, the restaurant's standard recipe includes salt that can be omitted when the chef prepares your order, and (2) Some chefs cook with salt "to taste," which means that they may add a pinch of salt here and there throughout the preparation. In both cases, if you want to minimize the amount of sodium consumed, it's important to specify very clearly that you want "no added salt."

Often items showing high sodium values contain soy sauce, teriyaki sauce, fish sauce, or other high sodium ingredients (see Chapter 9 for more information). These ingredients are included in the analyses unless specifically stated otherwise. You may be able to request less (or none) of these ingredients to reduce the sodium content. However, you should be aware that the taste will probably be altered.

Many items included in this book are listed as "moderate" (meaning 600 to 1000 mg sodium per entree) or "high" in sodium (meaning above 1000 mg sodium per entree) and are not recommended for those watching sodium intake.

> The double asterisk (**) next to the sodium values reminds you to specify "no added salt" to get the values as published.

How the check mark guidelines for sodium are set

Since no more than 2,400 mg of sodium is recommended per day, we consider a value of 960 mg (40% of maximum recommended daily intake) to be a reasonable maximum for a restaurant meal, and 600 mg to be a reasonable maximum for an entrée. Therefore, we set the guideline for sodium as follows:

✓✓ Excellent Choice = 0 to 300 mg sodium/entree
✓ Good Choice = 301 to 600 mg sodium/entree

Examples of "Excellent" and "Good" choices for sodium:

California Wok (Los Alamitos)
RAINBOW CHICKEN
Slices of chicken breast stir-fried with mixed vegetables in the chef's special white wine sauce.
✓✓ SODIUM: Excellent Choice (250 mg)**

Il Farro Caffe Trattoria (Newport Beach)
MISTO PESCE ALLA GRIGLIA AL SALMORIGLIO
Mix fish of the day, grilled, served simply with fresh lemon, extra virgin olive oil, parsley & a side of veggies.
✓✓ SODIUM: Excellent Choice (145 mg)**

McKenna's on the Bay (Long Beach)
LINGUINI WITH ROMA TOMATOES – SPECIAL REQUEST
with basil and sliced garlic. Request less oil (1 Tbs).
✓✓ SODIUM: Excellent Choice (15 mg)**

The Fish Market (Irvine)
LITE EATERS
Fresh fish, skewered, mesquite-grilled and seasoned.
✓✓ SODIUM: Excellent Choice (270 mg)**

** If you request no added salt

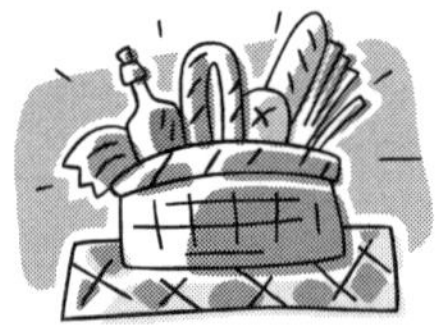

CHAPTER 7

Protein, Carbohydrates & Diabetic Exchanges

Protein: the building blocks

Protein is very important for a healthy body. Protein provides materials for growth, helps to maintain and repair tissues, manufactures the lipoproteins to carry fat and cholesterol, and assists in the maintenance of proper fluid levels.

Generally it's easy to get protein in your diet, and most Americans consume 2 - 3 times more than necessary. Excess protein does not create muscle, as many hope, but is stored as fat. Excess protein puts a strain on the liver and kidneys. In addition, some protein sources are also high in fat, calories and cholesterol, such as: beef, whole milk products, eggs, poultry with skin, cheese.

The best sources of protein are low-fat foods, including fish, poultry without skin, skim or low-fat milk products and tofu. Whole grains, vegetables and especially legumes (dried beans, peas and lentils) also contain some protein. Unless you are a very strict vegetarian, you probably get adequate protein with a balanced diet. If you are a strict vegetarian, a dietitian can analyze your present diet to make sure you're getting adequate amounts of protein.

Carbohydrates: energy

Total carbohydrates are made up of simple carbohydrates, complex carbohydrates, and fiber.

<u>Simple carbohydrates.</u> Sources of simple carbohydrates include table sugar, candies and other sweets, sodas and bakery goods. These foods contain little or no vitamins and minerals. They provide empty calories, i.e., calories that supply no nutrients and should therefore be minimized.

Fruits and some vegetables contain sugar naturally, and they also provide other nutrients, so they are valuable to a healthy diet. The sugar in simple carbohydrates is in a form that is absorbed quickly by the body, as opposed to the slower-digesting complex carbohydrates.

<u>Complex carbohydrates.</u> These carbohydrates contain many essential nutrients and are the body's most effective source of energy. It is recommended that 45% to 65% of total daily calories come from nutrient-dense carbohydrates (lower end of the range is recommended for those with diabetes). Foods high in complex carbohydrates include:

- breads and cereals
- rice and other grain products
- pasta
- dried beans, peas, and lentils
- vegetables

Because they contain more nutrients, whole grain breads, pasta, and rice are nutritionally superior to the processed "white" varieties. It is unusual for restaurants to offer whole grain pasta or rice, but you can often request "wheat" bread that contains at least some whole grain.

Dietary Fiber. The typical American diet is much too low in fiber. The American Cancer Society recommends 20 - 38 (depending on age and gender) grams of fiber daily. The average American consumes only 7 - 8 grams of fiber daily. Dietary fiber is a term used to describe parts of plant foods that are generally not digestible by humans. By increasing your intake of foods containing complex carbohydrates, and using whole grains, you will add dietary fiber to your diet.

There are two main types of fiber: soluble and insoluble. Soluble fiber may help lower blood cholesterol and control blood sugar and is found in oats, beans, carrots, apples and oranges. Insoluble fiber helps to move food through the body quickly and protect against colorectal cancer. Insoluble fiber is found in wheat bran and whole grains. Because both types of fiber have different functions for improving health, a variety of foods with fiber should be included in your diet. Fruits and vegetables are a significant source of nutrients and fiber. Thus, a diet rich in whole grains, breads, cereals, fruits and vegetables provides optimal amounts of nutrients, fiber and energy.

"Low-carb" diets

Recently, interest in low-carbohydrate diets has surged. Low-carb products are being promoted in supermarkets, and even restaurants are featuring low-carb selections on their menus. Most medical and nutrition experts agree that the long-term safety and effectiveness of low carbohydrate diets have not been demonstrated. Health professionals' concerns about such diets relate to the fact that in reducing the amount of carbohydrate, the amount of dietary fat (often saturated fat) and protein usually increases, potentially increasing the risk of heart, kidney and other diseases.

Reducing carbohydrates found in processed and "empty calorie" foods such as white flour and white sugar products is advisable. In contrast, complex carbohydrates found in whole grains, legumes, vegetables, etc., supply valuable nutrients, including vitamins, minerals, fiber, phytochemicals and antioxidants. Selecting dishes that supply these healthy nutrients and balance the amount of fat, calories, and protein is recommended, as discussed in more detail in Chapters 3 through 7.

Diabetic food exchanges

A well-balanced and carefully controlled diet is essential for those with diabetes. Recently carbohydrate counting has become common as a way of choosing foods and serving sizes. The grams of carbohydrate are listed on most menu items in this **Healthy Dining** book. The "diabetic exchanges" system traditionally recommended by the American Diabetes Association is also still used and is offered in this book. In this system, foods are grouped into the various exchange lists according to their similarities in calories, carbohydrate, protein and fat content, which influence how they are utilized by the body. Although carbohydrates have the largest influence on blood sugar levels, protein and fat also contribute calories and influence the rates of digestion, so they are important to the overall plan.

Even for those without diabetes, exchanges can give useful information about portion size and the overall balance between protein and simple and complex carbohydrates, as explained below.

One lean meat exchange is equivalent to approximately 7 grams of protein and 3 grams of fat. One bread (starch) exchange contains approximately 15 grams of carbohydrate and 3 grams of protein. Starchy vegetables (potatoes, corn, beans, etc.) are counted as bread (starch) exchanges rather than vegetable exchanges. Vegetable exchanges have less starch (5 grams of carbohydrate and 2 grams of protein) and lots of fiber. A fruit exchange contains approximately 15 grams of more easily digested (simple) carbohydrate. A milk exchange contains 12 grams of carbohydrate, 8 grams of protein, and only a trace of fat, assuming skim milk is used. A fat exchange represents 5 grams of fat.

Some diabetic exchange lists use separate categories for lean, medium-fat, and high-fat meats. The computerized system used for the **Healthy Dining** analysis uses the lean meat category, which assumes approximately 7 grams of protein and 3 grams of fat per meat exchange. In most entrees included in the book, the meat is very lean and the total fat from the meat is lower than the 3 grams of fat per meat exchange normally assumed. In these cases we have designated the meat exchanges as "extra lean," which indicates that the meat exchange contains less fat than the assumed standard of 3 grams of fat per meat exchange. Any added fat from additional ingredients (e.g., butter or oil used in preparation, sauces, spreads, etc.) is counted as separate fat exchanges. This means that the fat exchanges reflect additional fat added to the meat.

In many entrees shown in this book, extra fat (often unsaturated) is added, but with the very lean meat, the total grams of fat still come out very low. So you don't necessarily need to shy away from a selection that shows fat exchanges. Looking at the grams of fat probably gives better information about the overall fat content.

The food exchange system used by some weight loss programs is similar to the diabetic food exchange system. A dietitian can help you interpret these numbers to meet your own dietary needs.

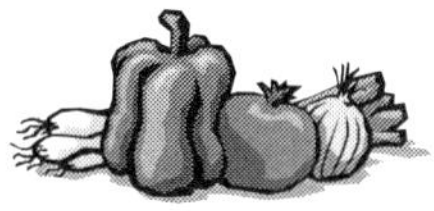

CHAPTER 8

Fruits & Vegetables—Nutrition Heavyweights

Science is finding that the saying "An apple a day keeps the doctor away" may be closer to the truth than most of us realize. And your mother was right — you should eat your vegetables! An abundance of research is in progress, and it is becoming increasingly clear that natural, whole foods such as fruits and vegetables contain more valuable substances than previously imagined, and certainly a more diverse range than available in nutrition supplements.

Fruits and vegetables deserve a special chapter in this book because of their importance in a healthy diet, and because their contributions overlap those of the other chapters so much. In addition to providing carbohydrates and high quality calories, they are packed full of other essentials — vitamins, minerals, fiber, antioxidants, and the more-recently discovered classes of compounds called phytochemicals (discussed in more detail below). Although numerical values are generally not available for these other substances, they are important and deserve special consideration as you make your food selections.

The World Health Organization, the National Cancer Institute, the American Cancer Society and other health organizations emphasize a clear relationship between the amounts of fruits and vegetables consumed and several diseases, especially cancer and cardiovascular diseases. These organizations encourage Americans to eat at least 5 servings of fruits and vegetables each day. Eating "5 a day" is important to ensure that your body gets a variety of health-promoting nutrients. Research has shown that people who eat at least 5 servings of fruits and vegetables a day have only half the cancer risk of those who eat only one or two servings a day.

Fruits and vegetables are nutritional powerhouses which:

- are excellent sources of vitamins and minerals
- contain fiber (most Americans don't eat enough fiber)
- are virtually fat-free (exceptions: coconut, olives and avocado) and cholesterol-free
- are particularly helpful in weight management, due to their high-fiber and low-fat content
- contain antioxidants and phytochemicals (discussed below)

Vitamins and minerals

Vitamins and minerals are essential for many bodily functions. They play a prominent role in maintaining the health of the brain, heart, bones, teeth and nerves, in making and repairing red blood cells, in regulating the body's balance of fluids, and in other vital functions. The absence of any one vitamin or mineral may result in a unique deficiency that can only be corrected by supplying that specific nutrient. In some cases, people who have a certain disease or condition may need to adjust their intake of a particular vitamin or mineral. However, consuming mega (large) doses of certain fat-soluble vitamins (particularly vitamins A and D) can be toxic. It's best to get most of your vitamins and minerals from natural, healthy foods.

It is important to consume a wide variety of fruits and vegetables in order to benefit fully from the antioxidants, vitamins and minerals they contain. For example, the following tables show fruits and vegetables that contain significant amounts of Vitamins A and C (the other major vitamins – B, D and E – come primarily from other food sources such as grains, seeds, nuts, dairy or meat):

Fruits and Vegetables High in Vitamin A:

Apricots (fresh or dried)	Broccoli	Carrots	Chinese cabbage
Cantaloupe & melons	Collards & other greens	Green onions	Mangoes
Papayas	Peaches & Nectarines	Persimmons	Spinach
Tomatoes	Sweet potatoes	Winter squash & pumpkins	

Fruits and Vegetables High in Vitamin C:

Bell peppers	Broccoli	Brussels sprouts	Cantaloupe & melons
Cauliflower	Grapefruit	Guavas	Kiwifruit
Lemons & other citrus	Mangoes	Oranges	Papayas
Raspberries	Strawberries		

Notice that there is little overlap among the fruits and vegetables that are high in vitamin A and C. Some fruits and vegetables that don't appear on either list may be high in other important nutrients. For example, bananas are high in potassium. Some fruits and vegetables, especially leafy green vegetables, citrus, berries, melons, and beans are high in folate, a B vitamin important in preventing heart disease, some types of anemia, and neural tube birth defects. There is no one food that "has it all." So be careful not to depend on a limited selection of fruits and vegetables to supply your nutrients. A glass of orange juice at breakfast and carrots at dinner, for example, move you toward your "5 a day" goal, but a wider variety of fruits and vegetables throughout the day is optimal.

Antioxidants

Antioxidants are disease-fighting compounds found in many foods. They neutralize free radicals, compounds that damage cells and lead to cardiovascular disease, cancer, cataracts, premature aging, and impaired immunity. Antioxidants include some vitamins (A, C, and E), beta carotene, some minerals (for example, selenium, copper, zinc, and manganese) and some of the phytochemicals discussed below. Fruits and vegetables are excellent sources of many of these antioxidants.

Phytochemicals

Phytochemicals are substances found in plant foods that are now recognized as powerful disease-fighting compounds. They have been shown to protect against cancer, cardiovascular disease, diabetes, and other medical conditions. "Phyto" means plant, and chemicals — well, not all chemicals are bad for you. Our bodies are made of chemicals, and some kinds are essential for good health. Fruits and vegetables contain thousands, perhaps tens or hundreds of thousands of different phytochemical compounds.

Scientists have grouped phytochemicals into at least 14 different classes, and still little is known about their functions and their interactions. Many appear to stimulate or block the effects of enzymes in the body, some of which can fight diseases such as cancer or cardiovascular disease. Some phytochemicals have received a great deal of media attention, such as resveratrol, a substance found in grapes that appears to lower blood cholesterol. The resveratrol in grapes may explain the initial studies showing a beneficial effect of wine in reducing the risk of cardiovascular disease. Soybeans contain genistein, which nutritionists now link to lowering hormone-related cancer risk and stimulating the immune system. Other examples include the vegetables from the cabbage family (cabbage, brussel sprouts and broccoli), which contain phytochemicals that interact with estrogens and prostaglandins in fighting cancer.

A phytochemical-rich diet includes lots of fruits, vegetables, legumes (beans, peas and lentils), herbs and spices, whole grains, soy products, and also tea and nuts. With literally thousands of different phytochemicals already identified, this area of nutrition continues to be a rich field for scientific study. The table below lists beneficial effects of some of the fruits and vegetables studied so far.

Food:	**Beneficial effects:**
Berries, melons, cucumbers, squash & pumpkins	Aids immune system and helps lower blood cholesterol
Broccoli & cabbage family and leafy green vegetables	Lowers risk of hormone-related cancers, boosts ability to fight cancer and protects DNA in cells
Carrots, apricots, other orange & deep yellow fruits & vegetables	Helps protect against cancer, plaque in arteries, blood clotting and loss of eyesight
Citrus (orange, grapefruit, lemon, lime)	Helps body resist carcinogens, and prevents blood clotting and blindness
Grapes (red)	Prevents blood clotting, protects DNA in cells and helps body resist carcinogens
Onions, garlic, leeks & chives	Controls cancer cells, blocks carcinogens, eliminates toxins and lowers blood cholesterol
Soybeans and soy foods	Helps block hormone-related cancers, slow tumor growth, and stimulate the immune system
Tomatoes & eggplant	Shields against carcinogens, reduces cancer and heart attack risk

The most effective approach is to eat as wide a variety of foods as possible to gain benefits from many sources. Studies have demonstrated that not all the foods listed above have the same cancer or blood cholesterol-fighting substances, and the phytochemicals may appear in different concentrations or be absorbed differently. Even different varieties of foods within the same category (such as various varieties of apples or lettuce) may have widely varying concentrations and kinds of phytochemicals. Unfortunately, there is no "magic pill" or supplement which can supply as much as whole foods can, or we would have long ago found an easier way to combat diet-related diseases such as cancer, heart disease, diabetes, and obesity.

What is considered one serving?

Fruits

1 medium whole fruit (apple, banana)
½ cup of canned or fresh fruit
6 oz. (or ¾ cup) 100% fruit juice
¼ cup of dried fruit

Vegetables

½ cup of raw or cooked vegetables
1 cup raw, leafy vegetables
6 oz. (or ¾ cup) vegetable juice

How can I get more fruits and vegetables in my diet?

For a snack or when you're on the go, select nectarines, plums, berries, apple wedges, baby carrots, broccoli spears, or cherry tomatoes. Also, dried fruit is a healthy option over candy. You can easily pack it in a bag and take it on the road or eat at your office.

At home, top your hot or cold cereal with fresh fruit, and drink a glass of 100% juice for breakfast. Smoothies made with fresh or frozen fruits and juices make a great breakfast or lunch choice. Fruit and vegetable juices are also delicious, sweet alternatives to soft drinks. At dinner, include a salad or raw vegetables with low-fat/non-fat dressing to reduce fat and calories. Steamed vegetables are always a good side dish, and you can also add vegetables to your favorite entrees, like tacos, lasagna, casseroles, and pasta dishes. Add pureed vegetables to sauces to fortify them and help get your "5 a day." Try more vegetarian meals, like tofu, rice or pasta with vegetables, or Oriental stir-fries. For dessert, bake apples, peaches, pears, or bananas, or make fruit cobblers.

Experiment with new recipes that emphasize fruits and vegetables, such as those starting on page 159 of this **Healthy Dining** book. Many cookbooks specialize in fruits, vegetables and other natural foods so you can try great-tasting dishes that will help you toward your "5 a day" goal.

When dining out, order meals that include vegetables or fruits as a major component. For example, Chicken with Vegetables at **Pick Up Stix** will provide better nutritional balance than a dish with chicken alone. **Round Table Pizza's** Gourmet Veggie Pizza, which includes artichoke hearts, zucchini, spinach, mushrooms and tomatoes, is a better choice than plain cheese pizza. For a quick meal and a great contribution to your "5 a day," try a blended fruit smoothie at **Jamba Juice**. You can also request substitutions for side dishes. For example, if French fries normally come as part of a meal, request a plain baked potato, steamed vegetables or seasonal fresh fruit instead. Most restaurants are happy to make substitutions if you ask.

> In choosing a restaurant meal from this book, you can determine if the meal contributes significantly to your "5 a day" goal. Look for the symbol next to the entrée's name. The indicates the dish provides at least 2 servings of fruits or vegetables (1 serving for side dishes).

Examples of restaurant meals with 2 or more fruit/vegetable servings:

Charo Chicken (multiple Orange County locations)

SMOKY BBQ RANCH CHICKEN SALAD 🍎

Juicy fire grilled chicken breast, lettuce, corn, cheese, pico de gallo, tortilla strips & BBQ ranch dressing.

✓ CALORIES: Good Choice (640) ✓ CHOLESTEROL: Good Choice (140 mg)
✓ FAT: Good Choice (19 g) SODIUM: High (2040 mg)
EXCHANGES: 6¾ Meat, ¾ Bread, 2 Veg, 2¼ Fruit, 2¼ Fat
PROTEIN: 54 g, CARBOHYDRATE: 67 g, FIBER: 7 g

Green Parrot Café (Santa Ana)

APPLE BRAISED SALMON 🍎

with fine herbs, served over spinach.

✓✓ CALORIES: Excellent Choice (370) ✓ CHOLESTEROL: Good Choice (90 mg)
✓ FAT: Good Choice (16 g)♥ ✓✓ SODIUM: Excellent Choice (150 mg)**
EXCHANGES: 4¼ Meat, 1¾ Veg, ½ Fruit, 1¼ Fat
PROTEIN: 37 g, CARBOHYDRATE: 16 g, FIBER: 4 g

Jamba Juice (multiple Orange County locations)

CARIBBEAN PASSION® SMOOTHIE *(16 oz.)* 🍎

Passion fruit juice blend, orange sherbet, frozen strawberries, frozen peaches and ice.

✓✓ CALORIES: Good Choice (290) ✓✓ CHOLESTEROL: Excellent Choice (5 mg)
✓✓ FAT: Excellent Choice (1½ g) ✓✓ SODIUM: Excellent Choice (40 mg)
PROTEIN: 2 g, CARBOHYDRATE: 67 g, FIBER: 3 g

Diho Siam (Costa Mesa and Mission Viejo)

FRESH PAPAYA SALAD (½ ORDER) 🍎

Papaya with chilies, carrots, green beans, tomatoes & green beans with Thai dressing. Analysis for ½ order.

✓✓ CALORIES: Excellent Choice (255) ✓✓ CHOLESTEROL: Excellent Choice (0 mg)
✓✓ FAT: Excellent Choice (7 g)♥ SODIUM: High (1160 mg)
EXCHANGES: 1 Meat, ½ Bread, 2¼ Veg, 1 Fruit, 1¼ Fat
PROTEIN: 12 g, CARBOHYDRATE: 40 g, FIBER: 8 g

Examples of side dishes with 1 or more fruit/vegetable servings:

The Back Bay Rowing & Running Club Restaurant (Costa Mesa)

VEGETABLE SOUP† *(12 oz. bowl)* 🍎

✓✓ CALORIES: Excellent Choice (70) ✓✓ CHOLESTEROL: Excellent Choice (5 mg)
✓✓ FAT: Excellent Choice (2 g)♥ SODIUM: High (1360 mg)
EXCHANGES: 1¾ Veg
PROTEIN: 4 g, CARBOHYDRATE: 11 g, FIBER: 3 g

The Health Emporium (Corona del Mar)

ORGANIC CARROT, CRANBERRY & WALNUT SALAD *(5 oz. serving)†* 🍎

✓ CALORIES: Good Choice (230) ✓✓ CHOLESTEROL: Excellent Choice (0 mg)
FAT: Moderate (11 g)♥ ✓✓ SODIUM: Excellent Choice (90 mg)**
EXCHANGES. 2 Veg, 1¼ Fruit, 2 Fat
PROTEIN: 3 g, CARBOHYDRATE: 33 g, FIBER: 5 g

Koo Koo Roo (Irvine)

BUTTERNUT SQUASH† *(6 oz.)* 🍎

✓✓ CALORIES: Excellent Choice (65) ✓✓ CHOLESTEROL: Excellent Choice (0 mg)
✓✓ FAT: Excellent Choice (0 g) ✓✓ SODIUM: Excellent Choice (5 mg)
EXCHANGES: ¾ Bread, 2½ Veg
PROTEIN: 2 g, CARBOHYDRATE: 17 g, FIBER: 4 g

🍎 at least 2 fruit/vegetable servings for entrees, 1 for side dishes

CHAPTER 9

Additional Tips for Healthy Dining

Here are some additional dining tips, adapted from "Eating Better When Eating Out," from the USDA Human Nutrition Information Service:

Appetizers: Enjoy raw vegetables dipped in salsa or low-calorie dressing, fruit or steamed seafood. Limit rich sauces, dips and batter-fried foods.

Soups: Choose broth or tomato-based soups rather than creamed soups. Lentil, bean and split pea soups are high in fiber. Most soups are high in sodium.

Breads: Whole grain bread is the best source of complex carbohydrates, vitamins, minerals, and fiber. Watch out for breads with added fat or sugar such as croissants, biscuits, cornbread, muffins (e.g., bran, corn, blueberry) and sweet rolls. Use toppings (butter, cream cheese and margarine) very sparingly.

Vegetables and Salads: Plain vegetables are high in fiber and nutrients and very low in calories, fat and sodium. However, butter, margarine and sauces increase the amount of calories, fat, cholesterol and sodium considerably. Look for vegetables seasoned with lemon, herbs or spices rather than fat and salt. Remember – salad dressings and toppings can add a lot of calories, fat and sodium.

Watch out for prepared salads that contain mayonnaise, salad dressing or oil, such as macaroni salad, potato salad, creamy coleslaw, tuna and chicken salad, and marinated vegetables. Some pasta salads are made with large amounts of oily dressing.

Main Entrees: Ask how meals are prepared and what ingredients are used. Is the fish or chicken broiled with butter or other fat? Is it served with a sauce? How large is the portion? Are vegetables fresh or canned, buttered or creamed?

Fish or poultry that is broiled, grilled, baked, steamed or poached is a good choice. However, entrees are often basted with large amounts of fat. Ask to have your entree prepared without added fat, and that chicken be prepared without skin (or remove the skin before eating). Request that lemon juice, wine or only a small amount of fat be used and that no salt be added.

Watch out for menu selections termed "light fare" or "light." "Light" may or may not mean lower in fat and calories. We have found restaurants in which "On the Light Side" means anything from smaller portions to lower prices!

Choose dishes flavored with herbs and spices rather than rich sauces, gravies, or dressings. If that's not an option, ask for gravies, sour cream, sauces, and other toppings to be served on the side and use sparingly. Limit your use of soy sauce, steak sauce, catsup, mustard, pickles and other condiments to help control sodium.

Portions are often very large. Ask for a take-home bag and eat the remaining portion the next day. Or share an entree with a friend and get an extra appetizer.

Many stir-fried entrees are prepared with very little oil, while some are prepared with too much. Request that yours be prepared with very little.

Pizza can be a low-fat, nutritious choice if you order yours with half the cheese and only vegetable toppings.

Sandwiches can be an excellent choice if you choose lean deli meats such as turkey or ham (but watch portion size!) instead of higher fat cold cuts, such as bologna or salami. Choose whole grain breads and go easy on or avoid oil, butter, avocado, and mayonnaise.

Desserts: Fruits are great! Sherbet, sorbet and low-fat frozen yogurt are much lower in fat than ice cream. If temptation gets to you, share the dessert with a dinner partner.

Words that signal *high fat* include:

buttered or buttery	creamed or creamy	rich
scalloped	fried	breaded
fritters	tempura	croquettes
crispy	with gravy	in cheese sauce
Hollandaise	au gratin	à la king
Béarnaise	Alfredo	Newburg

Words that signal *high sodium* include:

smoked	barbecued	pickled
broth	soy sauce	teriyaki
Creole sauce	marinated	cocktail sauce
tomato base	Parmesan	mustard sauce
fish sauce	hoisin sauce	chili paste

Appendix: Analysis Methods and Accuracy

How is the nutrition analysis done?

Using recipes supplied by the restaurant, a computerized nutritional analysis is performed with the Nutritionist IV and ESHA Food Processor computer programs. The programs use the U.S. Department of Agriculture (USDA) database. We regularly update our program with new data values published by the USDA. When values for recipe ingredients are not available from the USDA database, we contact the manufacturer for nutritional information. If the manufacturer does not have nutritional information, we match ingredients as closely as possible to another product that does have nutritional information.

The data coming from the USDA database and the computer analysis imply a high degree of accuracy. In reality, the USDA found that nutritional values of foods can vary between similar food samples by as much as 20%, and the numbers coming from their measurements represent their average data. As recommended by the FDA, we round the data as follows: for calories, cholesterol and sodium, to the nearest 5 (mg). For fat, protein, carbohydrates and fiber to the nearest whole number, and for diabetic exchanges to the nearest ¼ exchange. Therefore, it is important to note that the numerical values for the selected menu items published in this book are approximations only.

Notes about accuracy

One method to obtain nutritional information is a chemical analysis performed in a professional laboratory. That is, in fact, how the USDA obtained the information for its database. It is very expensive and time-consuming, and therefore not feasible for this project. Every effort was made to ensure accurate information from the computerized analysis and the USDA database.

Two main challenges were encountered with the computerized analysis. First, how much marinade do meats actually absorb? Second, how much oil is absorbed in flash-frying (a method commonly used in Chinese foods)? After numerous conversations with experts throughout the U.S., we found that there has been very little research in these areas. As recommended by nutritionists at the USDA and the Human Nutrition Information Service, we calculate that one gram per one ounce of marinade is absorbed, and that one teaspoon per six ounces of meat is absorbed with flash-frying.

Part II
Healthy Dining Menus

Arranged alphabetically

Also see indexes at back, arranged by cuisine, location, and alphabetically.

Summary of check mark system:

ENTRÉE GUIDELINES †

Calories	✓✓ Excellent Choice = 0 to 450 calories/entree ✓ Good Choice = 451 to 750 calories/entree
Fat	✓✓ Excellent Choice = 0 to 15 grams (g)/entree ✓ Good Choice = 16 to 25 grams (g)/entree
Cholesterol	✓✓ Excellent Choice = 0 to 75 milligrams (mg)/entree ✓ Good Choice = 76 to 150 milligrams (mg)/entree
Sodium	✓✓ Excellent Choice = 0 to 300 milligrams (mg)/entree ✓ Good Choice = 301 to 600 milligrams (mg)/entree

FOOTNOTES

♥ Primarily unsaturated fat
** If you request no added salt
† Side dish guidelines are ⅓ of entree guidelines
at least 2 fruit/vegetable servings

PRICE RANGE SYMBOLS

$ Average entree under $10
$$ Average entree $10 to $20
$$$ Average entree over $20

Special Request – modification of the usual restaurant recipe or preparation method. You must ask for the "Special Request" for the nutrient composition of the dish to correspond to the published nutrition information.

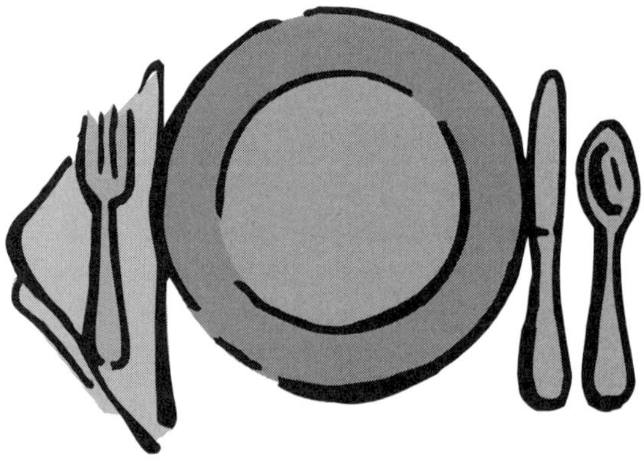

Acapulco offers California-style Mexican food and features traditional favorites – fajitas, burritos, enchiladas and combination platters as well as refreshing margaritas and seafood specialties reminiscent of fresh seafood enjoyed on the Mexican Riviera. Please visit www.acapulcorestaurants.com $

Acapulco Mexican Restaurants

Costa Mesa: 1565 Adams Ave.	(714) 241-0123	Orange: 1535 W. Katella	(714) 639-9550
Diamond Bar: 880 N. Diamond Bar Bl.	(909) 396-5330	Santa Ana: 1262 S.E. Bristol St.	(714) 754-6528
Laguna Niguel: 30100 Town Ctr. Dr.	(949) 495-3372	Stanton: 12765 Beach Blvd.	(714) 895-4444

Long Beach: 6270 E. Pacific Coast Hwy. (562) 596-3371

CHICKEN FAJITAS

Juicy chicken breast in our own special marinade on a sizzling skillet with sautéed onions and bell peppers. Served with rice, beans, pico de gallo, guacamole and your choice of warm corn or flour tortillas. Rice, beans and tortillas not included in analysis (see separate analyses below).

✓ CALORIES: Good Choice (565) CHOLESTEROL: Moderate (175 mg)
✓ FAT: Good Choice (25 g) SODIUM: High (1945 mg)
EXCHANGES: 8 Meat (extra lean), 3½ Veg, 3¾ Fat
PROTEIN: 60 g, CARBOHYDRATE: 25 g, FIBER: 6 g

FISH TACOS – SPECIAL REQUEST

We grill seasoned fish then roll it into two soft tortillas with crisp, fresh cabbage slaw and pico de gallo. Served with sautéed fresh vegetables and rice. Rice not included in analysis (see separate analysis below). Request corn tortillas.

✓ CALORIES: Good Choice (500) ✓✓ CHOLESTEROL: Excellent Choice (60 mg)
✓ FAT: Good Choice (24 g) SODIUM: High (1900 mg)
EXCHANGES: 2¼ Meat, 1¾ Bread, 2¾ Veg, 4¼ Fat
PROTEIN: 30 g, CARBOHYDRATE: 42 g, FIBER: 7 g

HALIBUT FILET WITH SALSA TOMATILLO

A light and flaky Alaskan halibut filet grilled with salsa tomatillo. Served with sautéed fresh vegetables and rice. Rice not included in analysis (see separate analysis below).

✓✓ CALORIES: Excellent Choice (420) ✓ CHOLESTEROL: Good Choice (100 mg)
✓ FAT: Good Choice (16 g) SODIUM: High (1850 mg)
EXCHANGES: 4½ Meat, ¼ Bread, 2¾ Veg, 2 Fat
PROTEIN: 51 g, CARBOHYDRATE: 18 g, FIBER: 4 g

RICE *(5 oz.)*

CAL: 170, FAT: 3♥, CHOL: <1, SOD: 675 mg; EXCH: 2 Bread, ¼ Veg, ½ Fat; PROTEIN: 3 g, CARB: 33 g, FIBER: 1 g

REFRIED BEANS *(5 oz.)*

CAL: 235, FAT: 7♥, CHOL: 0, SOD: 530 mg; EX: ½ Meat, 2¼ Bread, 1¼ Fat; PROTEIN: 11 g, CARB: 34 g, FIBER: 10 g

FLOUR TORTILLA *(6 inch)*

CAL: 90, FAT: 2♥, CHOL: 0, SOD: 160 mg; EXCH: 1 Bread, ½ Fat; PROTEIN: 2 g, CARB: 15 g, FIBER: 1 g

CORN TORTILLA *(6 inch)*

CAL: 60, FAT: 0, CHOL: 0, SOD: 25 mg; EXCH: ¾ Bread, ½ Fat; PROTEIN: 1 g, CARB: 12 g, FIBER: 1 g

♥ Primarily unsaturated fat
(apple icon) at least 2 fruit/vegetable servings

Angie's – "where friends and family meet to eat!" Originally opened about 25 years ago as a pizza parlor, Angie's now offers pasta, sandwiches, soups, salads, vegetarian dishes, appetizers, wines, espresso, cappuccino, and specialty desserts, as well as food to go and catering. Open from 11:30 am to 9:00 pm. $-$$.

Angie's Cuisine Italiano
14425 Newport Ave., Tustin, CA 92780 (714) 832-3434

MEDITERRANEAN SHRIMP

Shrimp sautéed lightly in olive oil, with roasted garlic & a hint of lemon, served on a fresh bed of linguine.

✓ CALORIES: Good Choice (645) CHOLESTEROL: Moderate (225 mg)
✓ FAT: Good Choice (17 g)♥ ✓✓ SODIUM: Excellent Choice (285 mg)**
EXCHANGES: 3½ Meat (extra lean), 5¼ Bread, 2¾ Fat
PROTEIN: 38 g, CARBOHYDRATE: 82 g, FIBER: 5 g

WHOLE EARTH CASSEROLE – SPECIAL REQUEST

Spaghetti in marinara with onions, mushrooms, zucchini, red and green bell peppers, black olives and tomatoes, covered with cheese and oven baked. Request less cheese (1 oz).

✓ CALORIES: Good Choice (610) ✓✓ CHOLESTEROL: Excellent Choice (20 mg)
✓ FAT: Good Choice (23 g) SODIUM: High (1080 mg)
EXCHANGES: ¾ Meat, 3¾ Bread, 3¼ Veg, 3¾ Fat
PROTEIN: 20 g, CARBOHYDRATE: 84 g, FIBER: 9 g

CAPELLINI POMODORO

Angel hair sautéed with olive oil, garlic, sweet basil and diced tomatoes.

✓✓ CALORIES: Excellent Choice (430) ✓✓ CHOLESTEROL: Excellent Choice (0 mg)
✓✓ FAT: Excellent Choice (15 g)♥ ✓✓ SODIUM: Excellent Choice (10 mg)**
EXCHANGES: 3¾ Bread, 1 Veg, 2¾ Fat
PROTEIN: 11 g, CARBOHYDRATE: 63 g, FIBER: 5 g

CHICKEN VEGETABLE PASTA

Skinless chicken breast with garden fresh steamed vegetables, served with angel hair pasta and marinara.

✓ CALORIES: Good Choice (600) ✓ CHOLESTEROL: Good Choice (85 mg)
✓✓ FAT: Excellent Choice (14 g) ✓ SODIUM: Good Choice (445 mg)**
EXCHANGES: 4½ Meat (extra lean), 3¾ Bread, 2½ Veg, 1¾ Fat
PROTEIN: 46 g, CARBOHYDRATE: 73 g, FIBER: 8 g

SPAGHETTI MARINARA

Our own secret recipe!

✓✓ CALORIES: Excellent Choice (370) ✓✓ CHOLESTEROL: Excellent Choice (0 mg)
✓✓ FAT: Excellent Choice (8 g) ♥ ✓ SODIUM: Good Choice (550 mg)**
EXCHANGES: 3¾ Bread, ½ Veg, 1¼ Fat
PROTEIN: 11 g, CARBOHYDRATE: 65 g, FIBER: 5 g

VEGETABLE BIN SANDWICH (½ SANDWICH)

Choose from any 5 veggies covered in marinara & melted cheese & served on a French roll. Analysis for ½ sandwich.

✓ CALORIES: Good Choice (465) ✓✓ CHOLESTEROL: Excellent Choice (45 mg)
✓ FAT: Good Choice (18 g) SODIUM: Moderate (805 mg)**
EXCHANGES: 1½ Meat, 2¾ Bread, 2¾ Veg, 2¼ Fat
PROTEIN: 22 g, CARBOHYDRATE: 58 g, FIBER: 4 g

♥ Primarily unsaturated fat
** If you request no added salt

In keeping with our tradition of physical fitness, The BBR&RC Restaurant strives to serve the finest and freshest foods possible. Our soups and chili are free of preservatives. Our eggs are fresh. Our tuna is packed in water. We don't add sulphites or MSG to anything, and our salad bar filled with fresh produce was chosen "Best Salad Bar of the Year" for 7 consecutive years by Orange County Magazine. $

The Back Bay Rowing & Running Club Restaurant

South Coast Plaza Mall, 3333 Bristol Street
Costa Mesa, CA 92626 (714) 641-0118

THAI TURKEY SALAD – SPECIAL REQUEST 🍎

Chunks of fresh-roasted turkey breast tossed with fresh iceberg lettuce, our unique Thai dressing with chopped peanuts, fresh cilantro and Japanese red peppers that create a superb sweet/hot flavor. With jicama strips, julienned red peppers and carrots. Request no crunchy noodles *(not included in analysis).*

✓✓ CALORIES: Excellent Choice (390) ✓ CHOLESTEROL: Good Choice (95 mg)
✓✓ FAT: Excellent Choice (8 g) ✓ SODIUM: Good Choice (470 mg)**
EXCHANGES: 5¼ Meat, 1¾ Bread, 1¼ Veg, 1 Fat
PROTEIN: 40 g, CARBOHYDRATE: 42 g, FIBER: 5 g

TURKEY BURGER – SPECIAL REQUEST

Ground turkey grilled the old fashioned way and served on a sesame bun, garnished with lettuce, thick slice of red tomato, shaved red onions and slice of pickle. Request dressing on the side *(not included in analysis).*

✓ CALORIES: Good Choice (540) ✓ CHOLESTEROL: Good Choice (115 mg)
✓ FAT: Good Choice (20 g) SODIUM: Moderate (705 mg)**
EXCHANGES: 3½ Meat, 3 Bread, ½ Veg, ½ Fruit, 1¾ Fat
PROTEIN: 35 g, CARBOHYDRATE: 55 g, FIBER: 5 g

VEGGIE HOT TUB – SPECIAL REQUEST 🍎

Fresh spinach, broccoli flowers, black beans, peppers, guacamole, carrots and roasted garlic with red onion rolled in a flour tortilla. Served with fabulous salsas. Request no cheese.

✓ CALORIES: Good Choice (490) ✓✓ CHOLESTEROL: Excellent Choice (0 mg)
✓ FAT: Good Choice (18 g)♥ SODIUM: High (1370 mg)
EXCHANGES: ¼ Meat, 3 Bread, 2½ Veg, 3½ Fat
PROTEIN: 15 g, CARBOHYDRATE: 69 g, FIBER: 9 g

WHOLE GRAIN VEGETARIAN BURGER – SPECIAL REQUEST

Whole grain vegetarian burger grilled the old fashioned way and served on a sesame bun, garnished with lettuce, tomato, red onions and slice of pickle. Request dressing on the side *(not included in analysis).*

✓ CALORIES: Good Choice (600) ✓✓ CHOLESTEROL: Excellent Choice (40 mg)
✓✓ FAT: Excellent Choice (8 g)♥ SODIUM: High (1020 mg)
EXCHANGES: 7 Bread, ¼ Veg, ½ Fruit, 1½ Fat
PROTEIN: 16 g, CARBOHYDRATE: 116 g, FIBER: 15 g

GRILLED CHICKEN SANDWICH – SPECIAL REQUEST

Skinless breast of chicken grilled and served on thick toasted sourdough with wedges of avocado, sprouts, lettuce, tomato and ranch style dressing. Request less avocado *(1 oz.)* and less dressing *(½ oz).*

✓ CALORIES: Good Choice (565) ✓ CHOLESTEROL: Good Choice (110 mg)
✓ FAT: Good Choice (18 g) SODIUM: Moderate (715 mg)**
EXCHANGES: 5¾ Meat (extra lean), 3 Bread, ¾ Veg, 2½ Fat
PROTEIN: 50 g, CARBOHYDRATE: 51 g, FIBER: 4 g

VEGETABLE SOUP† *(12 oz. bowl)* 🍎

✓✓ CALORIES: Excellent Choice (70) ✓✓ CHOLESTEROL: Excellent Choice (5 mg)
✓✓ FAT: Excellent Choice (2 g)♥ SODIUM: High (1360 mg)
EXCHANGES: 1¾ Veg
PROTEIN: 4 g, CARBOHYDRATE: 11 g, FIBER: 3 g

🍎 at least 2 servings fruits/vegetables for entrees, 1 for side dishes
† Side dish guidelines are ⅓ of entree guidelines

Baja Fresh is not your ordinary Mexican restaurant. All of our food is prepared fresh at each location. This ensures the FRESH, quality difference that you taste in our food. We believe we have developed recipes that provide you with the fullest and most pleasing FLAVORS for each of our offerings. While we have worked to develop products that reflect the best FLAVORS and quality for each of our items, many of our customers modify their orders to satisfy their individual taste or dietary needs (i.e., no onions, no sour cream, etc.). $

Baja Fresh Locations

Orange County locations in: Anaheim Hills, Brea, Buena Park, Corona Del Mar, Costa Mesa, Huntington Beach, Irvine, La Habra, Laguna Hills, Laguna Niguel, Lake Forest, Mission Viejo, Newport Beach, Rancho Santa Margarita, San Clemente, Santa Ana, and Seal Beach. For a complete list of all locations visit www.bajafresh.com.

ENCHILADAS VERANO

Charbroiled chicken, grilled peppers, chilis & onions, topped with salsa verde & shaved cheese, served with rice, beans, and pico de gallo.

✓ CALORIES: Good Choice (580) ✓✓ CHOLESTEROL: Excellent Choice (60 mg)
✓✓ FAT: Excellent Choice (9 g) SODIUM: High (2140 mg)
PROTEIN: 38 g, CARBOHYDRATE: 87 g, Fiber 21 g

BARE BURRITO (SERVED IN A BOWL, NO TORTILLA)

Charbroiled chicken, grilled peppers, chilis & onions, rice, beans, pico de gallo and salsa verde.

✓ CALORIES: Good Choice (650) ✓✓ CHOLESTEROL: Excellent Choice (75 mg)
✓✓ FAT: Excellent Choice (7 g) SODIUM: High (2410 mg)
PROTEIN: 45 g, CARBOHYDRATE: 99 g, Fiber 22 g

VEGETARIAN BARE BURRITO (SERVED IN A BOWL, NO TORTILLA)

Grilled peppers, chilis & onions, rice, beans, lettuce, jack cheese, pico de gallo and "Salsa Baja."

✓ CALORIES: Good Choice (560) ✓✓ CHOLESTEROL: Excellent Choice (10 mg)
✓✓ FAT: Excellent Choice (8 g) SODIUM: High (2040 mg)
PROTEIN: 20 g, CARBOHYDRATE: 102 g, Fiber 22 g

SHRIMP ENSALADA 🍎

Charbroiled "wild" gulf shrimp, romaine lettuce, pico de gallo salsa, and salsa verde, topped with tomato slices and cotija cheese. Dressing not included in analysis.

✓✓ CALORIES: Excellent Choice (180) CHOLESTEROL: Moderate (175 mg)
✓✓ FAT: Excellent Choice (4 g) SODIUM: High (1230 mg)
PROTEIN: 22 g, CARBOHYDRATE: 17 g, Fiber 6 g

BAJA MAHI MAHI TACO

Fresh mahi mahi, sliced avocado, cabbage, fresh pico de gallo salsa, and zesty avocado salsa.

✓✓ CALORIES: Excellent Choice (260) ✓✓ CHOLESTEROL: Excellent Choice (20 mg)
✓✓ FAT: Excellent Choice (10 g) ✓ SODIUM: Good Choice (460 mg)
PROTEIN: 13 g, CARBOHYDRATE: 32 g, Fiber 6 g

FRESH MAHI MAHI ENSALADA 🍎

Charbroiled mahi mahi, romaine lettuce, pico de gallo & salsa verde, topped with avocado, tomato slices and shaved cheese. Dressing not included in analysis.

✓✓ CALORIES: Excellent Choice (280) ✓✓ CHOLESTEROL: Excellent Choice (70 mg)
✓✓ FAT: Excellent Choice (9 g) SODIUM: High (1010 mg)
PROTEIN: 34 g, CARBOHYDRATE: 20 g, Fiber 7 g

Nutrition information provided by Baja Fresh.

🍎 at least 2 fruit/vegetable servings for entreés, 1 for side dishes

† Side dish guidelines are ⅓ of entrée guidelines

The Beach House

Established in 1968, the original Beach House recently celebrated its 35th year, and each night as the sun sets behind Catalina Island, diners at every table experience the same beauty that hundreds of thousands of others have enjoyed over the past three decades. The Beach House is an award-winning restaurant that offers a unique variety of dishes including fish, meat, fowl and pasta, and is open every day for breakfast, lunch and dinner. $$-$$$

The Beach House

619 Sleepy Hollow Lane, Laguna Beach, CA 92651 (949) 494-9707
25001 Dana Drive, Dana Point, CA 92629 (949) 496-7310

STUFFED ARTICHOKE – SPECIAL REQUEST†

Stuffed with crab meat. Request less butter (1 tsp.) in preparation.

✓ CALORIES: Good Choice (235) ✓ CHOLESTEROL: Good Choice (30 mg)
✓ FAT: Good Choice (6 g) SODIUM: High (435 mg)
EXCHANGES: ¾ Meat, 1½ Bread, 2½ Veg, 1 Fat
PROTEIN: 15 g, CARBOHYDRATE: 33 g, FIBER: 7 g

SAUTÉED BLUENOSE BASS

Served with fresh steamed vegetables.

✓✓ CALORIES: Excellent Choice (345) ✓ CHOLESTEROL: Good Choice (80 mg)
✓✓ FAT: Excellent Choice (11 g)♥ ✓ SODIUM: Good Choice (510 mg)**
EXCHANGES: 5¾ Meat (extra lean), 3¼ Veg, 1 Fat
PROTEIN: 41 g, CARBOHYDRATE: 17 g, FIBER: 5 g

BAKED GULF PRAWNS – SPECIAL REQUEST

Butterflied with parmesan cheese, sherry and garlic. Served with vegetables and wild rice pilaf (pilaf not included in analysis). Request less cheese (½ oz.) and less butter (1 Tbs.) in preparation, and vegetables steamed.

✓✓ CALORIES: Excellent Choice (425) CHOLESTEROL: Moderate (350 mg)
✓ FAT: Good Choice (20 g) SODIUM: High (1590 mg)
EXCHANGES: 2¾ Meat, 2 Veg, 6 Fat
PROTEIN: 52 g, CARBOHYDRATE: 14 g, FIBER: 5 g

BOUILLABAISSE

Fresh clams, catch of the day, mussels, prawns, scallops and Alaskan crab claw in a Mediterranean-style tomato saffron broth.

✓ CALORIES: Good Choice (480) CHOLESTEROL: Moderate (295 mg)
✓✓ FAT: Excellent Choice (7 g)♥ SODIUM: High (1990 mg)
EXCHANGES: 11½ Meat (extra lean), ¾ Veg, ½ Fat
PROTEIN: 86 g, CARBOHYDRATE: 12 g, FIBER: 1 g

♥ Primarily unsaturated fat
** If you request no added salt

What would the California coast be without crackling beach fires? A drive along the coast will bring you to the state-of-the-art restaurant, BeachFire Bar and Grill. Delectable coastal cuisine, patio dining, superior service, live music and an excellent wine program are the kindling for a truly unique experience. Awarded one of the top ten dining experiences by the Orange County Register, BeachFire boasts over 300 original pieces of artwork for sale by local artists, making the experience exciting for all the senses. Be sure to visit BeachFire for lunch and dinner seven days a week, happy hour weekdays, and live entertainment nightly. Visit BeachFire.com! $$

BeachFire

204 Avenida Del Mar Suite D, San Clemente, CA 92672 (949) 366-3232

AHI TACOS

Blackened sashimi tuna, wasabe crème, wakame salad, black beans, and rice.
Analysis does not include fried plantain.

✓ CALORIES: Good Choice (645) ✓✓ CHOLESTEROL: Excellent Choice (50 mg)
✓✓ FAT: Excellent Choice (15 g)♥ SODIUM: High (1335 mg)
EXCHANGES: 3¾ Meat (extra lean), 4¼ Bread, 1¼ Veg, 1¾ Fat
PROTEIN: 39 g, CARBOHYDRATE: 85 g, FIBER: 12 g

CARMELIZED HALIBUT – SPECIAL REQUEST

with carmelized shallot sauce and seasonal vegetables. Request only 2 oz. shallot sauce.
Garlic mashed potatoes not included in analysis.

✓ CALORIES: Good Choice (550) ✓ CHOLESTEROL: Good Choice (130 mg)
✓ FAT: Good Choice (25 g) ✓✓ SODIUM: Excellent Choice (155 mg)**
EXCHANGES: 5¾ Meat (extra lean), ¼ Bread, 1 Veg, 1¼ Other Carbs, 4¾ Fat
PROTEIN: 49 g, CARBOHYDRATE: 31 g, FIBER: 2 g

GRILLED CHICKEN TACO – SPECIAL REQUEST

Two corn tortillas, with grilled chicken, cilantro cumin cream and mixed cheese, black beans and rice.
Request less cheese (½ oz. per taco) and cilantro cumin cream on the side.
Analysis does not include cilantro cumin cream or fried plantain.

✓ CALORIES: Good Choice (675) ✓ CHOLESTEROL: Good Choice (135 mg)
✓ FAT: Good Choice (19 g) SODIUM: High (1170 mg)
EXCHANGES: 6 Meat (extra lean), 4 Bread, ½ Veg, 2¼ Fat
PROTEIN: 53 g, CARBOHYDRATE: 75 g, FIBER: 10 g

SWEET & SPICY CHICKEN SALAD – SPECIAL REQUEST

Fresh marinated Asian-style chicken, honey-lime vinaigrette and julienned lettuce mix.
Request less dressing (1 oz.) and fried wontons on the side. Analysis does not include fried wontons.

✓✓ CALORIES: Excellent Choice (300) ✓✓ CHOLESTEROL: Excellent Choice (70 mg)
✓ FAT: Good Choice (17 g) ✓✓ SODIUM: Excellent Choice (100 mg)**
EXCHANGES: 3¾ Meat (extra lean), ¾ Veg, 3 Fat
PROTEIN: 30 g, CARBOHYDRATE: 7 g, FIBER: 3 g

TORTILLA SOUP

Fresh vegetable and herb stock with grilled chicken, avocado, sour cream and tri-colored tortilla chips.
Analysis does not include tri-colored tortilla chips.

✓✓ CALORIES: Excellent Choice (200) ✓✓ CHOLESTEROL: Excellent Choice (60 mg)
✓✓ FAT: Excellent Choice (10 g) ✓ SODIUM: Good Choice (460 mg)
EXCHANGES: 2½ Meat, ¼ Bread, 1½ Veg, 1½ Fat
PROTEIN: 20 g, CARBOHYDRATE: 14 g, FIBER: 4 g

at least 2 fruit/vegetable servings

What is different about us is that our food is prepared homemade from scratch the way you would make it if you had the time. At the Blackboard Bistro we use only the freshest, highest quality ingredients and of course there are no preservatives. For example, we feature fresh ground Kona coffee and fresh squeezed juices, and our soups and salad dressings are made fresh from scratch every day. We have four different flavors of homemade preserves, made with the minimum of sugar, and we serve the freshest meats, and turkey, as well as offer Gardenburgers and other vegetarian choices. $-$$

Blackboard Bistro
1198 Pacific Coast Hwy., Seal Beach, CA 90740 (562) 596-9556
www.blackboardbistro.com

VEGETARIAN EGG WHITE OMELETTE – SPECIAL REQUEST

Three XL AA egg white omelette with mushroom, tomatoes, pepper and onions and avocado, served with brown rice. Request egg whites and less cheese *(½ oz). Sour cream and toast not included in analysis.*

✓ CALORIES: Good Choice (505) ✓✓ CHOLESTEROL: Excellent Choice (15 mg)
✓ FAT: Good Choice (23 g) ✓✓ SODIUM: Excellent Choice (275 mg)**
EXCHANGES: 2 Meat, 2¾ Bread, ¼ Fruit, 1 Veg, 4 Fat
PROTEIN: 21 g, CARBOHYDRATE: 54 g, FIBER: 7 g

BISTRO BURGER VEGGIE PATTY WITH SALAD – SPECIAL REQUEST

Gardenburger served with lettuce, tomato and salad for choice of side dish. Request salad dressing on the side *(pickles, salad dressing and croutons not included in analysis).*

✓ CALORIES: Good Choice (650) ✓✓ CHOLESTEROL: Excellent Choice (25 mg)
✓ FAT: Good Choice (16 g)♥ SODIUM: High (1145 mg)
EXCHANGES: 2¼ Meat, 5 Bread, 2¾ Veg, ½ Fruit, 1¾ Fat
PROTEIN: 29 g, CARBOHYDRATE: 101 g, FIBER: 17 g

CLASSIC TURKEY SANDWICH – SPECIAL REQUEST

Hand carved turkey with Swiss cheese, lettuce, tomato and mayo on squaw bread, served with seasonal fresh fruit. Request less Swiss cheese *(1 oz).*

✓ CALORIES: Good Choice (670) CHOLESTEROL: Moderate (155 mg)
✓ FAT: Good Choice (25 g) ✓ SODIUM: Good Choice (550 mg)**
EXCHANGES: 6¾ Meat, 1¾ Bread, 1 Veg, 1½ Fruit, 3¾ Fat
PROTEIN: 60 g, CARBOHYDRATE: 56 g, FIBER: 7 g

GOOD EARTH SANDWICH – SPECIAL REQUEST

Ripe tomatoes, red onion, alfalfa sprouts, spinach, cucumber, avocado and Jack cheese with 1000 Island on Squaw bread, served with seasonal fresh fruit. Request less cheese *(1 oz.)* and less dressing *(½ Tbs).*

✓ CALORIES: Good Choice (535) ✓✓ CHOLESTEROL: Excellent Choice (30 mg)
✓ FAT: Good Choice (25 g) SODIUM: Moderate (625 mg)**
EXCHANGES: ¾ Meat, 1¾ Bread, 2¼ Veg, 1¾ Fruit, 4¼ Fat
PROTEIN: 18 g, CARBOHYDRATE: 67 g, FIBER: 12 g

MUSHROOM JACK TURKEY BURGER – SPECIAL REQUEST

Turkey burger with fresh sautéed mushrooms and Jack cheese, served with a cup of vegetable soup. Request less Jack cheese *(½ oz). Analysis does not include pickles.*

✓ CALORIES: Good Choice (700) ✓ CHOLESTEROL: Good Choice (105 mg)
✓ FAT: Good Choice (21 g) SODIUM: High (1845 mg)
EXCHANGES: 4½ Meat, 3¼ Bread, 3¼ Veg, ½ Fruit, 1¾ Fat
PROTEIN: 47 g, CARBOHYDRATE: 73 g, FIBER: 8 g

ROSEMARY CHICKEN

A fresh double breast of chicken marinated in rosemary, herbs, and extra virgin olive oil, served with brown rice, veggies and a cup of vegetable soup.

✓ CALORIES: Good Choice (655) ✓ CHOLESTEROL: Good Choice (145 mg)
✓✓ FAT: Excellent Choice (12 g) SODIUM: High (1440 mg)
EXCHANGES: 7½ Meat (extra lean), 3¼ Bread, 2¾ Veg, 1 Fat
PROTEIN: 67 g, CARBOHYDRATE: 68 g, FIBER: 12 g

♥ Primarily unsaturated fat
** If you request no added salt

BLUEWATER GRILL

SEAFOOD RESTAURANT & OYSTER BAR

At the Bluewater Grill, the fish is so fresh the menu is printed daily! We feature over fifteen varieties of fresh fish which are prepared over a mesquite wood fired barbecue. In addition, we have numerous salads, pastas and an oyster bar with oysters, shrimp, crab, clams, mussels, sushi, sashimi, and much more. Our menu philosophy is to purchase the freshest fish possible and to serve it simply, without sauces filled with lots of calories. $$

Bluewater Grill

Newport Beach: 630 Lido Park Dr. (949) 675-3474
Santa Ana: 1621 W. Sunflower Ave. (714) 546-3474

FRESH FISH & SEAFOOD

Analyses for 8 oz. portions (unless noted otherwise) are listed in the table below.
Each is served with 2 side dishes – fresh broccoli and sliced tomatoes recommended (see analysis below).

Note: all carbohydrate values for fish and other seafood are essentially 0.

	Calories	Fat (g)	Cholesterol (mg)	Sodium (mg)	Protein (g)
Shrimp	✓✓ 225	✓✓ 2♥	445	✓ 505	47
Scallops	✓✓ 205	✓✓ 3♥	✓ 95	✓ 480	42
Oysters (6 med.)	✓✓ 60	✓✓ 2♥	✓✓ 45	✓✓ 95	6
Alaskan King Crab (1 lb.)	✓✓ 130	✓✓ 2♥	✓✓ 70	1435	26
Australian Lobster Tail *(without butter)*	✓✓ 265	✓✓ 2♥	195	1025	56
Maine Lobster *(without butter)*	✓✓ 445	✓✓ 3♥	325	1725	93
Orange Roughy	✓✓ 150	✓✓ 2♥	✓✓ 45	✓✓ 140	32
Lingcod	✓✓ 190	✓✓ 2♥	✓ 115	✓✓ 130	39
Mahi Mahi	✓✓ 195	✓✓ 2♥	165	✓✓ 200	42
Ahi Tuna	✓✓ 220	✓✓ 2♥	✓ 90	✓✓ 75	48
Monkfish	✓✓ 165	✓✓ 3♥	✓✓ 55	✓✓ 40	32
Red Snapper	✓✓ 225	✓✓ 3♥	✓ 85	✓✓ 100	47
Walleye Pike	✓✓ 270	✓✓ 4♥	250	✓✓ 150	56
Alaskan Halibut	✓✓ 245	✓✓ 5♥	✓✓ 75	✓✓ 125	47
Striped Bass	✓✓ 220	✓✓ 5♥	180	✓✓ 155	40
White Seabass	✓✓ 280	✓✓ 6♥	✓ 120	✓✓ 200	54
Rainbow Trout	✓✓ 270	✓✓ 8♥	✓ 130	✓✓ 60	47
Thresher Shark	✓✓ 265	✓✓ 9♥	✓ 105	✓✓ 160	43
Pacific Swordfish	✓✓ 275	✓✓ 9♥	✓ 90	✓✓ 205	45
Atlantic Salmon	✓✓ 315	✓✓ 14♥	✓ 120	✓✓ 95	44
Mississippi Catfish	✓✓ 345	✓ 18♥	✓ 145	✓✓ 180	42
King Salmon	✓✓ 365	✓ 21♥	✓ 135	✓✓ 95	41

SLICED TOMATOES AND FRESH BROCCOLI 🍎

CALORIES: 35, FAT: ½ g♥, CHOLESTEROL: 0 mg, SODIUM: 30 mg, FIBER: 3 g
EXCHANGES: 1¼ Veg; PROTEIN: 3 g, CARBOHYDRATE: 7 g

🍎 at least 2 fruit/vegetable servings for entrees, 1 for side dishes

† Side dish guidelines are ⅓ of entrée guidelines

CAFÉ Chin Chin ASIAN FAST CASUAL

"Chin Chin" not only means "to your health" but it is also known as a popular hotspot for Chinese and Asian food, offering generous portions served in a fast and friendly setting with a contemporary atmosphere. Café Chin Chin is committed to preparing nutritious, healthy food and offers "LITE" and "Low-Carb" stir-fry selections. **$**

Café Chin Chin

Lakewood Mall: Candlewood Restaurant Row (562) 616-7171
Tustin Market Place: 2945 El Camino Real (714) 689-3131

LITE FIERY SZECHUAN CHICKEN – SPECIAL REQUEST

Chicken with sweet chili hoisin sauce and zucchini, red bell peppers, water chestnuts, cloud ear mushrooms, and onions. Request LITE preparation.

✓ CALORIES: Good Choice (560) — CHOLESTEROL: Moderate (160 mg)
✓✓ FAT: Excellent Choice (10 g) — SODIUM: High (2595 mg)
EXCHANGES: 8 Meat (extra lean), ½ Bread, 3¾ Veg, ¼ Fruit, ½ Fat
PROTEIN: 61 g, CARBOHYDRATE: 45 g, FIBER: 8 g

LITE GINGER WINE SHRIMP – SPECIAL REQUEST

Classic light sauce with shrimp, ginger, snow peas, water chestnuts, carrots and Chinese wine. Request LITE preparation.

✓✓ CALORIES: Excellent Choice (435) — CHOLESTEROL: Moderate (290 mg)
✓✓ FAT: Excellent Choice (2 g)♥ — SODIUM: High (1785 mg)
EXCHANGES: 4½ Meat (extra lean), ¾ Bread, 5½ Veg, 1½ Fruit
PROTEIN: 35 g, CARBOHYDRATE: 67 g, FIBER: 13 g

LITE VEGETABLE BOWL WITH MANDARIN KUNG PAO SAUCE – SPECIAL REQUEST

Assorted vegetables stir-fried with Mandarin Kung Pao sauce and served over brown rice. Request LITE preparation

✓ CALORIES: Good Choice (705) — ✓✓ CHOLESTEROL: Excellent Choice (0 mg)
✓✓ FAT: Excellent Choice (4 g)♥ — SODIUM: High (2560 mg)
EXCHANGES: 5¾ Bread, 6¾ Veg, 1¾ Fruit, ½ Fat
PROTEIN: 20 g, CARBOHYDRATE: 153 g, FIBER: 21 g

LITE CHICKEN TERIYAKI RICE BOWL – SPECIAL REQUEST

Fresh vegetables topped with sweet teriyaki glazed chicken. Request LITE preparation, white meat chicken, and brown rice.

CALORIES: Moderate (855) — ✓ CHOLESTEROL: Good Choice (135 mg)
✓✓ FAT: Excellent Choice (11 g) — SODIUM: High (1650 mg)
EXCHANGES: 6¾ Meat (extra lean), 6 Bread, 3 Veg, 1 Fruit, ½ Fat
PROTEIN: 60 g, CARBOHYDRATE: 129 g, FIBER: 9 g

LITE CLASSIC CHICKEN SALAD – SPECIAL REQUEST

Roasted chicken, shredded lettuce, scallions, shredded carrots and toasted almonds in a LITE tart red ginger dressing. Request won ton crunchies on the side (not in analysis) and LITE dressing.

✓✓ CALORIES: Excellent Choice (440) — ✓✓ CHOLESTEROL: Excellent Choice (60 mg)
✓ FAT: Good Choice (16 g) — SODIUM: High (3570 mg)
EXCHANGES: 3 Meat (extra lean), 2 Bread, 1 Veg, 2½ Fat
PROTEIN: 31 g, CARBOHYDRATE: 43 g, FIBER: 5 g

STEAMED CHICKEN POTSTICKERS *(2)* – SPECIAL REQUEST†

Analysis for 2 potstickers and ½ serving of apricot sauce. Request potstickers steamed.

✓ CALORIES: Good Choice (175) — ✓ CHOLESTEROL: Good Choice (30 mg)
✓✓ FAT: Excellent Choice (5 g) — SODIUM: High (525 mg)**
EXCHANGES: 1 Meat, 1¼ Bread, ¼ Veg, ¼ Fat
PROTEIN: 10 g, CARBOHYDRATE: 22 g, FIBER: 1 g

♥ Primarily unsaturated fat
** If you request no added salt

Café de France has been a restaurant providing healthy and fresh food with the latest nutritional concepts and recipes that bring out the honest flavors in our French Cuisine. You will enjoy the finest food expertly prepared and beautifully presented. $

Café de France

4213 Campus Drive, Irvine, CA 92612 (949) 854-5002

CHICKEN SALAD

All white meat chicken breast, celery, onion, raisins, walnuts, crisp greens and a variety of garden vegetables. Dressing not included in analysis.

✓✓ CALORIES: Excellent Choice (415) ✓ CHOLESTEROL: Good Choice (100 mg)
✓✓ FAT: Excellent Choice (15 g) SODIUM: High (1305 mg)
EXCHANGES: 5 Meat (extra lean), 2½ Veg, ¾ Fruit, 1¾ Fat
PROTEIN: 44 g, CARBOHYDRATE: 29 g, FIBER: 10 g

CHICKEN DIJON

Marinated breast of chicken, topped with our own Dijon sauce and served with wild rice & steamed vegetables.

✓ CALORIES: Good Choice (490) ✓ CHOLESTEROL: Good Choice (145 mg)
✓ FAT: Good Choice (22 g) SODIUM: High (1915 mg)
EXCHANGES: 6¾ Meat (extra lean), ¼ Bread, 1¼ Veg, 2¾ Fat
PROTEIN: 56 g, CARBOHYDRATE: 16 g, FIBER: 4 g

SALMON WITH DILL SAUCE

Fresh salmon topped with roasted garlic, plum tomato, sweet onion and dill, served with wild rice and steamed vegetables.

✓ CALORIES: Good Choice (550) ✓ CHOLESTEROL: Good Choice (115 mg)
FAT: Moderate (29 g)♥ SODIUM: High (1755 mg)
EXCHANGES: 4¼ Meat, ¼ Bread, 3¾ Veg, 3¼ Fat
PROTEIN: 44 g, CARBOHYDRATE: 31 g, FIBER: 6 g

VEGETARIAN SANDWICH – SPECIAL REQUEST

Swiss cheese, sprouts, avocado and a variety of garden vegetables served on a baguette. Request no ranch dressing (not included in analysis).

✓ CALORIES: Good Choice (640) ✓✓ CHOLESTEROL: Excellent Choice (25 mg)
✓ FAT: Good Choice (22 g) SODIUM: Moderate (780 mg)**
EXCHANGES: 1 Meat, ¾ Bread, 1¾ Veg, 3¾ Fat
PROTEIN: 25 g, CARBOHYDRATE: 88 g, FIBER: 8 g

at least 2 fruit/vegetable servings

CAFÉ VIENNA CAFÉ HEIDELBERG

Café Vienna and Café Heidelberg feature an inviting dining experience for breakfast, lunch, and in-between meal treats. Unwind and relax on the outdoor patio or inside. Owner/chef Ferdinand Lettner is European-trained in cooking and baking. He has pleased the palates of diners the world over in numerous hotel restaurants. The popularity of Café Heidelberg and Café Vienna is evident by the many repeat customers and by the fact that finding a table on weekends can be a challenge! Come experience these delightful cafés for yourself! $

Café Heidelberg 1100 S. Coast Highway #116, Laguna Beach (949) 497-4594

Café Vienna 31542 S. Coast Highway, Laguna Beach (949) 499-3015

CALIFORNIA OMELETE – SPECIAL REQUEST

Egg whites, spinach, cheese, and sun-dried tomatoes topped with sliced avocado.
Request only ½ Tbs. oil/butter blend.

✓ CALORIES: Good Choice (530) ✓✓ CHOLESTEROL: Excellent Choice (45 mg)
✓ FAT: Good Choice (24 g) ✓ SODIUM: Good Choice (575 mg)**
EXCHANGES: 2¾ Meat, 8 Veg, ¼ Fruit, 4½ Fat
PROTEIN: 34 g, CARBOHYDRATE: 45 g, FIBER: 12 g

EGGS HEIDELBERG

Poached eggs, smoked Norwegian salmon & grilled cherry tomatoes served on top of 9-grain toast.

✓ CALORIES: Good Choice (610) CHOLESTEROL: High (465 mg)
✓ FAT: Good Choice (23 g) SODIUM: High (2400 mg)
EXCHANGES: 3½ Meat, 3½ Bread, ¼ Milk, 1 Veg, 2 Fat
PROTEIN: 41 g, CARBOHYDRATE: 60 g, FIBER: 8 g

POTATO PANCAKES – SPECIAL REQUEST

with apple sauce and fresh fruits. Request only 1 Tbs. butter/oil blend.

✓✓ CALORIES: Excellent Choice (395) ✓ CHOLESTEROL: Good Choice (100 mg)
✓✓ FAT: Excellent Choice (9 g) ✓✓ SODIUM: Excellent Choice (210 mg)**
EXCHANGES: ½ Meat, 2¼ Bread, 1¾ Fruit, ¼ Other Carb, 1½ Fat
PROTEIN: 8 g, CARBOHYDRATE: 73 g, FIBER: 7 g

CHICKEN BREAST SALAD – SPECIAL REQUEST

Grilled chicken breast over romaine lettuce with tomatoes and mushrooms.
Request only 1 Tbs. oil used in chicken preparation. Salad dressing not included in analysis.

✓✓ CALORIES: Excellent Choice (450) ✓ CHOLESTEROL: Good Choice (150 mg)
✓ FAT: Good Choice (20 g) ✓ SODIUM: Good Choice (435 mg)**
EXCHANGES: 8 Meat (extra lean), 1½ Veg, 3 Fat
PROTEIN: 59 g, CARBOHYDRATE: 7 g, FIBER: 3 g

TURKEY MELT

Turkey breast and melted Jack cheese on 7 grain bread.

✓✓ CALORIES: Excellent Choice (420) ✓ CHOLESTEROL: Good Choice (100 mg)
✓✓ FAT: Excellent Choice (13 g) SODIUM: Moderate (805 mg)**
EXCHANGES: 4¼ Meat, 2¼ Bread, ¾ Veg, 1½ Fat
PROTEIN: 39 g, CARBOHYDRATE: 36 g, FIBER: 5 g

♥ Primarily unsaturated fat
** If you request no added salt

CALIFORNIA WOK

Natural Chinese and Thai Cuisine

California Wok creatively captures the trend toward fresh food and Asian influence in Southern California. We emphasize the modern approach to Chinese and Thai cuisine, from the decor with dusty pink walls and black chairs, to the delicious flavors and crispness of the vegetables. We will gladly prepare any item on our menu without oil or salt upon your request. Each and every dish is prepared with tender loving care for your fullest enjoyment. After all, we are what we eat, and healthy hearts are happy hearts! We are a full service restaurant providing custom catering and banquet facilities. $

California Wok 4466 Cerritos Ave., Los Alamitos, CA 90720 (714) 527-0226

Sodium in most dishes can be reduced by up to ½ by requesting less soy sauce and/or fish sauce.

SHRIMP & LEMON GRASS SOUP

A hot, sour and spicy shrimp soup with lemon grass.

✓✓ CALORIES: Excellent Choice (225) CHOLESTEROL: Moderate (220 mg)
✓✓ FAT: Excellent Choice (2 g)♥ SODIUM: Moderate (890 mg)**
EXCHANGES: 3½ Meat (extra lean), 2¾ Veg
PROTEIN: 30 g, CARBOHYDRATE: 22 g, FIBER: 5 g

CHINESE CHICKEN SALAD

Chicken over lettuce and cabbage with carrots, water chestnuts, slivered almonds, sesame seeds and Chinese dressing. Crispy wontons not included in analysis.

✓ CALORIES: Good Choice (590) ✓ CHOLESTEROL: Good Choice (145 mg)
✓✓ FAT: Excellent Choice (14 g) SODIUM: High (2120 mg)
EXCHANGES: 7½ Meat (extra lean), 1¼ Bread, 3 Veg, ¾ Fruit, 1¼ Fat
PROTEIN: 59 g, CARBOHYDRATE: 57 g, FIBER: 7 g

RAINBOW CHICKEN

Slices of chicken breast stir-fried with mixed vegetables in the chef's special white wine sauce.

✓✓ CALORIES: Excellent Choice (375) ✓ CHOLESTEROL: Good Choice (130 mg)
✓✓ FAT: Excellent Choice (7 g) ✓✓ SODIUM: Excellent Choice (250 mg)**
EXCHANGES: 6¾ Meat (extra lean), ½ Bread, 3¼ Veg, ¼ Fat
PROTEIN: 52 g, CARBOHYDRATE: 26 g, FIBER: 6 g

TEPPANYAKI VEGETABLES AND TOFU

A mixture of vegetables – broccoli, red onions, fresh mushrooms, snow peas and bean sprouts, stir-fried with tofu and served with a delicate ginger, garlic and mustard sauce on the side (2 Tbs. included in analysis). Chicken or shrimp versions of this dish also available.

✓✓ CALORIES: Excellent Choice (255) ✓✓ CHOLESTEROL: Excellent Choice (<5 mg)
✓✓ FAT: Excellent Choice (12 g)♥ SODIUM: Moderate (795 mg)**
EXCHANGES: 1¼ Meat, ¼ Bread, 4 Veg, 1¾ Fat
PROTEIN: 18 g, CARBOHYDRATE: 25 g, FIBER: 7 g

SHRIMP IN GARLIC SAUCE

Shrimp sautéed with mixed vegetables in hot garlic sauce.

✓✓ CALORIES: Excellent Choice (270) CHOLESTEROL: Moderate (220 mg)
✓✓ FAT: Excellent Choice (7 g)♥ SODIUM: Moderate (625 mg)**
EXCHANGES: 2 Meat (extra lean), ½ Bread, 2¼ Veg, 1 Fat
PROTEIN: 27 g, CARBOHYDRATE: 24 g, FIBER: 4 g

LARB GAI – CHICKEN

Chopped chicken with ground rice grain, mint leaves, lime juice & chili, served with crisp cabbage leaves.

✓✓ CALORIES: Excellent Choice (425) ✓ CHOLESTEROL: Good Choice (130 mg)
✓✓ FAT: Excellent Choice (7 g) SODIUM: High (1065 mg)
EXCHANGES: 6¾ Meat (extra lean), 1 Bread, 2½ Veg, ¼ Fruit
PROTEIN: 52 g, CARBOHYDRATE: 39 g, FIBER: 5 g

♥ Primarily unsaturated fat
** If you request no added salt

Our mission is to provide the best tasting fast food anywhere. We do this by selecting the finest ingredients and preparing our delicious food hourly at each location. Our expert cooks combine the most expensive herbs and spices with the freshest produce available to give you an unforgettable dining experience. Please visit www.charochicken.com. $

Charo Chicken *WE DELIVER!*

Costa Mesa: 1170 Baker St., G1	(714) 540-9700	Long Beach: 4752 E. PCH	(562) 498-5600
Dana Point: 24831 Del Prado Av.	(949) 496-0044	Los Alamitos: 11105 Los Alamitos Bl.	(562) 598-7979
Foothill Ranch: 26696 Portola Pkwy	(949) 837-7800	Murrieta: 39252 Winchester Rd. #113	(909) 698-0080
Huntington Beach: 6531 Edinger Av.	(714) 892-2900	Redondo Bch: 1617 S. PCH, #101	(310) 792-0388
Irvine: 18040-A Culver Dr.	(949) 786-2000	San Clemente: 1021 Avenida Pico	(949) 366-2650
Lake Forest: 22611 Lake Forest Dr.	(949) 581-3770	Seal Beach: 333 Main St.	(562) 594-0909
Lakewood: 4846 Paramount Blvd.	(562) 216-9000	Tustin: 17612 E. 17th St.	(714) 832-1300

2 Pieces White Meat Chicken - Skinless

✓✓ Calories: Excellent Choice (185) ✓ Cholesterol: Good Choice (90 mg)
✓✓ Fat: Excellent Choice (5 g) ✓✓ Sodium: Excellent Choice (80 mg)**
Exchanges: 4¾ Meat
Protein: 33 g, Carbohydrate: 0 g, Fiber: 0 g

Fiesta Ensalada – Special Request 🍎

Juicy fire grilled chicken breast, lettuce, tomatoes, tortilla chips & cheese.
Request dressing on the side (not included in analysis).
✓✓ Calories: Excellent Choice (440) ✓ Cholesterol: Good Choice (120 mg)
✓ Fat: Good Choice (16 g) ✓ Sodium: Good Choice (535 mg)**
Exchanges: 6¼ Meat (extra lean), 1 Bread, 1½ Veg, 1¾ Fat
Protein: 51 g, Carbohydrate: 23 g, Fiber: 6 g

Smoky BBQ Ranch Chicken Salad 🍎

Juicy fire grilled chicken breast, lettuce, corn, cheese, pico de gallo salsa, tortilla strips and our own BBQ ranch dressing.
✓ Calories: Good Choice (640) ✓ Cholesterol: Good Choice (140 mg)
✓ Fat: Good Choice (19 g) Sodium: High (2040 mg)
Exchanges: 6¾ Meat, ¾ Bread, 2 Veg, 2¼ Fruit, 2¼ Fat
Protein: 54 g, Carbohydrate: 67 g, Fiber: 7 g

El Taco Grande

Corn tortillas with marinated chicken breast, cheddar cheese, lettuce, salsa, and dressing.
Tortilla chips not included in analysis.
✓✓ Calories: Excellent Choice (440) ✓ Cholesterol: Good Choice (90 mg)
✓ Fat: Good Choice (21 g) Sodium: High (1040 mg)
Exchanges: 3¾ Meat, 1½ Bread, 1 Veg, 3 Fat
Protein: 31 g, Carbohydrate: 32 g, Fiber: 2 g

Veggie Bowl

Generous portions of our critically acclaimed rice, pinto or black beans, and mild pico de gallo salsa.
✓ Calories: Good Choice (675) ✓✓ Cholesterol: Excellent Choice (0 mg)
✓ Fat: Good Choice (20 g)♥ Sodium: High (2565 mg)
Exchanges: 5¾ Bread, 1¾ Veg, 3¾ Fat
Protein: 21 g, Carbohydrate: 105 g, Fiber: 11 g

Rice (¾ cup serving) †

✓ Calories: Good Choice (175) ✓✓ Cholesterol: Excellent Choice (0 mg)
✓ Fat: Good Choice (6 g) Sodium: Moderate (325 mg)
Protein: 3 g, Carbohydrate: 28 g, Fiber: 1g; Exchanges: 1¾ Bread, 1 Fat

Corn on the Cob (3 inch cob) †

✓✓ Calories: Excellent Choice (40) ✓✓ Cholesterol: Excellent Choice (0 mg)
✓✓ Fat: Excellent Choice (0 g) ✓✓ Sodium: Excellent Choice (5 mg)**
Protein: 1 g, Carbohydrate: 10 g, Fiber: 1g; Exchanges: ½ Bread

🍎 at least 2 fruit/vegetable servings
† Side dish guidelines are ⅓ of entree guidelines

Our goal is to serve the freshest, tastiest Chinese food possible. To ensure quality, we have daily deliveries from our suppliers, including trips to the market to hand pick certain produce. Each dish is cooked to order and to the customer's specifications if requested. Any addition or deletion of ingredients such as salt, sugar, garlic, starch, etc., will be made upon request. $

Chin's Chinese Kitchen

13771 Newport Avenue, Tustin, CA 92780 (714) 838-0604

Analyses below are for ½ orders since dishes are often shared.

SNOWPEAS WITH SHRIMP (½ ORDER)

Shrimp, snowpeas and onion stir fired in special sauce.

✓✓ CALORIES: Excellent Choice (210) CHOLESTEROL: Moderate (165 mg)
✓✓ FAT: Excellent Choice (8 g)♥ ✓ SODIUM: Good Choice (485 mg)**
EXCHANGES: 2½ Meat (extra lean), 1¾ Veg, 1½ Fat
PROTEIN: 22 g, CARBOHYDRATE: 12 g, FIBER: 4 g

MIXED VEGETABLES (½ ORDER)

Broccoli, bamboo shoots, water chestnuts, carrots, bok choy, celery and bean sprouts.

✓✓ CALORIES: Excellent Choice (145) ✓✓ CHOLESTEROL: Excellent Choice (<1 mg)
✓✓ FAT: Excellent Choice (8 g)♥ ✓ SODIUM: Good Choice (350 mg)**
EXCHANGES: 2¾ Veg, 1½ Fat
PROTEIN: 7 g, CARBOHYDRATE: 16 g, FIBER: 5 g

BROCCOLI CHICKEN (½ ORDER)

Skinless chicken with broccoli and onions stir fried in special sauce.

✓✓ CALORIES: Excellent Choice (305) ✓ CHOLESTEROL: Good Choice (90 mg)
✓✓ FAT: Excellent Choice (14 g) ✓ SODIUM: Good Choice (405 mg)**
EXCHANGES: 4¼ Meat , 1½ Veg, 1½ Fat
PROTEIN: 35 g, CARBOHYDRATE: 10 g, FIBER: 4 g

CHICKEN CHOW MEIN (½ ORDER) – SPECIAL REQUEST

Skinless chicken with bamboo shoots, water chestnuts, celery and bean sprouts.
Request rice instead of crunchy noodles.

✓✓ CALORIES: Excellent Choice (435) ✓ CHOLESTEROL: Good Choice (90 mg)
✓✓ FAT: Excellent Choice (14 g) ✓ SODIUM: Good Choice (400 mg)**
EXCHANGES: 4¼ Meat, 1½ Bread, 3 Veg, 1½ Fat
PROTEIN: 39 g, CARBOHYDRATE: 38 g, FIBER: 5 g

at least 2 fruit/vegetable servings

The Culinary Wrap, where California Cuisine meets International Flare. "The greatest wraps around" – as many local and national publications have touted (i.e., Daily Pilot, Orange County Register and Orange County Weekly). Come in and taste what everyone is raving about—Healthy Food, Great Prices and Service amidst an Upbeat Atmosphere. $

The Culinary Wrap

Brea (Brea Union Plaza): 2435 E. Imperial Hwy., Suite E (714) 672-9727
Costa Mesa (Hillgren Square): 250 E. 17th St., Suite D (949) 548-4403
Cal State Long Beach on campus (49ER Shops): 6049 E. 7th St. (562) 494-9727

Wraps are served with choice of side dishes. Fruit, vegetables, or garden salad recommended.

THAI CHICKEN WRAP

Chicken, Thai lettuce mix, bean sprouts, cucumbers, cilantro and spicy peanut sauce.

✓✓ CALORIES: Excellent Choice (360) ✓✓ CHOLESTEROL: Excellent Choice (65 mg)
✓✓ FAT: Excellent Choice (10 g) SODIUM: Moderate (720 mg)**
EXCHANGES: 4 Meat (extra lean), 1¼ Bread, 1½ Veg, ½ Fruit, 1¼ Fat
PROTEIN: 37 g, CARBOHYDRATE: 36 g, FIBER: 4 g

SALMON WRAP

Blackened salmon, black bean and corn salsa, lettuce and chipotle chili sauce.

✓✓ CALORIES: Excellent Choice (415) ✓✓ CHOLESTEROL: Excellent Choice (45 mg)
✓ FAT: Good Choice (19 g)♥ SODIUM: High (1010 mg)
EXCHANGES: 2¼ Meat, 2 Bread, ½ Veg, ¼ Fruit, 2¾ Fat
PROTEIN: 24 g, CARBOHYDRATE: 37 g, FIBER: 5 g

GREEK WRAP

Roasted red peppers and eggplant, tomatoes, red onion, cucumbers, lettuce and feta tossed in a balsamic vinaigrette.

✓✓ CALORIES: Excellent Choice (365) ✓✓ CHOLESTEROL: Excellent Choice (25 mg)
✓ FAT: Good Choice (21 g) SODIUM: High (1435 mg)
EXCHANGES: ½ Meat, 1¼ Bread, 2¼ Veg, 3¾ Fat
PROTEIN: 10 g, CARBOHYDRATE: 37 g, FIBER: 5 g

SOUTHERN BOWL – SPECIAL REQUEST

Chicken, spinach and tomatoes over red beans and rice. Request no tortilla strips.

✓ CALORIES: Good Choice (715) ✓✓ CHOLESTEROL: Excellent Choice (65 mg)
✓✓ FAT: Excellent Choice (7 g) SODIUM: Moderate (905 mg)**
EXCHANGES: 4 Meat (extra lean), 7¼ Bread, 1½ Veg, ¾ Fat
PROTEIN: 42 g, CARBOHYDRATE: 119 g, FIBER: 4 g

THAI CHICKEN SALAD – HALF

Chicken, Thai lettuce mix, bean sprouts, cucumbers, cilantro and spicy peanut sauce, served with a pita wrapper.

✓✓ CALORIES: Excellent Choice (440) ✓✓ CHOLESTEROL: Excellent Choice (65 mg)
✓✓ FAT: Excellent Choice (11 g) SODIUM: Moderate (830 mg)**
EXCHANGES: 4 Meat (extra lean), 2 Bread, 1¾ Veg, ½ Fruit, 1½ Fat
PROTEIN: 40 g, CARBOHYDRATE: 50 g, FIBER: 6 g

♥ Primarily unsaturated fat
** If you request no added salt

One taste and you'll be hooked! With a climate comparable to Greece, Southern California is perfect for a Greek concept: freshly prepared, great tasting, reasonably priced healthy Greek food served in a casual, friendly atmosphere. Try our delicious Greek Lemon Chicken, Ka-Bobs, and our Famous Steak/Chicken/Shrimp pita Sandwiches. You'll also enjoy our vegetarian dishes: Greek salads, Falafel, Hummus, Spanakopita, and our popular Fire Feta® $

Daphne's Orange County locations:

Aliso Viejo: 26611 Aliso Creek Rd.	(949) 831-5004	Irvine: 14041 Jeffery Rd.	(949) 262-7260
Brea: 120 South Brea Blvd.	(714) 990-4790	La Habra: 1350 S. Beach Blvd.	(562) 690-5028
Costa Mesa: 3030 Harbor Blvd.	(714) 885-8945	Newport Beach: 1330 Bison Ave.	(949) 729-0671
Foothill Rch: 26612 Towne Ctr. Dr.	(949) 206-0049	R. Santa Margarita: 22245 El Paseo	(949) 766-4540
Fullerton: 1919 W. Malvern Ave.	(714) 446-7331	San Clemente: 979 Avenida Pico,	(949) 369-4611
Irvine: 5643 Alton Parkway	(949) 296-0188	Santa Ana: 2 E. Hutton Centre Dr.	(714) 689-0313
Irvine: 13250 Jamboree Rd.	(714) 832-5855	Santa Ana: 3941 Bristol St.	(714) 708-8430

CHICKEN BREAST PITA

Skewered chicken breast with veggies, flame broiled and wrapped in our delicious pita bread.

✓ CALORIES: Good Choice (565) ✓ CHOLESTEROL: Good Choice (130 mg)
✓ FAT: Good Choice (22 g) SODIUM: Moderate (865 mg)**
EXCHANGES: 7¼ Meat (extra lean), 2 Bread, ½ Veg, 3¼ Fat
PROTEIN: 52 g, CARBOHYDRATE: 34 g, FIBER: 2 g

SPICY CHICKEN SALAD – SPECIAL REQUEST

Greek salad topped with marinated flame broiled chicken breast and our spicy Fire Feta®.
Pita bread not include in analysis (see below).
Request less fire feta *(1 oz.)* and dressing on the side *(dressing not included in analysis, see below).*

✓ CALORIES: Good Choice (510) CHOLESTEROL: Moderate (160 mg)
✓ FAT: Good Choice (24 g) SODIUM: High (1050 mg)
EXCHANGES: 7¾ Meat (extra lean), 1¾ Veg, 3½ Fat
PROTEIN: 58 g, CARBOHYDRATE: 12 g, FIBER: 5 g

CHICKEN KA-BOB PLATE – SPECIAL REQUEST

Two flame broiled marinated chicken skewers with Greek salad.
Rice pilaf and pita bread not included in analysis (see below).
Request dressing on the side *(not included in analysis).*

✓✓ CALORIES: Good Choice (350) CHOLESTEROL: Moderate (160 mg)
✓✓ FAT: Good Choice (10 g) ✓ SODIUM: Good Choice (415 mg) **
EXCHANGES: 7¾ Meat (extra lean), 1 Veg, 1¼ Fat
PROTEIN: 56 g, CARBOHYDRATE: 5 g, FIBER: 2 g

RICE PILAF

CAL: 275, FAT: 7 g, CHOL: 20 mg, SOD: 880 mg; EXCH: 2¾ Bread, 1¼ Fat; PROTEIN: 5 g, CARB: 46 g, FIBER: 1 g

PITA BREAD

CAL: 200, FAT: 6 g, CHOL: 0 mg, SOD: 350 mg; EX: ½ Meat, 2 Bread; ¾ Fat; PROTEIN: 4 g, CARB: 30 g, FIBER: 1 g

SALAD DRESSING *(2 Tbs.)*

CAL: 140, FAT: 15 g, CHOL: 0 mg, SOD: 550 mg; EXCH: 3 Fat; PROTEIN: 0 g, CARB: 1 g, FIBER: <1 g

♥ Primarily unsaturated fat
** If you request no added salt

DIHO SIAM
Restaurant
THAI / CHINESE

THAI DISHES

"Sawatdee" – Welcome to Diho Siam family-style restaurants. In our native Thailand, we enjoy eating – the meal is a celebration. We are proud to offer the freshest ingredients, finest quality, and friendliest service. To provide the very best, all our food is cooked to order, and we have delightful selections for our vegetarian diners. Enjoy and thank you very much – "Khop Khun!" $

Diho Siam Thai Cuisine: Costa Mesa: 1835 Newport Blvd. (949) 645-3259
Lake Forest: 23600 Rockfield, Suite 2L (949) 859-4192
Mission Viejo: 27001 La Paz, Suite 100 (949) 597-1550

THAI DISHES: Fountain Valley: 10065 Garfield Ave. (at Brookhurst) (714) 962-1312

Analysis for each dish below is for ½ order, since meals are usually shared family-style.
Sodium values may be reduced by requesting less fish sauce, oyster sauce and/or curry paste.

GANG SOM PLA SALMON (½ ORDER) 🍎

Hot and sour tamarind flavor soup with salmon.

✓ CALORIES: Good Choice (470) — CHOLESTEROL: Moderate (185 mg)
✓ FAT: Good Choice (21 g) — SODIUM: High (2305 mg)
EXCHANGES: 4½ Meat, 3 Veg
PROTEIN: 63 g, CARBOHYDRATE: 30 g, FIBER: 8 g

FRESH PAPAYA SALAD (½ ORDER) 🍎

Papaya with chilies, carrots, green beans, tomatoes and peanuts with Thai spicy-lime dressing.
Not available at the Lake Forest location.

✓✓ CALORIES: Excellent Choice (255) — ✓✓ CHOLESTEROL: Excellent Choice (0 mg)
✓✓ FAT: Excellent Choice (7 g)♥ — SODIUM: High (1160 mg)
EXCHANGES: 1 Meat, ½ Bread, 2¼ Veg, 1 Fruit, 1¼ Fat
PROTEIN: 12 g, CARBOHYDRATE: 40 g, FIBER: 8 g

GRILLED ORANGE ROUGHY WITH MANGO SALSA (½ ORDER) 🍎

Grilled marinated orange roughy served with Thai ginger and mango salsa.

✓✓ CALORIES: Excellent Choice (375) — ✓✓ CHOLESTEROL: Excellent Choice (20 mg)
✓✓ FAT: Excellent Choice (11 g)♥ — SODIUM: High (1115 mg)
EXCHANGES: 1¾ Meat (extra lean), ½ Bread, 2¼ Veg, ¾ Fruit, 2 Fat
PROTEIN: 24 g, CARBOHYDRATE: 47 g, FIBER: 6 g

EGGPLANT WITH FRESH THAI BASIL (½ ORDER) – SPECIAL REQUEST 🍎

Asian eggplant, tofu, chili, Thai basil and black mushroom seasoned with house special sauce.
Request soft tofu (not fried) and less oil (1 Tbs).
Also available with chicken#, shrimp, scallops, or squid; nutrition data will vary.

✓✓ CALORIES: Excellent Choice (270) — ✓✓ CHOLESTEROL: Excellent Choice (0 mg)
✓✓ FAT: Excellent Choice (15 g)♥ — SODIUM: Moderate (900 mg)**
EXCHANGES: ½ Meat, ½ Bread, 3½ Veg, 3 Fat
PROTEIN: 7 g, CARBOHYDRATE: 30 g, FIBER: 5 g

GANG PA CHICKEN (WITHOUT COCONUT MILK) (½ ORDER) – SPECIAL REQUEST 🍎

Jungle red curry chicken# with Thai basil & assorted vegetables. Request less oil (1 Tbs.) & no coconut milk.
Also available with shrimp, scallops, or squid or as a vegetarian dish with tofu; nutrition data will vary.

✓✓ CALORIES: Excellent Choice (275) — ✓✓ CHOLESTEROL: Excellent Choice (75 mg)
✓✓ FAT: Excellent Choice (12 g) — SODIUM: Moderate (810 mg)**
EXCHANGES: 2½ Meat (extra lean), ¼ Bread, 2½ Veg, 1¼ Fat
PROTEIN: 28 g, CARBOHYDRATE: 23 g, FIBER: 5 g

MIXED VEGETABLES DELIGHT WITH SHRIMP (½ ORDER) – SPECIAL REQUEST 🍎

A variety of vegetables sautéed with garlic. Request less oil (1 Tbs) and no salt.
Chicken#, vegetarian, tofu, squid and scallops also available; nutrition data will vary.

✓✓ CALORIES: Excellent Choice (250) — CHOLESTEROL: Moderate (220 mg)
✓✓ FAT: Excellent Choice (8 g)♥ — SODIUM: Moderate (750 mg)**
EXCHANGES: 3¼ Meat (extra lean), ½ Bread, 1½ Veg, 1½ Fat
PROTEIN: 27 g, CARBOHYDRATE: 18 g, FIBER: 3 g

#Lake Forest location – please request white meat chicken.
🍎 at least 2 fruit/vegetable servings

El Pollo Loco offers a fresh, wholesome alternative to traditional fast food with real food you can feel good eating. Our chicken is marinated in a special blend of herbs, spices and fruit juices and then flame-grilled right before your eyes for flavor you won't find anywhere else. We serve our chicken with warm tortillas, fresh salsas and a wide variety of healthful sides, from fresh vegetables and salads to our famous pinto beans and Spanish rice. Complimenting our meals are signature entrees such as our famous Pollo Bowl®, that enable you to satisfy your appetite without sacrifice. Treat yourself to the delicious taste of El Pollo Loco, any way you like it.

El Pollo Loco has over 40 Orange County locations to serve you. For the one nearest you, please call 1-888-EPL-TOGO. $

FLAME-GRILLED SKINLESS CHICKEN BREAST – SPECIAL REQUEST

Request chicken skinless.

✓✓ CALORIES: Excellent Choice (155) ✓ CHOLESTEROL: Good Choice (95 mg)
✓✓ FAT: Excellent Choice (4 g) ✓ SODIUM: Good Choice (540 mg)
EXCHANGES: 4 Meat
PROTEIN: 29 g, CARBOHYDRATE: 0 g, FIBER: 0 g

POLLO CHOICE SKINLESS BREAST MEAL – SPECIAL REQUEST

Flame-grilled skinless chicken breast with vegetable blend, garden salad & house salsa. Salad dressing not included in analysis. Request chicken skinless.

✓✓ CALORIES: Excellent Choice (345) ✓ CHOLESTEROL: Good Choice (110 mg)
✓ FAT: Good Choice (16 g) SODIUM: High (1065 mg)
EXCHANGES: 4½ Meat, ¼ Bread, 2¼ Veg, 1¼ Fat
PROTEIN: 38 g, CARBOHYDRATE: 16 g, FIBER: 7 g

BRC BURRITO

Pinto beans, rice and cheese in a flour tortilla.

✓ CALORIES: Good Choice (530) ✓✓ CHOLESTEROL: Excellent Choice (15 mg)
✓✓ FAT: Excellent Choice (15 g) SODIUM: High (1395 mg)
EXCHANGES: ½ Meat, 5¼ Bread, 2½ Fat
PROTEIN: 17 g, CARBOHYDRATE: 79 g, FIBER: 6 g

POLLO BOWL®

Flame-grilled boneless skinless chicken breast with pinto beans, Spanish rice, pico de gallo, onion & cilantro.

✓ CALORIES: Good Choice (545) ✓✓ CHOLESTEROL: Excellent Choice (40 mg)
✓✓ FAT: Excellent Choice (10 g) SODIUM: High (2160 mg)
EXCHANGES: 2¾ Meat, 5¼ Bread, ½ Veg, 1 Fat
PROTEIN: 31 g, CARBOHYDRATE: 84 g, FIBER: 12 g

INDIVIDUAL SIDES:

FRESH VEGETABLES

CAL: 70, FAT: 4 g, CHOL: 0, SOD: 80 mg, PROT: 3 g, CARB: 6 g, FIB: 4 g; EXCH: 1¼ Veg, ¾ Fat

PINTO BEANS

CAL: 155, FAT: 4 g, CHOL: 0, SOD: 675 mg, PROT: 7 g, CARB: 24 g, FIB: 9 g; EXCH: ¼ Meat, 1½ Br, ½ Fat

SPANISH RICE

CAL: 160, FAT: 1 g, CHOL: 0, SOD: 420 mg, PROT: 3 g, CARB: 33 g, FIB: 1 g; EXCH: 2¼ Br, ¼ Fat

GARDEN SALAD (SMALL)

CAL: 110, FAT: 7 g, CHOL: 15, SOD: 270 mg, PROT: 5 g, CARB: 8 g, FIB: 2 g; EXCH: ½ Meat, ¼ Bread, ½ Veg, ½ Fat

 at least 2 fruit/vegetable servings for entrees, 1 for side dishes

Nobody else makes Mexican food taste this good. Come to El Torito where we serve traditional Mexican cuisine as well as unique specialties made only with the freshest ingredients. In addition to our Mexican favorites like sizzling fajitas and Mexican Caesar salad, our chefs have developed a variety of healthy and delicious items prepared daily to meet your nutritional needs. Join us at El Torito for lunch, dinner or Sunday brunch at any of our Southern California locations. $

El Torito Restaurants

With Orange County locations in Anaheim (2), Buena Park, Cypress, Dana Point, Fullerton, Irvine, Laguna Hills, Orange, Placentia, Tustin, Westminster and Yorba Linda.
Visit www.eltorito.com for a complete list of El Torito locations.

POLLO FRESCO – SPECIAL REQUEST

Tender chicken breast seasoned with adobo sauce and grilled to perfection. Served atop crispy tortilla strips, reduced-fat jack cheese and fresh spinach sautéed with garlic and herbs. Served with beans, fresh fruit relish and sweet corn cake (spinach, beans, fruit relish and sweet corn cake not included in analysis).

Request no tortilla strips.

✓✓ CALORIES: Excellent Choice (405) — CHOLESTEROL: Moderate (200 mg)
✓✓ FAT: Excellent Choice (14 g) — SODIUM: High (1370 mg)
EXCHANGES: 8¼ Meat, ¾ Veg, 1¼ Fat
PROTEIN: 58 g, CARBOHYDRATE: 7 g, FIBER: 1 g

GRILLED SOFT CHICKEN TACOS

Three freshly prepared soft tacos featuring grilled, fresh chicken breast. Accompanied by beans, rice, guacamole and sweet corn cake (beans, rice, guacamole and sweet corn cake not included in analysis).

✓ CALORIES: Good Choice (670) — CHOLESTEROL: Moderate (155 mg)
✓ FAT: Good Choice (23 g) — SODIUM: High (1470 mg)
EXCHANGES: 7¾ Meat, 2¾ Bread, 1 Veg, 3 Fat
PROTEIN: 63 g, CARBOHYDRATE: 49 g, FIBER: 3 g

SONORA BURRITO LITE

Tender, grilled chicken breast, pico de gallo, mild chiles and reduced-fat jack cheese are all wrapped in a large flour tortilla and topped with roasted tomatillo sauce. Served with fresh fruit and beans (beans not included in analysis).

✓ CALORIES: Good Choice (735) — CHOLESTEROL: High (330 mg)
✓ FAT: Good Choice (25 g) — SODIUM: High (2670 mg)
EXCHANGES: 8 Meat, 2½ Bread, 2½ Veg, ¾ Fruit, 3 Fat
PROTEIN: 65 g, CARBOHYDRATE: 64 g, FIBER: 8 g

GRILLED CHICKEN QUESADILLA LITE

Seasoned, tender chicken breast, reduced-fat jack cheese, fresh fruit relish and mild green chiles are all wrapped in a soft flour tortilla and lightly grilled and served with salsa picante and fresh fruit.

✓ CALORIES: Good Choice (615) — CHOLESTEROL: High (480 mg)
✓ FAT: Good Choice (24 g) — SODIUM: High (1380 mg)
EXCHANGES: 6¼ Meat, 2 Bread, ¾ Veg, 1 Fruit, 2¾ Fat
PROTEIN: 50 g, CARBOHYDRATE: 51 g, FIBER: 5 g

At the time of publication, recipes for spinach, rice and beans were being enhanced, so nutrition data was not available. Please check www.eltorito.com for up-to-date nutrition information.

Persian cuisine is one of the unexpected. While its basic ingredients (such as lamb and rice) are familiar, the ingredients that enhance it, while not unknown, are used infrequently in Western cuisine: pomegranates, pistachio nuts, saffron, dried lime, rosewater, yogurt, cardamon, cloves, barberry, fenugreek, the unique spice sumak – the list is endless. Gourmet Lunch Buffet every Monday and Friday. Come enjoy. $$

Ferdussi Taste of Persia

3605 S. Bristol St., Santa Ana, CA 92704 (714) 545-9096
at MacArthur Blvd., one block north of South Coast Plaza

SALMON ATASHI – SPECIAL REQUEST ♂

Charbroiled crushed tomato sauce with fresh pepper. Request less oil (½ Tbs).

✓✓ CALORIES: Excellent Choice (415) ✓ CHOLESTEROL: Good Choice (120 mg)
✓ FAT: Good Choice (21 g)♥ SODIUM: High (1275 mg)
EXCHANGES: 5¾ Meat, 1¼ Veg, 1¼ Fat
PROTEIN: 46 g, CARBOHYDRATE: 9 g, FIBER: 2 g

CHICKEN SHISH KABOB – SPECIAL REQUEST

Chunks of marinated chicken with grilled vegetables. Request less oil (1 Tbs).

✓ CALORIES: Good Choice (590) CHOLESTEROL: Moderate (220 mg)
✓ FAT: Good Choice (24 g) SODIUM: High (1370 mg)
EXCHANGES: 11¼ Meat, ¾ Veg, ¼ Fruit, 3 Fat
PROTEIN: 81 g, CARBOHYDRATE: 9 g, FIBER: 2 g

ADAS POLO (½ ORDER)

Basmati rice with dates, raisins and lentils. Analysis is for ½ order, assuming it is shared.

✓✓ CALORIES: Excellent Choice (330) ✓✓ CHOLESTEROL: Excellent Choice (0 mg)
✓✓ FAT: Excellent Choice (14 g)♥ ✓ SODIUM: Good Choice (585 mg)**
EXCHANGES: 1¾ Bread, 1½ Fruit, 2¾ Fat
PROTEIN: 4 g, CARBOHYDRATE: 49 g, FIBER: 3 g

WHITE FISH KABOB

Fresh filet of white fish dipped in saffron sauce and cooked on an open fire.
Analysis for basmati rice and saffron shown separately below.

✓✓ CALORIES: Excellent Choice (385) CHOLESTEROL: Moderate (165 mg)
✓ FAT: Good Choice (16 g)♥ ✓✓ SODIUM: Excellent Choice (145 mg)**
EXCHANGES: 3 Meat, ¼ Fruit, 1½ Fat
PROTEIN: 53 g, CARBOHYDRATE: 4 g, FIBER: 0 g

ALBALOO POLO

Simmered chicken covered with fluffy basmati rice mixed with sour black cherries and saffron.
Analysis for basmati rice and saffron shown separately below.

✓ CALORIES: Good Choice (525) CHOLESTEROL: Moderate (215 mg)
✓✓ FAT: Excellent Choice (14 g) ✓✓ SODIUM: Excellent Choice (195 mg)**
EXCHANGES: 11¼ Meat (extra lean), 1¼ Fruit, 1 Fat
PROTEIN: 80 g, CARBOHYDRATE: 18 g, FIBER: 1 g

BASMATI RICE AND SAFFRON

CAL: 265, FAT: 7 g♥, CHOL: 0 mg, SOD: 5 mg; EXCH: 3 BREAD, 1½ FAT; PROT: 4 g, CARB: 45 g

♂ at least 2 fruit/vegetable servings

Finbars Italian Kitchen – "A Not So Traditional Name... For A Not So Traditional Restaurant." The critics all agree – from the Southern California Restaurant Writers Association who voted Finbars the Winner of the Sterling Silver Medal Award, to the LA Times, the Orange County Register, and Elmer Dill, who rated "A" across the board on his report card. We offer a wide variety of pastas, pizza, soups, salads, sandwiches, and other specialties, and our entire menu is also available for take-out or delivery. $-$$

Finbars Italian Kitchen

Metro Pointe: 901-C South Coast Drive, Costa Mesa, CA 92626 (714) 641-3000
Bay City Center: 550 Pacific Coast Highway #111, Seal Beach, CA 90740 (562) 430-4303
www.finbars.com

All pasta dishes listed below are analyzed with low-carb pasta, which is higher in protein and fiber than regular pasta (regular pasta can be requested). Tell your server about your diet concerns. We can alter most of our dishes to your preference.

FIERY SHRIMP FETTUCINE

Sautéed tiger shrimp or chicken breast in a spicy tomato sauce laced with cayenne and chili pepper and served over low-carb pasta.

✓ CALORIES: Good Choice (565) | CHOLESTEROL: Moderate (230 mg)
✓✓ FAT: Excellent Choice (10 g) | ✓ SODIUM: Good Choice (405 mg)
EXCHANGES: 12¼ Meat (extra lean), 1½ Bread, 1 Veg, ¼ Other Carb, 1¼ Fat
PROTEIN: 87 g, CARBOHYDRATE: 48 g, FIBER: 18 g

PENNE MARSALA MARINARA – HEALTHY DINING CHOICE

Tomato herb and marsala wine sauce with garden vegetables & parmesan cheese.

✓ CALORIES: Good Choice (635) | ✓✓ CHOLESTEROL: Excellent Choice (25 mg)
✓ FAT: Good Choice (18 g) | SODIUM: Moderate (970 mg)
EXCHANGES: 8½ Meat (extra lean), 1¾ Bread, 3¾ Veg, ½ Other Carb, 3 Fat
PROTEIN: 67 g, CARBOHYDRATE: 66 g, FIBER: 24 g

CAPELLINI POMODORO – HEALTHY DINING CHOICE

Plum tomatoes with garlic, extra virgin olive oil and basil (prepared without oil if you prefer).

✓ CALORIES: Good Choice (500) | ✓✓ CHOLESTEROL: Excellent Choice (0 mg)
✓ FAT: Good Choice (16 g)♥ | ✓ SODIUM: Good Choice (395 mg)
EXCHANGES: 8 Meat (extra lean), 1¼ Bread, 2 Veg, 2¾ Fat
PROTEIN: 59 g, CARBOHYDRATE: 50 g, FIBER: 19 g

CHICKEN GIARDINA – HEALTHY DINING CHOICE

Bite size pieces of chicken breast sautéed with olive oil, garlic, onion, diced tomatoes, carrots, celery, oregano and fresh basil, served with a bouqettier of garden vegetables.

✓✓ CALORIES: Excellent Choice (405) | ✓ CHOLESTEROL: Good Choice (130 mg)
✓✓ FAT: Excellent Choice (11 g) | ✓ SODIUM: Good Choice (565 mg)
EXCHANGES: 6¾ Meat (extra lean), 3¾ Veg, 1¼ Fat
PROTEIN: 54 g, CARBOHYDRATE: 22 g, FIBER: 9 g

SHRIMP FRA DIAVOLO – HEALTHY DINING CHOICE

Tiger shrimp sautéed in a spicy garlic tomato sauce, served with a bouqettier of garden vegetables.

✓✓ CALORIES: Excellent Choice (400) | CHOLESTEROL: Moderate (260 mg)
✓ FAT: Good Choice (20 g)♥ | ✓ SODIUM: Good Choice (490 mg)
EXCHANGES: 5 Meat (extra lean), 3 Veg, 3¼ Fat
PROTEIN: 40 g, CARBOHYDRATE: 18 g, FIBER: 7 g

♥ Primarily unsaturated fat
** If you request no added salt

The Fish Market - casual style dining in a clean and comfortable atmosphere. The freshness and quality of our fish speaks for itself. We also offer a retail market where you can select from our extensive variety of fresh fish and menu items for take out. Our entire staff is committed to providing you, our guest, with the utmost in courteous, attentive service and superior seafood knowledge. Your experience is our number one priority; you are the most important person in our restaurants! $$-$$$

The Fish Market

85 Fortune Drive #329, Irvine, CA 92615 (949) 727-FISH (3474)

PASTA ANGELICA WITH SEAFOOD – SPECIAL REQUEST

Angel hair pasta tossed with scallops, pesto, garlic and tomatoes. Request less oil (¼ oz) and no cheese.

✓ CALORIES Good Choice (610) ✓✓ CHOLESTEROL: Excellent Choice (40 mg)
✓ FAT: Good Choice (17 g)♥ ✓ SODIUM: Good Choice (540 mg)**
EXCHANGES: 2¾ Meat (extra lean), 4¼ Bread, 2¼ Veg, 3 Fat
PROTEIN: 33 g, CARBOHYDRATE: 80 g, FIBER: 5 g

WARM SPINACH SALAD WITH FETA CHEESE – SPECIAL REQUEST

Request less oil (1 Tbs).

✓✓ CALORIES: Excellent Choice (305) ✓✓ CHOLESTEROL: Excellent Choice (25 mg)
✓ FAT: Good Choice (20 g) SODIUM: High (1325 mg)
EXCHANGES: ½ Meat, ¾ Bread, 1¼ Veg, 3½ Fat
PROTEIN: 8 g, CARBOHYDRATE: 24 g, FIBER: 4 g

SHELLFISH MARINARA (½ ORDER)

Linguine with clams topped with marinara sauce and grated romano cheese. Analysis is for ½ full order.

✓ CALORIES: Good Choice (480) ✓✓ CHOLESTEROL: Excellent Choice (45 mg)
✓✓ FAT: Excellent Choice (13 g) SODIUM: High (1445 mg)
EXCHANGES: 2 Meat (extra lean), 2¼ Bread, 4 Veg, 1½ Fat
PROTEIN: 26 g, CARBOHYDRATE: 63 g, FIBER: 7 g

CAJUN STYLE MEXICAN PRAWNS

Skewered and mesquite charbroiled. Served with choice of 2 side dishes (side dishes not included in analysis). Steamed vegetables & tomatoes recommended.

✓✓ CALORIES: Excellent Choice (320) CHOLESTEROL: High (390 mg)
✓✓ FAT: Excellent Choice (9 g)♥ ✓ SODIUM: Good Choice (470 mg)**
EXCHANGES: 7½ Meat (extra lean), 1¼ Fat
PROTEIN: 52 g, CARBOHYDRATE: 3 g, FIBER: 0 g

ASIAN STYLE HALIBUT – SPECIAL REQUEST

with black beans, garlic, ginger and soy sauce. Request halibut steamed or grilled & less sesame oil (1 Tbs). Served with choice of 2 side dishes (not included in analysis). Steamed vegetables & tomatoes recommended.

✓ CALORIES: Good Choice (495) ✓✓ CHOLESTEROL: Excellent Choice (75 mg)
✓ FAT: Good Choice (20 g)♥ SODIUM: High (1660 mg)
EXCHANGES: 6¾ Meat (extra lean), ¾ Bread, ¾ Veg, 3¼ Fat
PROTEIN: 54 g, CARBOHYDRATE: 17 g, FIBER: 5 g

LITE EATERS

Fresh fish, skewered, mesquite grilled and seasoned. Served with choice of 2 side dishes (side dishes not included in analysis). Steamed vegetables & tomatoes recommended.

✓✓ CALORIES: Excellent Choice (240) ✓✓ CHOLESTEROL: Excellent Choice (75 mg)
✓✓ FAT: Excellent Choice (7 g)♥ ✓✓ SODIUM: Excellent Choice (270 mg)**
EXCHANGES: 5¾ Meat (extra lean), ¾ Fat
PROTEIN: 41 g, CARBOHYDRATE: 0 g, FIBER: 0 g

♥ Primarily unsaturated fat
** If you request no added salt

"The best view in South Orange County," the Fisherman's Restaurant and Bar offers outside dining with Catalina sunsets and endless ocean vistas on the historic San Clemente Pier. The unique concept of family style dining, featuring Pacific Northwest seafood, originated from the owner's interest in fishing, digging for clams and catching crab and other seafood. The Fisherman's Restaurant has won numerous awards from Southern California Restaurant Writers and was also named "Best California Restaurant" by Sunset Magazine. $$

The Fisherman's Restaurant & Bar

611 Avenida Victoria, San Clemente, CA 92672 (949) 498-6390

FRESH FISH & SEAFOOD

Analyses below are for 8 oz. (except as noted) portions of basted, mesquite-grilled fish and seafood. Each meal is served with choice of side dishes (fresh vegetables, salad, and plain baked potato recommended, see analyses for vegetables and potato below) and bread, butter, and tartar sauce (not included in analyses).

Note: all carbohydrate values for fish and other seafood are essentially 0.

	Calories	Fat (g)	Cholesterol (mg)	Sodium (mg)**	Protein (g)
Ahi Tuna	✓✓ 305	✓✓ 9♥	✓ 120	✓✓ 190	56
Teriyaki Ahi	✓✓ 390	✓✓ 2♥	✓ 110	2010	59
Cajun Ahi Rare	✓✓ 330	✓✓10♥	✓ 110	735	57
Alaskan Halibut	✓✓ 305	✓✓12♥	✓ 90	✓✓ 230	50
Atlantic Salmon	✓✓ 370	✓21♥	✓ 140	✓✓ 200	47
Cajun Salmon	✓✓ 400	✓22♥	✓ 130	750	48
Mahi Mahi	✓✓ 250	✓✓ 8♥	185	✓310	45
Mako Shark	✓✓ 325	✓16♥	✓ 120	✓✓ 270	45
Cajun Shark	✓✓ 380	✓18♥	✓ 125	840	52
Pacific Swordfish	✓✓ 335	✓16♥	✓105	✓315	48
Striped Bass	✓✓ 275	✓✓12♥	205	✓✓ 265	43
White Seabass	✓✓ 275	✓✓11♥	✓110	✓✓ 260	45
Yellowtail	✓✓ 360	✓18♥	✓130	✓✓ 185	50
Prawns *(8 oz.)*#	✓✓ 290	✓✓ 9♥	510	610	53
Scallops *(7 oz.)*#	✓✓ 220	✓✓ 8♥	✓ 95	✓460	37

 # Does not include drawn butter served on the side.

SEASONED FRESH VEGETABLES – SPECIAL REQUEST – *Request no butter* 🍎

CALORIES: 30, FAT: ½ g♥, CHOL: 0 mg, SODIUM: 75 mg, PROTEIN: 2 g, CARBOHYDRATE: 6 g, FIBER: 3 g

BAKED POTATO *(½ plain 8 oz.)* 🍎

CALORIES: 250, FAT: ¼ g♥, CHOL: 0 mg, SODIUM: 20 mg, PROTEIN: 5 g, CARBOHYDRATE: 57 g, FIBER: 5 g

🍎 at least 2 fruit/vegetable servings for entrees, 1 for side dishes

Fitness Grill and Fitness Pizza put extraordinary effort into presenting culinary art at its healthiest and tastiest combination, in a pleasant, eclectic, yet relaxed atmosphere. We marinate and grill a selection of fresh lean meats, accompanied with a perfect balance of vegetables and grains. We offer organic greens in our salads. We use whole-wheat flour in our pastas and pizzas, add protein to the pizza crust, use lean meat and daily fresh vegetables along with low-fat and low-sodium sauces and low-fat cheese. Cheeseless pizza and ultra-thin crusts also available. $$

Fitness Grill 103-A W. Imperial Hwy., Brea (714) 672-0911
Fitness Pizza 18246 Imperial Hwy., Yorba Linda (714) 993-5421

Hockey Player Pizza (2 slices)

Marinated pieces of chicken breast and plenty of artichoke hearts topped with fresh pesto sauce. Nutrition information for 2 slices of pizza (½ pizza).

✓✓ Calories: Excellent Choice (325) ✓✓ Cholesterol: Excellent Choice (75 mg)
✓✓ Fat: Excellent Choice (10 g) ✓ Sodium: Good Choice (475 mg)**
Exchanges: 3¾ Meat, 1 Bread, 1 Veg, ½ Fat
Protein: 37 g, Carbohydrate: 23 g, Fiber: 5 g

Iron Man Pizza (2 slices)

Fresh spinach, sliced mushrooms, low-fat ricotta cheese and sliced black olives. A great source of iron and folic acid. Nutrition information for 2 slices of pizza (½ pizza).

✓✓ Calories: Excellent Choice (265) ✓✓ Cholesterol: Excellent Choice (35 mg)
✓✓ Fat: Excellent Choice (12 g) ✓ Sodium: Good Choice (500 mg)**
Exchanges: 1¾ Meat, 1 Bread, ½ Veg, 1 Fat
Protein: 18 g, Carbohydrate: 22 g, Fiber: 4 g

Seafood Brochette

Variety of marinated and grilled halibut, shrimp & scallops served over basmati wild rice & steamed spinach.

✓✓ Calories: Excellent Choice (345) Cholesterol: Moderate (155 mg)
✓✓ Fat: Excellent Choice (6 g)♥ ✓ Sodium: Good Choice (420 mg)**
Exchanges: 3¾ Meat (extra lean), 1½ Bread, 1½ Veg, ½ Fat
Protein: 41 g, Carbohydrate: 33 g, Fiber: 5 g

Chicken Lettuce Wrap

A flavorful high-protein minced chicken breast prepared fitness-chang style, served with chilled romaine hearts.

✓✓ Calories: Excellent Choice (335) ✓ Cholesterol: Good Choice (95 mg)
✓✓ Fat: Excellent Choice (13 g) ✓ Sodium: Good Choice (575 mg)**
Exchanges: 5¾ Meat (extra lean), ½ Bread, ½ Veg, 1¼ Fat
Protein: 42 g, Carbohydrate: 10 g, Fiber: 1 g

Halibut Salad

Cajun-blackened halibut over a cooked mixture of diced tomatoes and variety of beans in our special vinegar sauce over field greens, garnished with steamed asparagus, fresh papaya and feta cheese.

✓ Calories: Good Choice (490) ✓ Cholesterol: Good Choice (90 mg)
✓ Fat: Good Choice (16 g) ✓ Sodium: Good Choice (595 mg)**
Exchanges: 4¼ Meat, ½ Bread, 2¼ Veg, ½ Fruit, 2 Fat
Protein: 49 g, Carbohydrate: 37 g, Fiber: 9 g

Grilled Veggie Platter

Grilled eggplant, zucchini, mushrooms, onions, green and red bell pepper and artichoke hearts served over steamed spinach and basmati wild rice, and served with feta cheese

✓✓ Calories: Excellent Choice (280) ✓✓ Cholesterol: Excellent Choice (15 mg)
✓✓ Fat: Excellent Choice (9 g) ✓✓ Sodium: Excellent Choice (265 mg)**
Exchanges: ¼ Meat, 1½ Bread, 3½ Veg, 1¼ Fat
Protein: 12 g, Carbohydrate: 43 g, Fiber: 10 g

at least 2 fruit/vegetable servings

The Flame Broiler

Always Good, Always Guaranteed

At The Flame Broiler, you get delicious, low fat, no frying, no skin, no bone, no MSG, all served with one-of-a-kind sauce. We are a healthy quick service Korean-style restaurant, where you can view the chefs as they prepare your food. Please come and enjoy your meal! $

The Flame Broiler

Costa Mesa: 204 E. 17th St. #103 (949) 650-6939
Fullerton: 1203 E. Chapman Ave. (714) 526-1128
Carson: 17535 Central Ave. (310) 537-6575
Orange: 2316 W. Chapman Ave. (714) 938-1156
Stanton: 12700 Beach Blvd. (714) 899-1863
La Jolla: 8867 Villa La Jolla Dr. #606 (858) 587-8989

CHICKEN BOWL

Teriyaki chicken served over steamed rice and topped with teriyaki sauce and green onions.

✓✓ CALORIES: Excellent Choice (450)
✓ CHOLESTEROL: Good Choice (115 mg)
✓✓ FAT: Excellent Choice (12 g)
SODIUM: Moderate (650 mg)**

EXCHANGES: 4¾ Meat, 3 Bread
PROTEIN: 37 g, CARBOHYDRATE: 46 g, FIBER: 1 g

BEEF BOWL

Teriyaki beef served over steamed rice and topped with teriyaki sauce and green onions.

✓✓ CALORIES: Excellent Choice (435)
✓✓ CHOLESTEROL: Excellent Choice (70 mg)
✓✓ FAT: Excellent Choice (10 g)
SODIUM: Moderate (705 mg)**

EXCHANGES: 4 Meat, 3 Bread, ¼ Fat
PROTEIN: 36 g, CARBOHYDRATE: 48 g, FIBER: 1 g

VEGGIE BOWL

Broccoli, cabbage and carrots served over steamed rice and topped with teriyaki sauce and green onions.

✓✓ CALORIES: Excellent Choice (175)
✓✓ CHOLESTEROL: Excellent Choice (0 mg)
✓✓ FAT: Excellent Choice (1 g)♥
✓ SODIUM: Good Choice (585 mg)**

EXCHANGES: 1¾ Bread, 2 Veg
PROTEIN: 6 g, CARBOHYDRATE: 39 g, FIBER: 5 g

CHICKEN VEGGIE BOWL

Teriyaki chicken with broccoli, cabbage and carrots served over steamed rice and topped with teriyaki sauce.

✓ CALORIES: Good Choice (485)
✓ CHOLESTEROL: Good Choice (115 mg)
✓✓ FAT: Excellent Choice (12 g)
SODIUM: Moderate (675 mg)**

EXCHANGES: 4¾ Meat, 3 Bread, 1½ Veg
PROTEIN: 39 g, CARBOHYDRATE: 54 g, FIBER: 4 g

BEEF VEGGIE BOWL

Teriyaki beef with broccoli, cabbage and carrots served over steamed rice and topped with teriyaki sauce.

✓✓ CALORIES: Excellent Choice (390)
✓✓ CHOLESTEROL: Excellent Choice (70 mg)
✓✓ FAT: Excellent Choice (10 g)
SODIUM: Moderate (735 mg)**

EXCHANGES: 4 Meat, 2 Bread, 1½ Veg
PROTEIN: 36 g, CARBOHYDRATE: 39 g, FIBER: 3 g

HALF & HALF BOWL

Teriyaki chicken & beef served over steamed rice and topped with teriyaki sauce and green onions.

✓✓ CALORIES: Excellent Choice (445)
✓ CHOLESTEROL: Good Choice (90 mg)
✓✓ FAT: Excellent Choice (11 g)
SODIUM: Moderate (675 mg)**

EXCHANGES: 4½ Meat, 3 Bread
PROTEIN: 36 g, CARBOHYDRATE: 47 g, FIBER: 1 g

♥ Primarily unsaturated fat
** If you request no added salt

GELSON'S THE *Super* MARKET *Gelson's was founded in 1951 by brothers Bernard and Eugene Gelson as an extraordinary grocery shopping experience for discerning consumers. Long recognized as one of the nation's premier supermarket chains, Gelson's is known for superior produce, highest quality meat, seafood and deli, an unmatched selection of wine and liquor, and exceptional service. You know you will find what you're looking for at Gelson's, whether it be an unusual ingredient, special spice, gourmet prepared foods from our Service Deli, or scrumptious delights from one of our exquisite bakeries.* $

Gelson's Orange County locations:

Irvine: 5521 Alton Parkway, Irvine, CA 92618 (949) 551-6093
Dana Point: 24 Monarch Bay Plaza, Dana Pt., CA 92629 (949) 488-8147
Newport Beach: 1660 San Miguel Dr., Newport Beach, CA 92660 (949) 644-8660

SPICY GRILLED SALMON *(6 oz.)*

✓✓ CALORIES: Excellent Choice (290) ✓ CHOLESTEROL: Good Choice (80 mg)
✓✓ FAT: Excellent Choice (15 g)♥ SODIUM: Moderate (605 mg)
PROTEIN: 27 g, CARBOHYDRATE: 11 g, FIBER: 0 g

JESSICA'S SESAME EDAMAME SALAD *(4 oz.)*†

✓✓ CALORIES: Excellent Choice (90) ✓✓ CHOLESTEROL: Excellent Choice (0 mg)
✓✓ FAT: Excellent Choice (4 g)♥ ✓ SODIUM: Good Choice (110 mg)
PROTEIN: 5 g, CARBOHYDRATE: 8 g, FIBER: 3 g

GRILLED VEGETABLES *(4 oz.)*† 🍎

✓✓ CALORIES: Excellent Choice (55) ✓✓ CHOLESTEROL: Excellent Choice (0 mg)
✓✓ FAT: Excellent Choice (3 g)♥ ✓✓ SODIUM: Excellent Choice (10 mg)
PROTEIN: 1 g, CARBOHYDRATE: 6 g, FIBER: 2 g

CALORIE COOL COLE SLAW *(4 oz.)*† 🍎

✓✓ CALORIES: Excellent Choice (130) ✓✓ CHOLESTEROL: Excellent Choice (5 mg)
✓ FAT: Good Choice (6 g) ✓ SODIUM: Good Choice (195 mg)
PROTEIN: 1 g, CARBOHYDRATE: 18 g, FIBER: 2 g

CHOPPED VEGETABLE & BARLEY SALAD *(4 oz.)*†

✓✓ CALORIES: Excellent Choice (60) ✓✓ CHOLESTEROL: Excellent Choice (<1 mg)
✓✓ FAT: Excellent Choice (<1 g) ✓✓ SODIUM: Excellent Choice (70 mg)
PROTEIN: 3 g, CARBOHYDRATE: 11 g, FIBER: 3 g

FRESH FRUIT SALAD *(4 oz.)*† 🍎

✓✓ CALORIES: Excellent Choice (45) ✓✓ CHOLESTEROL: Excellent Choice (0 mg)
✓✓ FAT: Excellent Choice (<1 g)♥ ✓✓ SODIUM: Excellent Choice (5 mg)
PROTEIN: 1 g, CARBOHYDRATE: 11 g, FIBER: 1 g

SPINACH & GRAPE SALAD *(4 oz.)*†

✓ CALORIES: Good Choice (160) ✓✓ CHOLESTEROL: Excellent Choice (5 mg)
FAT: Moderate (12 g) SODIUM: Moderate (265 mg)
PROTEIN: 5 g, CARBOHYDRATE: 10 g, FIBER: 4 g

Nutrition information provided by Gelson's Markets.

🍎 at least 2 fruit/vegetable serving for entrées, 1 for side dishes
† Side dish guidelines are ⅓ of entrée guidelines

Enjoy fine dining in the courtyard! The Green Parrot Café serves California bistro-style cuisine in our enchanting Spanish style courtyard, complete with a fountain and an intimate café. There are private rooms seating up to 50, where you will dine surrounded by works of art available for purchase through the Calafia Art Gallery. This is the perfect atmosphere for your wedding reception, birthday, anniversary party, graduation, or any special event. Lunch served Monday through Friday 11 am to 2:30 pm, dinner Tuesday through Friday, beginning at 4 pm. $$

Green Parrot Café

2035 North Main Street, Santa Ana, CA 92706
(714) 550-6040

APPLE BRAISED SALMON

with fine herbs, served over spinach.

✓✓ CALORIES: Excellent Choice (370) ✓ CHOLESTEROL: Good Choice (90 mg)
✓ FAT: Good Choice (16 g)♥ ✓✓ SODIUM: Excellent Choice (150 mg)**
EXCHANGES: 4¼ Meat, 1¾ Veg, ½ Fruit, 1¼ Fat
PROTEIN: 37 g, CARBOHYDRATE: 16 g, FIBER: 4 g

SAUTÉED SHRIMP SALAD – SPECIAL REQUEST

with avocado, watermelon and fine herbs. Request less oil (2 tsp.) and less avocado (¼ avocado).

✓✓ CALORIES: Excellent Choice (315) ✓ CHOLESTEROL: Good Choice (150 mg)
✓ FAT: Good Choice (22 g)♥ ✓✓ SODIUM: Excellent Choice (185 mg)**
EXCHANGES: 2¼ Meat (extra lean), ½ Fruit, 4¼ Fat
PROTEIN: 18 g, CARBOHYDRATE: 13 g, FIBER: 1 g

WIDE NOODLES WITH PORTABELLO MUSHROOMS

with pinenuts and spinach.

✓ CALORIES: Good Choice (495) ✓✓ CHOLESTEROL: Excellent Choice (35 mg)
✓ FAT: Good Choice (20 g) ✓ SODIUM: Good Choice (590 mg)**
EXCHANGES: 1¾ Meat, 2½ Bread, 1 Veg, 2¼ Fat
PROTEIN: 29 g, CARBOHYDRATE: 51 g, FIBER: 5 g

FRESH MARINATED SALMON – SPECIAL REQUEST

with citrus vinaigrette, potato blini and spring greens. Request less vinaigrette (1 oz.).

✓✓ CALORIES: Excellent Choice (375) ✓ CHOLESTEROL: Good Choice (150 mg)
✓ FAT: Good Choice (19 g) SODIUM: High (4620 mg)
EXCHANGES: 3¼ Meat, 1 Bread, ¼ Fruit, 2¼ Fat
PROTEIN: 28 g, CARBOHYDRATE: 21 g, FIBER: 2 g

♥ Primarily unsaturated
** If you request no added salt

The first Gypsy Den was established in 1994 in Costa Mesa. With plush chairs, funky fixtures, thriftstore treasures in every nook and cranny, and prayer rugs hanging from the multi-colored walls, the Gypsy Den offers a unique Bohemian retreat, with warm lights and an eclectic décor indoors and lots of plants, trees, climbing ivy and a fountain outdoors. Owners Catherine Graziano and musician-artist-handyman-waiter husband Joe Ongie opened their second location in the summer of 1999 in the Artist's Village in downtown Santa Ana with a larger space, bakery, performance stage, and an expanded menu. The Gypsy Den is one of Orange County's great hangs, and it doesn't hurt that the food is also very, very good! $

The Gypsy Den

Costa Mesa: 2930 Bristol Street (LAB anti-mall) (714) 549-7012
Santa Ana: 125 N. Broadway (Artist's Village) (714) 835-8840
www.gypsyden.com

Mandarin Chicken Salad – Special Request 🍎

Request less fried wontons (1 oz.) and dressing on the side (dressing not included in analysis).

✓ Calories: Good Choice (630) ✓ Cholesterol: Good Choice (135 mg)
✓ Fat: Excellent Choice (24 g) Sodium: Moderate (655 mg)
Exchanges: 7¼ Meat (extra lean), 2½Veg, 1 Fruit, 2 Fat
Protein: 57 g, Carbohydrate: 46 g, Fiber: 8 g

Lowfat Apple Oatmeal Muffin:

✓✓ Calories: Excellent Choice (445) ✓✓ Cholesterol: Excellent Choice (<1 mg)
✓✓ Fat: Excellent Choice (2 g)♥ ✓ Sodium: Good Choice (470 mg)
Exchanges: ¼ Meat, 2¾ Bread, ¼ Fruit, ¼ Milk, 2½ Other Carb
Protein: 11 g, Carbohydrate: 98 g, Fiber: 6 g

Lentil soup *(8 oz. cup)*†

✓✓ Calories: Excellent Choice (130) ✓✓ Cholesterol: Excellent Choice (0 mg)
✓✓ Fat: Excellent Choice (½ g)♥ Sodium: Moderate (280 mg)
Exchanges: 1¼ Bread, ¾ Veg
Protein: 9 g, Carbohydrate: 24 g, Fiber: 6 g

Acorn squash soup *(8 oz. cup)*† 🍎

✓✓ Calories: Excellent Choice (80) ✓✓ Cholesterol: Excellent Choice (5 mg)
✓✓ Fat: Excellent Choice (3 g)♥ Sodium: Moderate (330 mg)
Exchanges: 1¾ Veg, ½ Fat
Protein: 2 g, Carbohydrate: 13 g, Fiber: 2 g

Creamless Cream of Tomato Soup *(8 oz. cup)*† 🍎

✓✓ Calories: Excellent Choice (60) ✓✓ Cholesterol: Excellent Choice (0 mg)
✓✓ Fat: Excellent Choice (1 g)♥ Sodium: Moderate (350 mg)
Exchanges: 1¾ Veg, ¼ Other Carb
Protein: 3 g, Carbohydrate: 11 g, Fiber: 3 g

Reduced fat brownie *(5 oz.)* Cal: 485, Fat: 13 g♥, Chol: 0, Sod: 180 mg;
Exch: ¾ Meat, 1¾ Bread, 2¾ Other Carb, 2¼ Fat; Protein: 10 g, Carb: 83 g, Fiber: 4 g

🍎 at least 2 fruit/vegetable servings for entrees, 1 for side dishes
† Side dish guidelines are ⅓ of entree guidelines

THE HEALTH EMPORIUM MARKET & GRILLE

Open from 8 am to 8 pm, 7 days a week, The Health Emporium in Corona del Mar is a full-service gourmet natural food market and fully organic grille, deli, café, bakery, catering house and juice bar. As part of the market, we feature an exclusively organic produce department, full-service vitamin, herb, sports nutrition, homeopathy, aroma therapy, essential oil, personal care and natural cosmetic store in a store. We cater simple platters-to-go, full-service seated and staffed dining & large-scale corporate events. $

The Health Emporium

3347 East Pacific Coast Hwy, Corona del Mar, CA 92625 (949) 673-2244

WILD SALMON AND VEGETABLE SKEWER

✓✓ CALORIES: Excellent Choice (260) ✓ CHOLESTEROL: Good Choice (85 mg)
✓✓ FAT: Excellent Choice (10 g)♥ ✓✓ SODIUM: Excellent Choice (90 mg)**
EXCHANGES: 4 Meat, ¼ Bread, 1¾ Veg
PROTEIN: 32 g, CARBOHYDRATE: 11 g, FIBER: 3 g

ORGANIC MEXICAN CORN CHOWDER *(16 oz. bowl)*

✓✓ CALORIES: Excellent Choice (355) ✓✓ CHOLESTEROL: Excellent Choice (0 mg)
✓✓ FAT: Excellent Choice (3 g)♥ SODIUM: Moderate (750 mg)
EXCHANGES: 4½ Bread, 1 Veg
PROTEIN: 11 g, CARBOHYDRATE: 81 g, FIBER: 9 g

FRESH ALBACORE TUNA SALAD *(5 oz. serving)*

✓✓ CALORIES: Excellent Choice (205) ✓✓ CHOLESTEROL: Excellent Choice (50 mg)
✓✓ FAT: Excellent Choice (10 g)♥ ✓✓ SODIUM: Excellent Choice (225 mg)
EXCHANGES: 3 Meat, ¼ Veg, ¼ Fruit, 1¾ Fat
PROTEIN: 22 g, CARBOHYDRATE: 6 g, FIBER: <1 g

ORGANIC ITALIAN TOFU SALAD *(5 oz. serving)†*

✓✓ CALORIES: Excellent Choice (60) ✓✓ CHOLESTEROL: Excellent Choice (0 mg)
✓✓ FAT: Excellent Choice (2 g)♥ ✓ SODIUM: Good Choice (115 mg)
EXCHANGES: ¼ Meat, 1 Veg
PROTEIN: 4 g, CARBOHYDRATE: 8 g, FIBER: 2 g

HERBED TABOULI SALAD *(5 oz. serving)†*

✓✓ CALORIES: Excellent Choice (105) ✓✓ CHOLESTEROL: Excellent Choice (0 mg)
✓✓ FAT: Excellent Choice (1 g)♥ ✓✓ SODIUM: Excellent Choice (80 mg)
EXCHANGES: 1¼ Bread, ¼ Veg
PROTEIN: 4 g, CARBOHYDRATE: 23 g, FIBER: 6 g

BROWN RICE & BLACK BEANS *(5 oz. serving)†*

✓✓ CALORIES: Excellent Choice (140) ✓✓ CHOLESTEROL: Excellent Choice (0 mg)
✓✓ FAT: Excellent Choice (1 g)♥ ✓ SODIUM: Good Choice (145 mg)
EXCHANGES: ¼ Meat, 1½ Bread, ¼ Veg
PROTEIN: 6 g, CARBOHYDRATE: 27 g, FIBER: 5 g

ORGANIC CARROT, CRANBERRY & WALNUT SALAD *(5 oz. serving)†*

✓ CALORIES: Good Choice (230) ✓✓ CHOLESTEROL: Excellent Choice (0 mg)
FAT: Moderate (11 g)♥ ✓✓ SODIUM: Excellent Choice (90 mg)
EXCHANGES: 2 Veg, 1¼ Fruit, 2 Fat
PROTEIN: 3 g, CARBOHYDRATE: 33 g, FIBER: 5 g

♥ Primarily unsaturated fat
** If you request no added salt

Ho Sum Bistro is a locally renowned neighborhood restaurant located on the Balboa Peninsula in Newport Beach. Famous for its fabulous Ho Sum Chicken Salad, it also serves an array of other "Califoriental" delicacies. Set in a bright and casual atmosphere, our food and helpful friendly staff promise to make your visit to Ho Sum a memorable one! $

Ho Sum Bistro

(949) 675-0896

3112 Newport Blvd., Newport Beach, CA 92663

HO SUM CHICKEN SALAD – SPECIAL REQUEST

Roasted and shredded chicken breast with lettuce and red ginger dressing.
Request no wontons (not included in analysis).

✓✓ CALORIES: Excellent Choice (335) | ✓ CHOLESTEROL: Good Choice (120 mg)
✓✓ FAT: Excellent Choice (9 g) | SODIUM: High (1085 mg)
EXCHANGES: 6¼ Meat (extra lean), ¼ Bread, 1 Veg, ¾ Fat
PROTEIN: 47 g, CARBOHYDRATE: 14 g, FIBER: 4 g

HO SUM DUMPLINGS

Five delectable chicken dumplings in a spicy cilantro sauce.

✓ CALORIES: Good Choice (460) | ✓ CHOLESTEROL: Good Choice (100 mg)
✓ FAT: Good Choice (20 g) | SODIUM: High (1730 mg)
EXCHANGES: 3½ Meat (extra lean), 1½ Bread, 1¾ Veg, 1½ Fat
PROTEIN: 31 g, CARBOHYDRATE: 37 g, FIBER: 2 g

SESAME STEAMED VEGETABLES

An array of fresh garden vegetables steamed to perfection.
Served with a delicate soy-ginger sauce and sprinkled with sesame seeds.

✓✓ CALORIES: Excellent Choice (125) | ✓✓ CHOLESTEROL: Excellent Choice (0 mg)
✓✓ FAT: Excellent Choice (2 g)♥ | SODIUM: High (1140 mg)
EXCHANGES: ¼ Bread, 3 Veg
PROTEIN: 8 g, CARBOHYDRATE: 21 g, FIBER: 7 g

CALIFORIENTAL RICE

Pot-steamed with chicken and vegetables. The aroma of this rice will drive you wild.

✓ CALORIES: Good Choice (595) | ✓✓ CHOLESTEROL: Excellent Choice (65 mg)
✓✓ FAT: Excellent Choice (4 g) | SODIUM: High (1680 mg)
EXCHANGES: 3¼ Meat (extra lean), 6¼ Bread, 1¾ Veg, ¼ Fat
PROTEIN: 34 g, CARBOHYDRATE: 103 g, FIBER: 3 g

CHINESE PEPPER CHICKEN

Tender julienned chicken breast, bell pepper, celery, mushroom, and onion
stir fried in a spicy sauce, and served over brown rice.

✓✓ CALORIES: Excellent Choice (405) | ✓ CHOLESTEROL: Good Choice (85 mg)
✓✓ FAT: Excellent Choice (9 g) | SODIUM: Moderate (730 mg)**
EXCHANGES: 4½ Meat (extra lean), 2¼ Bread, 1 Veg, 1 Fat
PROTEIN: 36 g, CARBOHYDRATE: 42 g, FIBER: 1 g

QUENELLES

Five dumplings stuffed with a light blend of chicken, vegetables and its own sauce.

✓✓ CALORIES: Excellent Choice (230) | ✓✓ CHOLESTEROL: Excellent Choice (30 mg)
✓✓ FAT: Excellent Choice (3 g) | SODIUM: High (2025 mg)
EXCHANGES: 1½ Meat, 1½ Bread, ¾ Veg, ¼ Fat
PROTEIN: 17 g, CARBOHYDRATE: 32 g, FIBER: 2 g

at least 2 fruit/vegetable servings

il Farro Caffe Trattoria offers a fun, casual atmosphere serving authentic Italian Mediterranean cuisine. The name is inspired by the unique grain "Farro," which is considered an "elixir of long life." You can indulge in everything from a formal dinner to a light fare or simply a late night dessert and cocktail. Our food is fresh and authentic. We grill or roast our meats and fish whenever possible and remove all skin and visible fat. We are concerned with good taste and good health because we care and know that you, "our guests," expect it of us. Farro products are available retail at our restaurant and website, www.ilfarro.com. $$

il Farro Caffe Trattoria

111 21st Place, Newport Beach, CA 92663 (949) 723-5711

MISTO PESCE ALLA GRIGLIA AL SALMORIGLIO

Mix fish of the day, grilled, served simply with fresh lemon, extra virgin olive oil, parsley & a side of veggies.

✓✓ CALORIES: Excellent Choice (440) ✓ CHOLESTEROL: Good Choice (95 mg)
✓ FAT: Good Choice (23 g)♥ ✓✓ SODIUM: Excellent Choice (145 mg)**
EXCHANGES: 5 Meat, 1¼ Veg, 2¾ Fat
PROTEIN: 49 g, CARBOHYDRATE: 8 g, FIBER: 4 g

FARRILLI V.I.P.

Farro spiral pasta with fresh asparagus, tiger shrimp, green onions, fresh tomato and basil.

✓ CALORIES: Good Choice (695) CHOLESTEROL: Moderate (275 mg)
✓ FAT: Good Choice (18 g)♥ ✓ SODIUM: Good Choice (430 mg)**
EXCHANGES: 5 Meat (extra lean), 4½ Bread, 2 Veg, 3¼ Fat
PROTEIN: 51 g, CARBOHYDRATE: 82 g, FIBER: 11 g

FILI DELLA CASA

Farro tubular pasta with chicken, sun dried tomatoes, fresh tomatoes, extra virgin olive oil and garlic.

CALORIES: Moderate (925) ✓ CHOLESTEROL: Good Choice (85 mg)
✓ FAT: Good Choice (20 g) ✓✓ SODIUM: Excellent Choice (290 mg)**
EXCHANGES: 5¼ Meat (extra lean), 4½ Bread, 4¾ Veg, 3 Fat
PROTEIN: 61 g, CARBOHYDRATE: 133 g, FIBER: 14 g

FARROTTO FORESTIERA

Farro risotto with chicken, spinach, mushrooms, asparagus, fresh tomatoes and red onion.

CALORIES: Moderate (770) ✓ CHOLESTEROL: Good Choice (85 mg)
✓ FAT: Good Choice (21 g) ✓ SODIUM: Good Choice (325 mg)**
EXCHANGES: 4½ Meat (extra lean), 6 Bread, 1¾ Veg, 3½ Fat
PROTEIN: 45 g, CARBOHYDRATE: 100 g, FIBER: 10 g

CASARECCIA TOSCANA

Spiral pasta with broccoli, chicken, artichokes, farro grain and garlic.

✓ CALORIES: Good Choice (715) ✓ CHOLESTEROL: Good Choice (90 mg)
✓✓ FAT: Excellent Choice (15 g) ✓✓ SODIUM: Excellent Choice (270 mg)**
EXCHANGES: 4½ Meat (extra lean), 5¾ Bread, 1½ Veg, 1¾ Fat
PROTEIN: 49 g, CARBOHYDRATE: 96 g, FIBER: 9 g

♥ Primarily unsaturated fat
** If you request no added salt

Located on Katella Avenue across from the Arrowhead Pond, J.T. Schmid's encompasses 17,500 sq. feet of indoor and outdoor dining and provides a palm tree lit patio, private banquet facilities and incredible dining atmosphere for business lunches, social gatherings or a romantic dinner for two. We offer gourmet food and quality microbrews at moderate prices as well as live music on the patio. $$

J T Schmid's Brewhouse & Eatery

2610 E. Katella Avenue, Anaheim, CA 92806 (714) 634-9200

GRILLED BANGKOK CHICKEN

Grilled chicken breast glazed with teriyaki and served over steamed rice and mixed vegetables.

✓ CALORIES: Good Choice (690) — CHOLESTEROL: Moderate (175 mg)
✓ FAT: Good Choice (17 g) — SODIUM: High (1855 mg)
EXCHANGES: 9 Meat (extra lean), 3 Bread, ¾ Veg
PROTEIN: 76 g, CARBOHYDRATE: 56 g, FIBER: 3 g

TUSCAN SWORDFISH – SPECIAL REQUEST

Grilled swordfish braised with lemon pepper, cumin and coriander seeds, served over a chilled white bean salad with a sundried tomato relish and a mango mint sauce *Request grilled without oil.*

✓ CALORIES: Good Choice (625) — ✓ CHOLESTEROL: Good Choice (80 mg)
✓ FAT: Good Choice (25 g)♥ — SODIUM: High (1860 mg)
EXCHANGES: 4¾ Meat, 1½ Bread, 2 Veg, ½ Fruit, 3 Fat
PROTEIN: 50 g, CARBOHYDRATE: 52 g, FIBER: 9 g

AHI TUNA WRAP – SPECIAL REQUEST

Ahi tuna slightly blackened with cilantro and steamed rice, wrapped in a spinach tortilla and served with wasabi sour cream and our homemade mango sauce. Request less pesto sauce (½ oz).

✓ CALORIES: Good Choice (740) — ✓✓ CHOLESTEROL: Excellent Choice (70 mg)
✓ FAT: Good Choice (21 g)♥ — SODIUM: Moderate (885 mg)**
EXCHANGES: 4½ Meat, 5¾ Bread, 1½ Veg, ¼ Fruit, 3¾ Fat
PROTEIN: 49 g, CARBOHYDRATE: 98 g, FIBER: 6 g

CHINESE CHICKEN SALAD – SPECIAL REQUEST

Mixed greens, tri-colored peppers, bean sprouts, fried wontons, roasted peanuts and mandarin oranges, tossed in our wasabi vinaigrette. Request less dressing (1 oz).

✓ CALORIES: Good Choice (570) — ✓ CHOLESTEROL: Good Choice (130 mg)
✓ FAT: Good Choice (23 g) — ✓ SODIUM: Good Choice (545 mg)**
EXCHANGES: 7 Meat (extra lean), ¾ Bread, 1½ Veg, ½ Fruit, 3¼ Fat
PROTEIN: 54 g, CARBOHYDRATE: 36 g, FIBER: 5 g

GRILLED TERIYAKI SALMON SALAD – SPECIAL REQUEST

Grilled teriyaki salmon topped with toasted sesame seeds, served over mixed field greens with peppers, onions, sprouts and water chestnuts, and tossed in our wasabi vinaigrette. Request less dressing (1 oz).

✓ CALORIES: Good Choice (475) — ✓ CHOLESTEROL: Good Choice (90 mg)
✓ FAT: Good Choice (23 g)♥ — SODIUM: High (1725 mg)
EXCHANGES: 4¼ Meat, 2¼ Veg, ¼ Fruit, 1½ Fat
PROTEIN: 40 g, CARBOHYDRATE: 29 g, FIBER: 4 g

♥ Primarily unsaturated fat
** If you request no added salt

Jamba Juice is a leading retail purveyor of blended-to-order smoothies and fresh squeezed juices. Our mission is to enrich the active daily experience of our customers, community & team members through the life-nourishing qualities of fruits & vegetables. All smoothies include one FREE Juice Boost & are available in our 16 oz., 24 oz., or 32 oz. sizes. Also try our nutritious breads and pretzels. $

Jamba Juice

Orange County locations: Anaheim at Downtown Disney, Brea, Costa Mesa, Fullerton, Huntington Beach, Irvine, Irvine Spectrum, Laguna Beach, Long Beach, Newport Beach, Orange at the Block, Seal Beach, Tustin & Westminster.
Call 1-888-JAMBA12 or visit www.jambajuice.com for your nearest location.

STRAWBERRY NIRVANA® SMOOTHIE *(16 oz.)* 🍎

Enlightened base, frozen strawberries, apple strawberry juice blend, ice, and frozen bananas.

✓✓ CALORIES: Good Choice (160) ✓✓ CHOLESTEROL: Excellent Choice (5 mg)
✓✓ FAT: Excellent Choice (0 g) ✓✓ SODIUM: Excellent Choice (230 mg)
PROTEIN: 6 g, CARBOHYDRATE: 34 g, FIBER: 3 g

MANGO MANTRA® SMOOTHIE *(16 oz.)* 🍎

Enlightened base, frozen mangos, fresh orange juice, ice, and frozen peaches.

✓✓ CALORIES: Good Choice (170) ✓✓ CHOLESTEROL: Excellent Choice (5 mg)
✓✓ FAT: Excellent Choice (½ g) ✓✓ SODIUM: Excellent Choice (230 mg)
PROTEIN: 7 g, CARBOHYDRATE: 36 g, FIBER: 2 g

CARIBBEAN PASSION® SMOOTHIE *(16 oz.)* 🍎

Passion fruit juice blend, orange sherbet, frozen strawberries, frozen peaches and ice.

✓✓ CALORIES: Good Choice (290) ✓✓ CHOLESTEROL: Excellent Choice (5 mg)
✓✓ FAT: Excellent Choice (1½ g) ✓✓ SODIUM: Excellent Choice (40 mg)
PROTEIN: 2 g, CARBOHYDRATE: 67 g, FIBER: 3 g

PROTEIN BERRY PIZZAZZ™ SMOOTHIE *(16 oz.)* 🍎

Soymilk, frozen strawberries, frozen bananas, ice and Protein Boost.

✓✓ CALORIES: Excellent Choice (280) ✓✓ CHOLESTEROL: Excellent Choice (0 mg)
✓✓ FAT: Excellent Choice (1 g)♥ ✓✓ SODIUM: Excellent Choice (170 mg)
PROTEIN: 15 g, CARBOHYDRATE: 56 g, FIBER: 4 g

STRAWBERRIES WILD® SMOOTHIE *(16 oz.)* 🍎

Apple strawberry juice blend, nonfat vanilla frozen yogurt, frozen strawberries, frozen bananas, and ice.

✓✓ CALORIES: Good Choice (290) ✓✓ CHOLESTEROL: Excellent Choice (0 mg)
✓✓ FAT: Excellent Choice (0 g) ✓✓ SODIUM: Excellent Choice (115 mg)
PROTEIN: 4 g, CARBOHYDRATE: 69 g, FIBER: 3 g

GRIN & CARROT BREAD *(1 mini loaf) Packed with shreds of carrots, raisins, walnuts, pineapple & hints of cinnamon.*
CAL: 250, FAT: 10 g♥, CHOL: 25 mg, SOD: 250 mg; PROT: 5 g, CARB: 36 g, FIBER: 1 g

HONEY BERRY BRAN BREAD *(1 mini loaf) with raisins, blueberries & spices. Good source of protein, fiber & iron!*
CAL: 320, FAT: 12 g♥, CHOL: 30 mg, SOD: 360 mg; PROT: 6 g, CARB: 48 g, FIBER: 6 g

Nutrition information supplied by Jamba Juice.

🍎 at least 2 fruit/vegetable servings

KOO·KOO·ROO® GOOD FOR YOO.™

Koo Koo Roo California Kitchen features Original Skinless Flame-Broiled Chicken,™ fresh oven-roasted turkey breast, garlic & country herb rotisserie chicken, salads, and a wide assortment of freshly prepared gourmet side dishes. Food is made fresh throughout the day and appeals to those who appreciate delicious, high quality, fresh food that can be enjoyed on the premises or as a home meal replacement. Take out and catering available. $

Koo Koo Roo 13792 Jamboree Rd., Irvine, CA 92612 (714) 508-9900

KOO KOO ROO SKINLESS CHICKEN BREAST *(4.2 oz.)*

✓✓ CALORIES: Excellent Choice (195) ✓ CHOLESTEROL: Good Choice (120 mg)
✓✓ FAT: Excellent Choice (6 g) ✓ SODIUM: Good Choice (435 mg)
EXCHANGES: 5 Meat (extra lean)
PROTEIN: 35 g, CARBOHYDRATE: 0 g, FIBER: 0 g

ORIGINAL CHICKEN SANDWICH – SPECIAL REQUEST

Request no dressing.
✓✓ CALORIES: Excellent Choice (375) ✓ CHOLESTEROL: Good Choice (90 mg)
✓✓ FAT: Excellent Choice (6 g) SODIUM: Moderate (710 mg)
EXCHANGES: 3¾ Meat (extra lean), 2¾ Bread, ½ Veg, ¼ Fat
PROTEIN: 35 g, CARBOHYDRATE: 45 g, FIBER: 3 g

TURKEY SANDWICH – SPECIAL REQUEST

Request no mayo.
✓✓ CALORIES: Excellent Choice (445) ✓ CHOLESTEROL: Good Choice (120 mg)
✓✓ FAT: Excellent Choice (3 g) ✓✓ SODIUM: Excellent Choice (270 mg)
EXCHANGES: 6¼ Meat (extra lean), 3¼ Bread, ¼ Veg, ½ Fat
PROTEIN: 49 g, CARBOHYDRATE: 52 g, FIBER: 3 g

Side Dishes:

VEGETABLE SOUP† *(8 oz.)* 🍎

✓✓ CALORIES: Excellent Choice (120) ✓✓ CHOLESTEROL: Excellent Choice (0 mg)
✓✓ FAT: Excellent Choice (3 g)♥ SODIUM: High (620 mg)
EXCHANGES: ½ Bread, 1¾ Veg, ½ Fat; PROTEIN: 3 g, CARBOHYDRATE: 21 g, FIBER: 4 g

BUTTERNUT SQUASH† *(6 oz.)* 🍎

✓✓ CALORIES: Excellent Choice (65) ✓✓ CHOLESTEROL: Excellent Choice (0 mg)
✓✓ FAT: Excellent Choice (0 g) ✓✓ SODIUM: Excellent Choice (5 mg)
EXCHANGES: ¾ Bread, 2½ Veg; PROTEIN: 2 g, CARBOHYDRATE: 17 g, FIBER: 4 g

STEAMED VEGETABLES† *(4 oz.)* 🍎

✓✓ CALORIES: Excellent Choice (35) ✓✓ CHOLESTEROL: Excellent Choice (0 mg)
✓✓ FAT: Excellent Choice (0 g) ✓✓ SODIUM: Excellent Choice (30 mg)
EXCHANGES: 1½ Veg; PROTEIN: 2 g, CARBOHYDRATE: 7 g, FIBER: 2 g

GREEN BEANS† *(4 oz.)* 🍎

✓✓ CALORIES: Excellent Choice (60) ✓✓ CHOLESTEROL: Excellent Choice (5 mg)
✓✓ FAT: Excellent Choice (3 g) ✓ SODIUM: Good Choice (170 mg)
EXCHANGES: 1½ Veg, ½ Fat; PROTEIN: 2 g, CARBOHYDRATE: 8 g, FIBER: 2 g

ROASTED GARLIC POTATOES† *(5 oz.)* 🍎

✓✓ CALORIES: Excellent Choice (145) ✓✓ CHOLESTEROL: Excellent Choice (5 mg)
✓✓ FAT: Excellent Choice (3 g) ✓ SODIUM: Good Choice (145 mg)
EXCHANGES: 1¾ Bread, ½ Fat; PROTEIN: 2 g, CARBOHYDRATE: 28 g, FIBER: 2 g

🍎 at least 2 fruit/vegetable servings for entrees, 1 for side dishes
† Side dish guidelines are ⅓ of entree guidelines

La Salsa FRESH MEXICAN GRILL®

The Original Made-to-Order Fresh Mexican Restaurant! At La Salsa you'll find a variety of delicious Mexican recipes and tastes all prepared individually to your order and liking. A fresh salsa bar also allows you to garnish with a wide variety of salsas and trimmings. No prepackaged burritos, no MSG, no microwaves. Tell us what you want...we'll make it fresh! For more info & locations, visit www.lasalsa.com. $

La Salsa Orange County locations:

Irvine: 3850 Baranca Parkway (949) 786-7692
8673 Irvine Center Drive (949) 450-8511
14171 Jeffrey Road (949) 551-6680
Newport Beach: Fashion Island Mall (949) 640-4289
Laguna Hills: 25912 La Paz Rd. (949) 672-0027
Tustin: 535 E. Main Street (714) 838-8253
Newport Beach: 4341 MacArthur Blvd. (949) 475-2506

Chips not included in analyses below.

CHICKEN TACO LA SALSA

Two soft corn tortillas filled with charbroiled chicken, Jack and Cheddar cheeses, lettuce and tomatoes.

✓✓ CALORIES: Excellent Choice (270)
✓✓ FAT: Excellent Choice (8 g)
✓✓ CHOLESTEROL: Excellent Choice (65 mg)
✓ SODIUM: Good Choice (330 mg)
PROTEIN: 17 g, CARBOHYDRATE: 32 g, FIBER: 2 g

SONORA MAHI MAHI TACO

Flour tortilla taco filled with grilled Mahi Mahi, lettuce, tomatoes, Jack and Cheddar cheeses and topped with our Sonora sauce and a squeeze of lime.

✓✓ CALORIES: Excellent Choice (200)
✓✓ FAT: Excellent Choice (8 g)
✓✓ CHOLESTEROL: Excellent Choice (30 mg)
SODIUM: Moderate (640 mg)
PROTEIN: 13 g, CARBOHYDRATE: 17 g, FIBER: 0 g

VEGGIE TACO

Two soft corn tortillas filled with fajita vegetables, black beans, Jack & Cheddar cheeses, lettuce & tomatoes.

✓✓ CALORIES: Excellent Choice (280)
✓✓ FAT: Excellent Choice (10 g)
✓✓ CHOLESTEROL: Excellent Choice (25 mg)
✓ SODIUM: Good Choice (420 mg)
PROTEIN: 12 g, CARBOHYDRATE: 37 g, FIBER: 4 g

CHILE-LIME SALAD – SPECIAL REQUEST

Chicken, Romaine, Cotija cheese, tomatoes & avocado, with our own Chile-Lime dressing. Request no tortilla strips and dressing on the side (neither included in analysis). Mango Salsa is an excellent dressing alternative.

✓ CALORIES: Good Choice (495)
✓✓ FAT: Excellent Choice (15 g)
✓ CHOLESTEROL: Good Choice (95 mg)
SODIUM: Moderate (820 mg)
PROTEIN: 29 g, CARBOHYDRATE: 19 g, FIBER: 5 g

LOS CABOS SHRIMP BURRITO – SPECIAL REQUEST

Grilled shrimp, Sonora sauce, fire-roasted fajita veggies, rice, cabbage, crema & avocado in a flour tortilla. Request no cheese.

✓ CALORIES: Good Choice (555)
✓ FAT: Good Choice (21 g)
✓✓ CHOLESTEROL: Excellent Choice (60 mg)
SODIUM: High (1995 mg)
PROTEIN: 21 g, CARBOHYDRATE: 77 g, FIBER: 4 g

CHICKEN, BEAN & CHEESE BURRITO

With freshly made beans and Jack and Cheddar cheese in a flour tortilla.

✓ CALORIES: Good Choice (725)
✓ FAT: Good Choice (22 g)
✓ CHOLESTEROL: Good Choice (100 mg)
SODIUM: High (1545 mg)
PROTEIN: 43 g, CARBOHYDRATE: 88 g, FIBER: 9 g

½ RICE & ½ BEANS: CAL: 235, FAT: 4 g♥, CHOL: 0 mg, SOD: 775 mg; PROT: 10 g, CARB: 45 g, FIBER: 9 g

Nutrition information supplied by La Salsa.

♥ Primarily unsaturated fat
** If you request no added salt

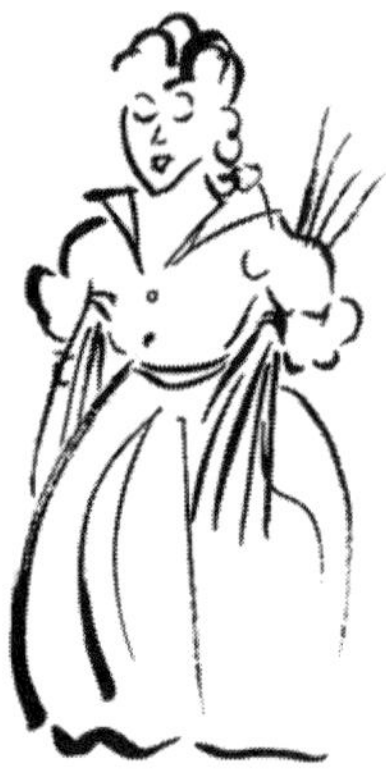

Located in a historical home in the resort town of Dana Point, Luciana's Ristorante has been serving the Orange County community for over 22 years. The décor is reminiscent of a cozy European style inn, establishing it as one of Orange County's most romantic restaurants. Awarded the Southern California Restaurant Writers gold medal since 1991, three stars from the California Restaurant Writers, Zagat Survey and an Award of Excellence for its wine list, Luciana's has been setting the standard for classic as well as innovative Italian cuisine. Whether visiting our cozy restaurant or our Bed and Breakfast and Cooking School in Tuscany, Italy, you are sure to experience the best and freshest combination of the old and new worlds. $$

Luciana's Ristorante

24312 Del Prado (PCH), Dana Point, CA 92629 (949) 661-6500

SPIDINI (APPETIZER)

Tiger shrimp with couscous, olives, cucumber & drizzled herb vinaigrette.

✓✓CALORIES: Excellent Choice (205) ✓ CHOLESTEROL: Good Choice (110 mg)
✓✓FAT: Excellent Choice (6 g)♥ ✓ SODIUM: Good Choice (430 mg)**
EXCHANGES: 1¾ Meat (extra lean), 1¼ Bread, 1¼ Fat
PROTEIN: 15 g, CARBOHYDRATE: 21 g, FIBER: 1 g

GRILLED VEGETABLE PLATTER

✓✓ CALORIES: Excellent Choice (210) ✓✓ CHOLESTEROL: Excellent Choice (0 mg)
✓✓ FAT: Excellent Choice (14 g)♥ ✓✓ SODIUM: Excellent Choice (10 mg)**
EXCHANGES: 3½ Veg, 2¾ Fat
PROTEIN: 5 g, CARBOHYDRATE: 20 g, FIBER: 5 g

CALAMARI AL SALTO

Calamari sautéed with fresh tomatoes, scallions, Kalamata olives and capers in a lemon white wine sauce.

✓✓ CALORIES: Excellent Choice (195) CHOLESTEROL: Moderate (240 mg)
✓✓ FAT: Excellent Choice (9 g)♥ SODIUM: Moderate (820 mg)**
EXCHANGES: 2¼ Meat (extra lean), ½ Veg, 3¾ Fat
PROTEIN: 17 g, CARBOHYDRATE: 9 g, FIBER: 1 g

CIOPPINO

✓ CALORIES: Good Choice (460) CHOLESTEROL: High (405 mg)
✓ FAT: Good Choice (20 g)♥ ✓ SODIUM: Good Choice (505 mg)**
EXCHANGES: 7 Meat (extra lean), ½ Veg, 3 Fat
PROTEIN: 58 g, CARBOHYDRATE: 10 g, FIBER: 1 g

FETTUCCINE BOSCAIOLA

Fettuccini pasta, sautéed tiger prawns, mushrooms, spinach and sun-dried tomatoes in a light garlic white wine sauce.

✓ CALORIES: Good Choice (485) CHOLESTEROL: Moderate (195 mg)
✓✓ FAT: Excellent Choice (10 g)♥ ✓✓ SODIUM: Excellent Choice (280 mg)**
EXCHANGES: 3 Meat (extra lean), 3¼ Bread, 2¼ Veg, 1¾ Fat
PROTEIN: 34 g, CARBOHYDRATE: 62 g, FIBER: 6 g

CHICKEN VERMICELLI

Glass noodles with chicken breast, asparagus, carrots and red onion.

✓ CALORIES: Good Choice (720) ✓ CHOLESTEROL: Good Choice (100 mg)
✓✓ FAT: Excellent Choice (9 g) ✓✓ SODIUM: Excellent Choice (110 mg)**
EXCHANGES: 5 Meat (extra lean), 7½ Bread, 1¼ Veg, 1 Fat
PROTEIN: 37 g, CARBOHYDRATE: 119 g, FIBER: 4 g

at least 2 fruit/vegetable servings

For over 20 years, Luigi's has been a favorite of the locals. You will enjoy the friendly, lively atmosphere created by this family owned and operated Italian restaurant. An extensive menu includes delicious chicken and baked specialties, pizza, sandwiches, salads, veal, seafood, a catch of the day, and Luigi's famous pasta specialties. $$

Luigi's D'Italia

801 S. State College, Anaheim, CA 92806
(714) 490-0990 (714) 533-1300

HALIBUT LIVORNESE – SPECIAL REQUEST

Halibut poached in a tomato garlic and wine sauce. Request less oil (1 Tbs).

✓ CALORIES: Good Choice (465) ✓✓ CHOLESTEROL: Excellent Choice (75 mg)
✓ FAT: Good Choice (20 g)♥ SODIUM: High (1735 mg)
EXCHANGES: 4½ Meat (extra lean), 2 Veg, 3 Fat
PROTEIN: 50 g, CARBOHYDRATE: 14 g, FIBER: 3 g

NEW ZEALAND MUSSELS WITH RED SAUCE – SPECIAL REQUEST

Served over linguine with freshly prepared red sauce. Request less oil (1 Tbs).

✓ CALORIES: Good Choice (515) ✓ CHOLESTEROL: Good Choice (80 mg)
✓ FAT: Good Choice (18 g)♥ SODIUM: High (1895 mg)
EXCHANGES: 2½ Meat (extra lean), 2½ Bread, 1½ Veg, 2¾ Fat
PROTEIN: 29 g, CARBOHYDRATE: 55 g, FIBER: 5 g

LINGUINI AGLIO E OLIO – SPECIAL REQUEST

With fresh garlic, basil, olive oil and Italian seasonings. Request less oil (1 Tbs).

✓✓ CALORIES: Excellent Choice (450) ✓✓ CHOLESTEROL: Excellent Choice (0 mg)
✓✓ FAT: Excellent Choice (15 g)♥ ✓✓ SODIUM: Excellent Choice (15 mg)**
EXCHANGES: 2½ Bread, ¼ Veg, 2¾ Fat
PROTEIN: 12 g, CARBOHYDRATE: 69 g, FIBER: 4 g

PENNE PRIMAVERA WITH TOMATO SAUCE – SPECIAL REQUEST

Carrots, broccoli, zucchini, cauliflower and garlic in tomato sauce. Request less oil (1 Tbs).

✓✓ CALORIES: Excellent Choice (420) ✓✓ CHOLESTEROL: Excellent Choice (0 mg)
✓ FAT: Good Choice (16 g)♥ ✓ SODIUM: Good Choice (520 mg)**
EXCHANGES: 2½ Bread, 3¾ Veg, 2¾ Fat
PROTEIN: 12 g, CARBOHYDRATE: 62 g, FIBER: 9 g

VEGETARIAN CHEESELESS PIZZA (⅓ MEDIUM PIZZA)

✓ CALORIES: Good Choice (600) ✓✓ CHOLESTEROL: Excellent Choice (0 mg)
✓ FAT: Good Choice (22 g)♥ ✓ SODIUM: Good Choice (305 mg)**
EXCHANGES: 4½ Bread, 3½ Veg, 4 Fat
PROTEIN: 15 g, CARBOHYDRATE: 90 g, FIBER: 10 g

♥ Primarily unsaturated fat
** If you request no added salt

A splash of Morocco in Southern California, this exquisitely decorated restaurant is authentic from its inlaid tables to its superb gourmet Moroccan cuisine. Enjoy a fun and exotic feast in the Moroccan tradition featuring belly dancing. Open for dinner from 5 to 11 pm. Reservations suggested. $$$

Marrakesh 1976 Newport Blvd., Costa Mesa, CA 92627 (949) 645-8384

Analyses below are for individual portions, although several portions are served family-style on platters.

SHRIMP KABOB WITH SAFFRON RICE

Grilled shrimp served over saffron sauce rice with harisa (hot sauce) on the side (harisa not included in analysis).

✓✓ CALORIES: Excellent Choice (210) ✓ CHOLESTEROL: Good Choice (115 mg)
✓✓ FAT: Excellent Choice (5 g)♥ ✓✓ SODIUM: Excellent Choice (175 mg)**
EXCHANGES: 2¼ Meat (extra lean), 1¼ Bread, ¾ Fat
PROTEIN: 17 g, CARBOHYDRATE: 22 g, FIBER: 0 g

COUS COUS VEGETABLES

Traditional dish of Morocco, a bed of steamed cracked wheat covered with cooked vegetables and raisins.

✓ CALORIES: Good Choice (670) ✓✓ CHOLESTEROL: Excellent Choice (0 mg)
✓ FAT: Good Choice (19 g)♥ ✓✓ SODIUM: Excellent Choice (270 mg)**
EXCHANGES: 5½ Bread, 2¾ Veg, 3½ Fat
PROTEIN: 18 g, CARBOHYDRATE: 107 g, FIBER: 10 g

FISH TANGINE – SPECIAL REQUEST

Fillet of fish (choice of halibut or swordfish) sautéed with tomatoes, garlic, cumin, olive oil & paprika. Request less oil (2 tsp. per person). Analysis for halibut; swordfish slightly higher in fat.

✓✓ CALORIES: Excellent Choice (395) ✓✓ CHOLESTEROL: Excellent Choice (50 mg)
✓✓ FAT: Excellent Choice (15 g)♥ ✓ SODIUM: Good Choice (390 mg)**
EXCHANGES: 4½ Meat (extra lean), ¾ Bread, 2¼ Veg, ¼ Fruit, 2¼ Fat
PROTEIN: 36 g, CARBOHYDRATE: 31 g, FIBER: 7 g

SPICED CARROTS SALAD †

Delightfully spiced carrots.

✓✓ CALORIES: Excellent Choice (110) ✓✓ CHOLESTEROL: Excellent Choice (0 mg)
✓✓ FAT: Excellent Choice (5 g)♥ ✓✓ SODIUM: Excellent Choice (100 mg)**
EXCHANGES: 3 Veg, 1 Fat
PROTEIN: 2 g, CARBOHYDRATE: 16 g, FIBER: 5 g

CUCUMBER AND TOMATO SALAD †

✓ CALORIES: Good Choice (155) ✓✓ CHOLESTEROL: Excellent Choice (0 mg)
FAT: Moderate (9 g)♥ ✓ SODIUM: Good Choice (115 mg)**
EXCHANGES: 3¼ Veg, 1¾ Fat
PROTEIN: 5 g, CARBOHYDRATE: 16 g, FIBER: 5 g

HARIRA SOUP †

✓✓ CALORIES: Excellent Choice (90) ✓✓ CHOLESTEROL: Excellent Choice (0 mg)
✓✓ FAT: Excellent Choice (1 g)♥ SODIUM: High (505 mg)**
EXCHANGES: ½ Bread, 2¼ Veg
PROTEIN: 5 g, CARBOHYDRATE: 18 g, FIBER: 6 g

at least 2 fruit/vegetable servings for entrees, 1 for side dishes
† Side dish guidelines are ⅓ of entrée guidelines

McCormick & Schmick's Seafood Restaurant is one of Orange County's most popular dining and gathering spots. Our menu features fresh seafood from the Pacific Northwest and other regional favorites. Salads, pastas, poultry and steak entrees are also available. Enjoy the timeless and traditional presentation and décor. Happy hour 4-6:30 pm and 9:30 to midnight Monday thru Friday. Dinner served daily from 5 pm. Reservations recommended. $$

McCormick & Schmick's Seafood Restaurant

2000 Main Street, Irvine, CA 92614 (949) 756-0505

GRILLED MAHI MAHI

with mango-orange barbeque glaze and served with seasonal vegetables.

✓ CALORIES: Good Choice (510) ✓ CHOLESTEROL: Good Choice (125 mg)
✓✓ FAT: Excellent Choice (12 g)♥ ✓ SODIUM: Good Choice (430 mg)**
EXCHANGES: 2¾ Meat, 2¼ Veg, 3½ Fruit, 2 Fat
PROTEIN: 37 g, CARBOHYDRATE: 66 g, FIBER: 7 g

GRILLED HALIBUT WITH FRESH SALSA

Topped with the Chef's special salsa-of-the-day and served with seasonal vegetables.

✓✓ CALORIES: Excellent Choice (375) ✓✓ CHOLESTEROL: Excellent Choice (65 mg)
✓✓ FAT: Excellent Choice (13 g)♥ ✓✓ SODIUM: Excellent Choice (225 mg)**
EXCHANGES: 4 Meat (extra lean), 2¼ Veg, ½ Fruit, 1¾ Fat
PROTEIN: 45 g, CARBOHYDRATE: 18 g, FIBER: 7 g

SEARED BLACKENED AHI

served rare with Cajun spices, pickled ginger and wasabi.

✓✓ CALORIES: Excellent Choice (255) ✓✓ CHOLESTEROL: Excellent Choice (75 mg)
✓✓ FAT: Excellent Choice (4 g)♥ SODIUM: High (2905 mg)
EXCHANGES: 5½ Meat (extra lean), ¼ Fat
PROTEIN: 44 g, CARBOHYDRATE: 15 g, FIBER: 1 g

NICOISE SALAD – SPECIAL REQUEST

with seared rare Ahi tuna. Request dressing on the side and use sparingly (dressing not included in analysis).

✓✓ CALORIES: Excellent Choice (235) ✓ CHOLESTEROL: Good Choice (105 mg)
✓✓ FAT: Excellent Choice (4 g) ✓✓ SODIUM: Excellent Choice (180 mg)**
EXCHANGES: 3¾ Meat, ¾ Bread, 1¼ Veg, ¼ Fat
PROTEIN: 31 g, CARBOHYDRATE: 19 g, FIBER: 3 g

PACIFIC SEAFOOD STEW

with mussels, crab, clams and prawns.

✓✓ CALORIES: Excellent Choice (415) CHOLESTEROL: Moderate (260 mg)
✓✓ FAT: Excellent Choice (14 g)♥ SODIUM: High (1305 mg)
EXCHANGES: 6½ Meat (extra lean), 2 Veg, 1¼ Fat
PROTEIN: 58 g, CARBOHYDRATE: 17 g, FIBER: 2 g

ATLANTIC SALMON – SPECIAL REQUEST

baked on a cedar plank and served with a Pinot Noir sauce and seasonal vegetables. Request sauce on the side and use sparingly (sauce not included in analysis).

✓✓ CALORIES: Excellent Choice (430) ✓ CHOLESTEROL: Good Choice (105 mg)
✓ FAT: Good Choice (24 g)♥ ✓✓ SODIUM: Excellent Choice (135 mg)**
EXCHANGES: 5 Meat, 2¼ Veg, 2¼ Fat
PROTEIN: 42 g, CARBOHYDRATE: 12 g, FIBER: 6 g

♥ Primarily unsaturated fat
** If you request no added salt

McKenna's specializes in seafood, and we offer an ever-changing selection, grilled and prepared to enhance the natural flavors. We also offer piping hot sourdough bread, fresh every 15 minutes from our ovens, as well as steaks and other favorites. No matter what your occasion, McKenna's will meet or exceed your expectations for service, style, and quality of food. As long as friendships flourish and conversations flow, we will cherish the opportunity to set your table and help set the mood. $$-$$$

McKenna's on the Bay

190 Marina Drive, Long Beach, CA 90803 (562) 342-9411

JOE'S SEAFOOD CIOPPINO

CALORIES: Moderate (845) — CHOLESTEROL: Moderate (205 mg)
✓ FAT: Good Choice (23 g)♥ — SODIUM: High (2045 mg)
EXCHANGES: 6¾ Meat (extra lean), 3¾ Bread, 2½ Veg, 3¾ Fat
PROTEIN: 71 g, CARBOHYDRATE: 76 g, FIBER: 6 g

WOOD GRILLED VEGETABLE SALAD – SPECIAL REQUEST

Fresh in-season grilled vegetables over greens with goat cheese.
Request dressing and avocado on the side (not included in analysis).
✓✓ CALORIES: Excellent Choice (360) — ✓✓ CHOLESTEROL: Excellent Choice (45 mg)
FAT: Moderate (26 g) — ✓ SODIUM: Good Choice (330 mg)**
EXCHANGES: 1¾ Meat, ½ Bread, 1½ Veg, 4 Fat
PROTEIN: 17 g, CARBOHYDRATE: 19 g, FIBER: 5 g

WOOD GRILLED HAWAIIAN MAHI MAHI

with soy shiitake mushroom glaze and served with mashed potatoes and fresh in-season vegetables.
✓ CALORIES: Good Choice (530) — CHOLESTEROL: Moderate (205 mg)
✓ FAT: Good Choice (18 g) — SODIUM: High (1140 mg)
EXCHANGES: 3¾ Meat, 1½ Bread, 1¼ Veg, ¼ Fruit, 3 Fat
PROTEIN: 49 g, CARBOHYDRATE: 43 g, FIBER: 5 g

LINGUINI WITH ROMA TOMATOES – SPECIAL REQUEST

with basil and sliced garlic. Request less oil (1 Tbs).
✓ CALORIES: Good Choice (470) — ✓✓ CHOLESTEROL: Excellent Choice (0 mg)
✓✓ FAT: Excellent Choice (15 g)♥ — ✓✓ SODIUM: Excellent Choice (15 mg)**
EXCHANGES: 3¾ Bread, 1¾ Veg, 2¾ Fat
PROTEIN: 12 g, CARBOHYDRATE: 72 g, FIBER: 5 g

HAWAIIAN AHI TUNA – SPECIAL REQUEST

with spinach and bell pepper coulis. Request no dill oil or fried wontons.
✓✓ CALORIES: Excellent Choice (405) — ✓ CHOLESTEROL: Good Choice (80 mg)
✓ FAT: Good Choice (17 g)♥ — SODIUM: Moderate (695 mg)**
EXCHANGES: 5½ Meat (extra lean), 2 Veg, 3 Fat
PROTEIN: 48 g, CARBOHYDRATE: 14 g, FIBER: 7 g

♥ Primarily unsaturated fat
** If you request no added salt

Mother's Market & Kitchen

Mother's Market & Kitchen is dedicated to the high values of holistic and healthful living. The restaurant offers abundant portions and low prices that complement the beautiful presentation and friendly service, and caters to specialized diets. Zagat chose Mother's for the 2000/2001 Award of Distinction. Stop by our store. Mother's offers organic produce, grocery, bulk foods and the freshest juices in town, as well as the largest selection of discounted vitamins, sports nutrition, supplements and herbs in Orange County. Many loyal fans consider Mother's a second home. They enjoy being able to eat and shop for food at the same place. $

Mother's Market & Kitchen Restaurant, Deli & Fresh Juice Bar

Costa Mesa: 225 E. 17th St. (949) 631-4741 Huntington Beach: 19770 Beach Blvd. (714) 963-6667
Irvine: 2963 Michelson Dr. (949) 752-6667 Laguna Wds: 24165 Paseo De Valencia (949) 768-6667

TOFU SCRAMBLE

Tofu sautéed with bell peppers, onions & arame seaweed, served with organic brown rice. Toast not in analysis.

✓ CALORIES: Good Choice (510) ✓✓ CHOLESTEROL: Excellent Choice (0 mg)
✓ FAT: Good Choice (25 g)♥ ✓✓ SODIUM: Excellent Choice (60 mg)
PROTEIN: 23 g, CARBOHYDRATE: 52 g

BLACK BEAN TACOS – SPECIAL REQUEST

Two corn tortillas stuffed with lettuce, tomato, fresh cilantro, and black beans. Request no cheese. Mexican organic basmati rice and salsa not included in analysis.

✓ CALORIES: Good Choice (570) ✓✓ CHOLESTEROL: Excellent Choice (0 mg)
✓✓ FAT: Excellent Choice (10 g)♥ ✓ SODIUM: Good Choice (340 mg)
PROTEIN: 22 g, CARBOHYDRATE: 104 g

SPRINGTIME SALAD 🍎

A colorful selection of broccoli, cauliflower, grated beets and carrots, tomato, cucumber, mushrooms and avocado slices atop organic mixed greens.

✓✓ CALORIES: Excellent Choice (240) ✓✓ CHOLESTEROL: Excellent Choice (0 mg)
✓ FAT: Good Choice (16 g)♥ ✓✓ SODIUM: Excellent Choice (70 mg)
PROTEIN: 11 g, CARBOHYDRATE: 22 g

PENNE PASTA WITH TOMATO-BASIL-GARLIC

8 oz. penne pasta topped with 4 oz tomato basil garlic.

✓✓ CALORIES: Excellent Choice (280) ✓✓ CHOLESTEROL: Excellent Choice (0 mg)
✓✓ FAT: Excellent Choice (6 g)♥ ✓✓ SODIUM: Excellent Choice (10 mg)
PROTEIN: 8 g, CARBOHYDRATE: 46 g

FRESH SEASONAL FRUIT WITH NON-FAT YOGURT OR COTTAGE CHEESE 🍎

A refreshing medley of seasonal fruit topped with non-fat yogurt and raw trail mix.

✓✓ CALORIES: Excellent Choice (245) ✓✓ CHOLESTEROL: Excellent Choice (<5 mg)
✓✓ FAT: Excellent Choice (9 g)♥ ✓✓ SODIUM: Excellent Choice (150 mg)
PROTEIN: 11 g, CARBOHYDRATE: 36 g

Seasonal fruit topped with cottage cheese and raw trail mix.

✓✓ CALORIES: Excellent Choice (285) ✓✓ CHOLESTEROL: Excellent Choice (15 mg)
✓✓ FAT: Excellent Choice (9 g)♥ ✓✓ SODIUM: Excellent Choice (285 mg)
PROTEIN: 26 g, CARBOHYDRATE: 31 g

MA'S VEGETARIAN CHILI *(8 oz.)*†

Ma's homemade high-protein remedy in an authentic zesty sauce, made with organic kidney beans.

✓✓ CALORIES: Excellent Choice (120) ✓✓ CHOLESTEROL: Excellent Choice (0 mg)
✓✓ FAT: Excellent Choice (1 g)♥ SODIUM: High (985 mg)
PROTEIN: 10 g, CARBOHYDRATE: 22 g

Nutrition information supplied by Mother's Market & Kitchen.

† Side dish guidelines are ⅓ of entree guidelines
🍎 at least 2 fruit/vegetable servings

Since 1995, the Newport Beach Brewing Company has occupied the old Delaney's Seafood Market building in the historic Cannery Village. Our logo depicts the Dory Fleet, John Wayne's Wild Goose, and the Wedge, all historical landmarks of Newport Beach. Today, after several brew awards and glowing food reviews, the Newport Beach Brewing Co. still offers the best patio dining and largest on-site parking lot on the Balboa Peninsula, while maintaining a socially comfortable environment. You can watch your favorite sports on our new 50-inch plasma TV or projection TV, watch food being barbequed in front of you, or just enjoy the company of family and friends. Open every day from 11:30 am to 11:30 pm. $-$$

Newport Beach Brewing Co. 2920 Newport Blvd., Newport Beach (949) 675-8449

Brewery Lettuce Wraps

Broiled chicken, sesame seeds, lettuce leaves, carrots, bean sprouts and sides of Thai, plum and curry sauces (see separate analyses for sauces below).

✓✓ Calories: Excellent Choice (395) ✓ Cholesterol: Good Choice (150 mg)
✓✓ Fat: Excellent Choice (7 g) ✓✓ Sodium: Excellent Choice (180 mg)**
Exchanges: 8 Meat (extra lean), 4¼ Veg
Protein: 61 g, Carbohydrate: 22 g, Fiber: 7 g

Cioppino – Special Request

Snow crab, gulf shrimp, fresh fish and clams, in an Italian broth. Request less oil (1 Tbs.) and no butter.

Calories: Moderate (775) Cholesterol: High (380 mg)
✓ Fat: Good Choice (24 g)♥ Sodium: High (1830 mg)
Exchanges: 10 Meat (extra lean), 3½ Veg, 2¾ Fat
Protein: 107 g, Carbohydrate: 38 g, Fiber: 5 g

Seared Ahi Tuna Salad – Special Request

Rare seared Ahi tuna with baby greens and wasabi vinaigrette. Request less oil (½ Tbs). Soy sauce on side not included in analysis.

✓ Calories: Good Choice (510) ✓✓ Cholesterol: Excellent Choice (65 mg)
✓ Fat: Good Choice (23 g)♥ Sodium: High (1375 mg)
Exchanges: 4½ Meat (extra lean), 1 Bread, 1¾ Veg, ½ Fruit, 4 Fat
Protein: 40 g, Carbohydrate: 38 g, Fiber: 5 g

Veggie Pizza (½ Pizza)

Mushrooms, artichoke, tomatoes, onions, and peppers. Analysis for one half pizza.

✓ Calories: Good Choice (690) ✓✓ Cholesterol: Excellent Choice (45 mg)
✓ Fat: Good Choice (18 g) Sodium: High (1595 mg)
Exchanges: 1½ Meat, 3¾ Bread, 4 Veg, 2¼ Fat
Protein: 54 g, Carbohydrate: 81 g, Fiber: 18 g

Spaghetti Marinara

Served with mushrooms and parmesan cheese.

✓ Calories: Good Choice (700) ✓✓ Cholesterol: Excellent Choice (15 mg)
Fat: Moderate (30 g) Sodium: Moderate (700 mg)**
Exchanges: ¼ Meat, 3¾ Bread, 4¼ Veg, 5 Fat
Protein: 20 g, Carbohydrate: 94 g, Fiber: 8 g

Plum Sauce *(2 Tbs.)*

Cal: 45, Fat: 1 g, Chol: 0, Sodium: 245 mg, Prot: 0, Carb: 9 g, Fiber: 0, Exch: ¼ Bread, ¼ Fruit, ¼ Fat

Thai Sauce *(2 Tbs.)*

Cal: 100, Fat: 6 g, Chol: 0, Sod: 830 mg, Prot: 4 g, Carb: 9 g, Fiber: 1 g, Exch: ¼ Meat, ¼ Br, ¼ Veg, 1 Fat

Curry Sauce *(2 Tbs.)*

Cal: 135, Fat: 12 g, Chol: 25 mg, Sodium: 285 mg, Protein: 1 g, Carb: 6 g, Fiber: 0, Exch: ¼ Fruit, 2½ Fat

** If you request no added salt
at least 2 fruit/vegetable servings

For more than a generation, families and friends have been coming to Old Spaghetti Factories, located across the United States, to enjoy our delicious food, charming atmosphere and friendly service. We invite you to dine amidst old world antiques, collected from around the world, while savoring perfectly cooked pasta and spaghetti sauces, freshly made using only the finest ingredients. $

The Old Spaghetti Factory

Newport Beach: 2110 Newport Blvd., Newport Beach, CA 92663 (949) 675-8654
Fullerton: 110 East Santa Fe Ave., Fullerton, CA 92832 (714) 526-6801
Riverside: 3191 Mission Inn Ave., Riverside, CA 92507 (909) 784-4417
Rancho Cucamonga: 11896 Foothill Blvd., Rancho Cucamonga, CA 91730 (909) 980-3585

Analyses below do not include bread, salad and ice cream served with the entrée.

SPAGHETTI WITH TOMATO SAUCE

Italians would say "Marinara."

✓✓ CALORIES: Excellent Choice (450) ✓✓ CHOLESTEROL: Excellent Choice (0 mg)
✓✓ FAT: Excellent Choice (6 g)♥ SODIUM: Moderate (820 mg)**
EXCHANGES: 5 Bread, 1¾ Veg, ¾ Fat
PROTEIN: 14 g, CARBOHYDRATE: 85 g, FIBER: 7 g

SPAGHETTI WITH MUSHROOM SAUCE

Fresh tender mushrooms, swimming in authentic Italian tomato sauce.

✓ CALORIES: Good Choice (455) ✓✓ CHOLESTEROL: Excellent Choice (0 mg)
✓✓ FAT: Excellent Choice (7 g)♥ SODIUM: Moderate (625 mg)**
EXCHANGES: 4¾ Bread, 1¾ Veg, 1 Fat
PROTEIN: 14 g, CARBOHYDRATE: 84 g, FIBER: 6 g

SPINACH & CHEESE RAVIOLI

Tender pillows of pasta stuffed with spinach and three kinds of cheese, topped with our savory tomato sauce.

✓✓ CALORIES: Excellent Choice (450) ✓✓ CHOLESTEROL: Excellent Choice (60 mg)
✓✓ FAT: Excellent Choice (13 g) SODIUM: Moderate (935 mg)**
EXCHANGES: 2 Meat, 3¾ Bread, 1 Veg, 2½ Fat
PROTEIN: 21 g, CARBOHYDRATE: 63 g, FIBER: 4 g

SPINACH TORTELLINI WITH MUSHROOM SAUCE – SPECIAL REQUEST

Hat shaped pasta, stuffed with a delicious blend of meat & cheese.
Request Mushroom Sauce instead of Alfredo Sauce.

✓ CALORIES: Good Choice (560) ✓✓ CHOLESTEROL: Excellent Choice (55 mg)
✓✓ FAT: Excellent Choice (14 g) SODIUM: High (1420 mg)
EXCHANGES: 1 Meat, 5¼ Bread, 1 Veg, 2 Fat
PROTEIN: 24 g, CARBOHYDRATE: 84 g, FIBER: 4 g

SPAGHETTI WITH RICH MEAT SAUCE

For purists – our recipe comes straight from Naples.

✓ CALORIES: Good Choice (505) ✓✓ CHOLESTEROL: Excellent Choice (25 mg)
✓✓ FAT: Excellent Choice (10 g) SODIUM: Moderate (955 mg)**
EXCHANGES: ¾ Meat, 5 Bread, 1¼ Veg, 1¼ Fat
PROTEIN: 19 g, CARBOHYDRATE: 83 g, FIBER: 6 g

HOUSE SALAD WITH HONEY MUSTARD FAT FREE DRESSING †

✓✓ CALORIES: Excellent Choice (50) ✓✓ CHOLESTEROL: Excellent Choice (0 mg)
✓✓ FAT: Excellent Choice (0 g)♥ ✓ SODIUM: Good Choice (170 mg)**
EXCHANGES: ½ Veg, ½ Fruit
PROTEIN: 1 g, CARBOHYDRATE: 11 g, FIBER: 1 g

♥ Primarily unsaturated fat
† Side dish guidelines are ⅓ of entrée guidelines

At Pane e Vino we have developed what we feel is the ultimate Italian dining experience. Our focus is providing you, as our valued guests, with delicious freshly prepared meals. We take pride in our prompt, professional staff, as well as our warm atmosphere and great location in the heart of Orange County. $$

Pane e Vino

240 S. Brea Blvd., Brea, CA 92821
(714) 256-7779   www.panevino.biz

CAPELLINI AL POMODORO FRESCO – SPECIAL REQUEST 🍎

Angel hair pasta, fresh tomatoes, basil, garlic, and extra virgin olive oil.
Request less oil (½ oz).

✓ CALORIES: Good Choice (480)   ✓✓ CHOLESTEROL: Excellent Choice (0 mg)
✓ FAT: Good Choice (16 g)♥   ✓✓ SODIUM: Excellent Choice (20 mg)**

EXCHANGES: 4 Bread, 1¼ Veg, 2¾ Fat
PROTEIN: 12 g, CARBOHYDRATE: 71 g, FIBER: 4 g

ZITI ALLA PUTANESCA – SPECIAL REQUEST

Short tube pasta, capers, pitted Kalamata olives, oregano, and tomato sauce.
Request less oil (½ oz.) and no butter.

✓ CALORIES: Good Choice (520)   ✓✓ CHOLESTEROL: Excellent Choice (10 mg)
✓ FAT: Good Choice (24 g)♥   SODIUM: High (1825 mg)

EXCHANGES: 3 Bread, ¼ Other Carb, 1 Veg, 4¼ Fat
PROTEIN: 12 g, CARBOHYDRATE: 64 g, FIBER: 5 g

PAILLARD DI POLLO CON RUCCOLA E ASIAGO - SPECIAL REQUEST

Charcoal grilled double breast of chicken, pounded thin, plenty of arrugula, and shaved Asiago cheese.
Request less oil (½ Tbs.) and vinaigrette on the side (vinaigrette not included in analysis).

✓ CALORIES: Good Choice (590)   CHOLESTEROL: Moderate (240 mg)
✓ FAT: Good Choice (24 g)   SODIUM: Moderate (830 mg)**

EXCHANGES: 12¼ Meat , ¼ Veg, 3 Fat
PROTEIN: 87 g, CARBOHYDRATE: 3 g, FIBER: 1 g

CARPACCIO†

Thin slices of raw beef, lemon juice, and mustard sauce.

✓✓ CALORIES: Excellent Choice (130)   ✓ CHOLESTEROL: Good Choice (30 mg)
FAT: Moderate (9 g)   ✓ SODIUM: Good Choice (190 mg)**

EXCHANGES: 1½ Meat (extra lean), 1½ Fat
PROTEIN: 12 g, CARBOHYDRATE: 1 g, FIBER: 0 g

MOZZARELLA E POMODORO – SPECIAL REQUEST†

Fresh mozzarella, tomatoes, basil, and cold pressed olive oil. Request less oil (½ Tbs.) and no added salt.

✓✓ CALORIES: Excellent Choice (100)   ✓✓ CHOLESTEROL: Excellent Choice (25 mg)
✓ FAT: Good Choice (8 g)   ✓✓ SODIUM: Excellent Choice (40 mg) **

EXCHANGES: ¾ Meat, ¼ Veg, ¼ Fat
PROTEIN: 5 g, CARBOHYDRATE: 1 g, FIBER: 0 g

† Side dish guidelines are ⅓ of entrée guidelines
🍎 at least 2 fruit/vegetable servings

Pascal Restaurant and Pascal Epicerie & Wine are proud to serve unique cuisine to our discerning clientele. Our menu is prepared with the freshest, best quality ingredients offered and cooked daily with care and professionalism on these premises. Remember, we are here to make your life easier and healthier. $$

Pascal Epicerie & Wine: 1000 Bristol Street, Newport Beach (949) 261-9041
Pascal Restaurant: 1000 Bristol Street, Newport Beach (949) 752-0107

AVAILABLE AT PASCAL EPICERIE & WINE

SALADE NICOISE – SPECIAL REQUEST

Butter lettuce, fresh albacore tuna, bell peppers and green beans.
Request dressing on the side (not included in analysis).

✓✓ CALORIES: Excellent Choice (325) CHOLESTEROL: Moderate (245 mg)
✓✓ FAT: Excellent Choice (8 g) ✓✓ SODIUM: Excellent Choice (265 mg)**
EXCHANGES: 4¾ Meat (extra lean), ¾ Bread, 2 Veg, 1 Fat
PROTEIN: 39 g, CARBOHYDRATE: 23 g, FIBER: 4 g

SPINACH CHICKEN SALAD – SPECIAL REQUEST

Chicken breast, baby spinach, roasted peppers and mushrooms.
Request dressing on the side (not included in analysis).

✓✓ CALORIES: Excellent Choice (230) ✓ CHOLESTEROL: Good Choice (95 mg)
✓✓ FAT: Excellent Choice (5 g) ✓✓ SODIUM: Excellent Choice (155 mg)**
EXCHANGES: 5 Meat (extra lean), 1½ Veg, ¼ Fat
PROTEIN: 39 g, CARBOHYDRATE: 8 g, FIBER: 4 g

SALMON SALAD – SPECIAL REQUEST

Mixed greens, poached salmon, asparagus and capers.
Request dressing on the side (not included in analysis).

✓✓ CALORIES: Excellent Choice (250) ✓ CHOLESTEROL: Good Choice (80 mg)
✓✓ FAT: Excellent Choice (9 g)♥ ✓✓ SODIUM: Excellent Choice (195 mg)**
EXCHANGES: 3¾ Meat, 1¾ Veg
PROTEIN: 32 g, CARBOHYDRATE: 9 g, FIBER: 4 g

AVAILABLE AT PASCAL RESTAURANT & OCCASIONALLY AT PASCAL EPICERIE & WINE

FREE RANGE CHICKEN BREAST PROVENCAL

Roasted breast of chicken served with olives, sweet garlic and tomatoes. Garnished with steamed asparagus.

✓ CALORIES: Good Choice (530) CHOLESTEROL: Moderate (180 mg)
✓ FAT: Good Choice (19 g) SODIUM: Moderate (840 mg)**
EXCHANGES: 9 Meat (extra lean), 1½ Veg, ¼ Other Carbs, 2¾ Fat
PROTEIN: 69 g, CARBOHYDRATE: 18 g, FIBER: 5 g

BRAISED SEABASS WITH THYME CRUST – SPECIAL REQUEST

Pascal's #1 specialty served with tomato concassé.
Request less butter (½ oz). Buerre blanc sauce not included in analysis.

✓ CALORIES: Good Choice (530) ✓ CHOLESTEROL: Good Choice (90 mg)
✓ FAT: Good Choice (22 g)♥ SODIUM: Moderate (610 mg)**
EXCHANGES: 3¾ Meat (extra lean), 2¼ Bread, 1¾ Veg, ¼ Other Carbs, 3 ½ Fat
PROTEIN: 34 g, CARBOHYDRATE: 48 g, FIBER: 6 g

♥ Primarily unsaturated fat
** If you request no added salt

Pat & Oscar's started out in San Diego over 10 years ago as a single take-out restaurant. Today our restaurants total 23, stretching throughout Southern California and into Arizona. And to think, we built it all on breadsticks! But we're also committed to serving other great foods like the ones listed below – in a clean, relaxed and friendly atmosphere. Please come by soon and see for yourself! $

Pat & Oscar's

Buena Park: 8386 La Palma Avenue (714) 484-9861
Irvine at the Marketplace: 13786 Jamboree Road, Suite A (714) 505-6070
Lake Forest: 26771 Rancho Parkway (949) 707-3900
Orange Town & Country: 763 S. Main Street (714) 836-5500

BARBEQUE CHICKEN PIZZA (2 SLICES)

BBQ chicken, red onions, cilantro & BBQ sauce. Analysis is for 2 slices (⅓ pizza).

✓✓ CALORIES: Excellent Choice (440) ✓✓ CHOLESTEROL: Excellent Choice (50 mg)
✓✓ FAT: Excellent Choice (14 g) SODIUM: Moderate (765 mg)**
EXCHANGES: 2 Meat, 3 Bread, ¼ Veg, ¼ Fruit, 1½ Fat
PROTEIN: 21 g, CARBOHYDRATE: 56 g, FIBER: 2 g

GOURMET VEGETARIAN PIZZA (2 SLICES)

Feta, broccoli, tomatoes, carrots, spinach & pesto. Analysis is for 2 slices (⅓ pizza).

✓ CALORIES: Good Choice (475) ✓✓ CHOLESTEROL: Excellent Choice (45 mg)
✓ FAT: Good Choice (20 g) SODIUM: Moderate (800 mg)**
EXCHANGES: 1¼ Meat, 3¼ Bread, ¾ Veg, 3 Fat
PROTEIN: 18 g, CARBOHYDRATE: 55 g, FIBER: 3 g

TURKEY POCKET SANDWICH

Roasted turkey breast with roma tomatoes and shredded lettuce on fresh homemade bread.

✓ CALORIES: Good Choice (645) ✓ CHOLESTEROL: Good Choice (130 mg)
✓✓ FAT: Excellent Choice (7 g) SODIUM: High (2530 mg)
EXCHANGES: 5½ Meat, 5¼ Bread, 1 Veg, 6¼ Fat
PROTEIN: 49 g, CARBOHYDRATE: 95 g, FIBER: 5 g

VEGGIE POCKET SANDWICH – SPECIAL REQUEST

Provolone cheese, mushrooms, red onions, green peppers, olives, roma tomatoes & shredded lettuce on fresh homemade bread. Request less cheese (1 oz. included in analysis) and fat-free dressing (not included in analysis).

✓ CALORIES: Good Choice (680) ✓✓ CHOLESTEROL: Excellent Choice (20 mg)
✓ FAT: Good Choice (23 g) SODIUM: High (1175 mg)
EXCHANGES: ¼ Meat, 6¼ Bread, 2¾ Veg, 3¼ Fat
PROTEIN: 23 g, CARBOHYDRATE: 101 g, FIBER: 9 g

GREEK SALAD – SPECIAL REQUEST

Tomatoes, olives, cucumbers, beets, red onions, feta cheese and peppers. Request fat-free dressing (not included in analysis).

✓✓ CALORIES: Excellent Choice (265) ✓✓ CHOLESTEROL: Excellent Choice (55 mg)
✓✓ FAT: Excellent Choice (15 g) SODIUM: Moderate (820 mg)**
EXCHANGES: 1¼ Meat, 2¾ Veg, 2 Fat
PROTEIN: 13 g, CARBOHYDRATE: 21 g, FIBER: 6 g

LEMON CHICKEN SANDWICH

Lemon marinated chicken with lemon seasoning, roma tomatoes and shredded lettuce on fresh homemade bread.

CALORIES: Moderate (820) ✓ CHOLESTEROL: Good Choice (145 mg)
✓ FAT: Good Choice (19 g) SODIUM: High (1455 mg)
EXCHANGES: 7½ Meat, 5½ Bread, 1½ Veg, 2¼ Fat
PROTEIN: 66 g, CARBOHYDRATE: 92 g, FIBER: 6 g

** If you request no added salt
at least 2 fruit/vegetable servings

Pick Up Stix takes the best traditional Asian food and adapts it to American tastes by reducing the oils and adding wine, vinegar and soy sauce to create a more flavorful dish. The food is prepared in an open-style kitchen, treating guests to a show of the art of Chinese cooking as they watch their meals wok'd fresh (cooked-to-order). Pick Up Stix continues to receive numerous awards for "Best Chinese Food," "Best Take Out" and "Best Chinese Restaurant" from the Orange County Register and other regional publications. $

Pick Up Stix has 23 Orange County locations. Please visit www.pickupstix.com for details.

CALIFORNIA ROLL *(2 pieces)*†

Made fresh throughout the day! With shaved ginger and Japanese wasabi mustard. Analysis is for 2 pieces.

✓✓ CALORIES: Excellent Choice (145) ✓✓ CHOLESTEROL: Excellent Choice (10 mg)
✓ FAT: Good Choice (8 g) SODIUM: Moderate (325 mg)
EXCHANGES: ½ Meat, ½ Bread, ¼ Veg, 1½ Fat
PROTEIN: 4 g, CARBOHYDRATE: 15 g, FIBER: <1 g

CHINESE CHICKEN SALAD

Oven roasted marinated white meat chicken over fresh greens, Mandarin oranges, sprinkled with sunflower and sesame seeds and topped with Chinese croutons.

✓ CALORIES: Good Choice (530) ✓ CHOLESTEROL: Good Choice (90 mg)
✓ FAT: Good Choice (16 g) SODIUM: High (1980 mg)
EXCHANGES: 4¾ Meat (extra lean), 1¾ Bread, 1½ Veg, ½ Fruit, 2 Fat
PROTEIN: 42 g, CARBOHYDRATE: 57 g, FIBER: 7 g

CHICKEN WITH VEGETABLES

Steamed white meat chicken with broccoli, carrots, zucchini, mushrooms and water chestnuts in a sauce of white wine, garlic and soy. Analysis does not include rice (see separate analysis below).

✓ CALORIES: Good Choice (650) CHOLESTEROL: Moderate (165 mg)
✓✓ FAT: Excellent Choice (10 g) SODIUM: High (1770 mg)
EXCHANGES: 8¾ Meat (extra lean), 2¼ Bread, 5¼ Veg, ¾ Fat
PROTEIN: 68 g, CARBOHYDRATE: 69 g, FIBER: 7 g

SZECHWAN CHICKEN

Chicken in a blend of seared red chili peppers mixed with green and white onions, carrots and celery. Analysis does not include rice (see separate analysis below).

✓ CALORIES: Good Choice (590) CHOLESTEROL: Moderate (165 mg)
✓✓ FAT: Excellent Choice (10 g) SODIUM: High (2210 mg)
EXCHANGES: 8¾ Meat (extra lean), 1¼ Bread, 4 Veg, ¾ Fat
PROTEIN: 67 g, CARBOHYDRATE: 56 g, FIBER: 8 g

SZECHWAN SHRIMP – SPECIAL REQUEST

Shrimp in a blend of seared red chili peppers mixed with green and white onions, carrots and celery. Request shrimp steamed with no oil. Analysis does not include rice (see separate analysis below).

✓ CALORIES: Good Choice (555) CHOLESTEROL: High (340 mg)
✓✓ FAT: Excellent Choice (15 g)♥ SODIUM: High (2340 mg)
EXCHANGES: 5½ Meat, 1¾ Bread, 4 Veg, 2¾ Fat
PROTEIN: 44 g, CARBOHYDRATE: 60 g, FIBER: 9 g

BUDDHA'S FEAST

Analysis does not include rice (see separate analysis below).

✓✓ CALORIES: Excellent Choice (370) ✓✓ CHOLESTEROL: Excellent Choice (5 mg)
✓✓ FAT: Excellent Choice (1 g)♥ SODIUM: High (1645 mg)
EXCHANGES: ¼ Meat, 2 Bread, 7¾ Veg, ¼ Fat
PROTEIN: 11 g, CARBOHYDRATE: 80 g, FIBER: 10 g

RICE *(6 oz.)* CAL: 220, FAT: ½ g♥, CHOL: 0, SOD: <5 mg; EXCH: 3¼ Bread; PROTEIN: 5 g, CARB: 48 g, FIBER: 1 g

♥ Primarily unsaturated fat

Red Rock Chili mania focuses very simply on a bowl of chili. It is a craving, a passion, an obsession for a simmered combination of meat and chile peppers whose distinctive aroma makes an indelible imprint on the senses. Even the words "Red Rock Chili" are exciting to a chili lover, for it evokes the memories of a dish that warms the heart and embraces the body in an aura of sensuous satisfaction. Red Rock Chili is the ambrosia of modern man. Please visit us in person and at www.redrockchili.com $

Red Rock Chili Co.

401 Newport Center Dr. A106 (Fashion Island), Newport Beach, CA 92660 (949) 760-0752

REGULAR RED ROCK CHILI *(8 oz.)*

✓✓ CALORIES: Excellent Choice (220) ✓✓ CHOLESTEROL: Excellent Choice (40 mg)
✓✓ FAT: Excellent Choice (12 g) SODIUM: Moderate (740 mg)
EXCHANGES: 1¼ Meat, ½ Bread, 1 Veg, 1¼ Fat
PROTEIN: 13 g, CARBOHYDRATE: 16 g, FIBER: 5 g

HOT ROCK CHILI *(8 oz.)* 🍎

✓✓ CALORIES: Excellent Choice (185) ✓✓ CHOLESTEROL: Excellent Choice (25 mg)
✓✓ FAT: Excellent Choice (8 g) SODIUM: Moderate (840 mg)
EXCHANGES: ¾ Meat, ½ Bread, 1¾ Veg, 1 Fat
PROTEIN: 10 g, CARBOHYDRATE: 17 g, FIBER: 5 g

WHITE ROCK CHILI *(8 oz.)*

✓✓ CALORIES: Excellent Choice (150) ✓✓ CHOLESTEROL: Excellent Choice (20 mg)
✓✓ FAT: Excellent Choice (2 g) ✓ SODIUM: Good Choice (445 mg)
EXCHANGES: 1½ Meat (extra lean), ½ Bread, 1¼ Veg
PROTEIN: 12 g, CARBOHYDRATE: 23 g, FIBER: 5 g

TOFU VEGGIE CHILI *(8 oz.)*

✓✓ CALORIES: Excellent Choice (150) ✓✓ CHOLESTEROL: Excellent Choice (0 mg)
✓✓ FAT: Excellent Choice (4 g)♥ ✓ SODIUM: Good Choice (480 mg)
EXCHANGES: ½ Meat, ¾ Bread, ¾ Veg, ½ Fat
PROTEIN: 9 g, CARBOHYDRATE: 22 g, FIBER: 5 g

CHICKEN SOUP *(8 oz.)*

✓✓ CALORIES: Excellent Choice (150) ✓✓ CHOLESTEROL: Excellent Choice (50 mg)
✓✓ FAT: Excellent Choice (2 g) ✓ SODIUM: Good Choice (485 mg)
EXCHANGES: 2½ Meat (extra lean), ¾ Bread, ¼ Veg
PROTEIN: 19 g, CARBOHYDRATE: 12 g, FIBER: 1 g

LENTIL SOUP *(8 oz.)*

✓✓ CALORIES: Excellent Choice (125) ✓✓ CHOLESTEROL: Excellent Choice (<1 mg)
✓✓ FAT: Excellent Choice (<1 g) ✓ SODIUM: Good Choice (455 mg)
EXCHANGES: ½ Meat (extra lean), 1¼ Bread, ½ Veg
PROTEIN: 9 g, CARBOHYDRATE: 23 g, FIBER: 1 g

VEGETARIAN SOUP *(8 oz.)*

A great blend of fresh veggies, cooked and flavored to perfection!

✓✓ CALORIES: Excellent Choice (50) ✓✓ CHOLESTEROL: Excellent Choice (0 mg)
✓✓ FAT: Excellent Choice (1 g)♥ ✓ SODIUM: Good Choice (515 mg)
EXCHANGES: ½ Bread, ¾ Veg
PROTEIN: 2 g, CARBOHYDRATE: 11 g, FIBER: 1

🍎 at least 2 fruit/vegetable servings
♥ Primarily unsaturated fat

We offer pizzas with a variety of sauces, a blend of whole milk mozzarella, cheddar and provolone cheeses, superior meats, fresh vegetables, and dough rolled fresh daily in our restaurants. There are many locations in Orange County for your convenience. For more information, please visit our website: www.roundtablepizza.com. $

Participating Round Table Pizza locations in Orange County:

Costa Mesa: 204 East 17th St. #102	(949) 722-8888	Lake Forest: 22722 Lambert St. #1705	(949) 859-8888
Costa Mesa: 1175 Baker St. #A	(714) 549-2101	Lakewood: 5250 Faculty Avenue	(562) 408-1914
Dana Point: 32525B Golden Lantern	(949) 496-9800	Long Beach: CSULB Student Union	(562) 494-1194
Fountain Valley: 11095 Warner Ave.	(714) 839-0276	Mission Viejo: 25290 Marguerite Pk. #D	(949) 951-3403
Huntington Beach: 19750 Beach Bl.	(714) 963-9877	Newport Beach: 4551 Jamboree Rd. #B	(949) 261-2222
Irvine: 3851 Alton Parkway	(949) 476-3030	San Clemente: 612 Camino de los Mares	(949) 496-7701
Irvine: 3953 Irvine Blvd.	(714) 508-9800		

Analyses below are for thin crust pizza; pan crust adds approx. ½ g fat & 50 calories per slice.

GUINEVERE'S GARDEN DELIGHT® PIZZA (2 SLICES)

Our classic red sauce, three cheeses, mushrooms, black olives, Roma tomatoes, yellow onions, and green peppers. Analysis for 2 slices large pizza.

✓✓ CALORIES: Excellent Choice (420) ✓✓ CHOLESTEROL: Excellent Choice (40 mg)
✓✓ FAT: Excellent Choice (14 g) SODIUM: High (1100 mg)
PROTEIN: 18 g, CARBOHYDRATE: 50 g, FIBER: 4 g

GOURMET VEGGIE™ PIZZA (2 SLICES)

Creamy garlic sauce, three cheeses, artichoke hearts, zucchini, spinach, mushrooms, Roma tomatoes, red & green onions, Italian herb seasoning & lots of chopped garlic. Analysis for 2 slices large pizza.

✓✓ CALORIES: Excellent Choice (440) ✓✓ CHOLESTEROL: Excellent Choice (40 mg)
✓ FAT: Good Choice (18 g) SODIUM: Moderate (960 mg)
PROTEIN: 18 g, CARBOHYDRATE: 50 g, FIBER: 4 g

CHICKEN & GARLIC GOURMET™ PIZZA (2 SLICES)

Creamy garlic sauce, three cheeses, roasted chicken, mushrooms, Roma tomatoes, red & green onions, Italian herb seasoning & lots of chopped garlic. Analysis for 2 slices large pizza.

✓ CALORIES: Good Choice (460) ✓✓ CHOLESTEROL: Excellent Choice (60 mg)
✓ FAT: Good Choice (18 g) SODIUM: High (1180 mg)
PROTEIN: 22 g, CARBOHYDRATE: 48 g, FIBER: 2 g

HAWAIIAN PIZZA (2 SLICES)

Tender slices of ham and juicy pineapple tidbits. Baked with a blend of 3 cheeses on our zesty red sauce. Analysis for 2 slices large pizza.

✓✓ CALORIES: Excellent Choice (420) ✓✓ CHOLESTEROL: Excellent Choice (50 mg)
✓✓ FAT: Excellent Choice (14 g) SODIUM: High (1240 mg)
PROTEIN: 20 g, CARBOHYDRATE: 50 g, FIBER: 2 g

Nutrition information supplied by Round Table Pizza

Royal Khyber features the finest in Indian cuisine, which is universally known for its distinctive flavorings. It was the lure of spices that brought explorers to the Indian coast, and it is the use of selected spices to bring out the flavors of dishes that is the special art practiced at Royal Khyber. Tandoori oven cooking is also recognized for its flavorful and healthy cuisine, where meats, poultry or fish is skinned and defatted and marinated for hours in home-made yogurt, ginger, garlic paste and delicate blend of spices, then cooked in the imported clay oven at 450 F degrees-plus temperature, fired with mesquite charcoals. The intimate atmosphere and spectacularly presented dishes at Royal Khyber create an ultimate dining experience. $$-$$$

Royal Khyber (714) 436-1010

South Coast Village Plaza, 1621 W. Sunflower Ave. Ste. D-53, Santa Ana, CA 92704

Analyses for all items below is for ½ order, since they are usually shared.

TANDOORI CHICKEN (½ ORDER)

Marinated in homemade yogurt, with a blend of flavorful spices, then cooked in a traditional Tandoori clay oven.

✓✓ CALORIES: Excellent Choice (245) ✓ CHOLESTEROL: Good Choice (115 mg)
✓✓ FAT: Excellent Choice (8 g) ✓ SODIUM: Good Choice (450 mg)**
EXCHANGES: 5¼ Meat
PROTEIN: 38 g, CARBOHYDRATE: 2 g, FIBER: 0 g

TANDOORI FISH TIKKA (½ ORDER)

Marinated in homemade yogurt, with a blend of flavorful spices, then cooked in a traditional Tandoori clay oven.

✓✓ CALORIES: Excellent Choice (190) ✓✓ CHOLESTEROL: Excellent Choice (60 mg)
✓✓ FAT: Excellent Choice (6 g)♥ SODIUM: Moderate (770 mg)**
EXCHANGES: 4¼ Meat
PROTEIN: 30 g, CARBOHYDRATE: 2 g, FIBER: 0 g

KARAHI CHICKEN (½ ORDER)

Chicken breast with a light Karahi sauce of garlic, tomatoes, olive oil and herbs.

✓✓ CALORIES: Excellent Choice (235) ✓ CHOLESTEROL: Good Choice (100 mg)
✓✓ FAT: Excellent Choice (6 g) ✓✓ SODIUM: Excellent Choice (170 mg)**
EXCHANGES: 5¼ Meat, ½ Veg, ¼ Fat
PROTEIN: 38 g, CARBOHYDRATE: 4 g, FIBER: 1 g

CURRIED SEAFOOD (½ ORDER)

Prawns, scallops, fish, mussels & lobster tail in a light Karahi sauce cooked with white wine.

✓✓ CALORIES: Excellent Choice (270) CHOLESTEROL: Moderate (170 mg)
✓✓ FAT: Excellent Choice (8 g)♥ ✓ SODIUM: Good Choice (550 mg)**
EXCHANGES: 4 Meat, ¼ Veg, 1 Fat
PROTEIN: 37 g, CARBOHYDRATE: 6 g, FIBER: 1 g

FISH MALABAR (½ ORDER)

Fresh fish cooked with mustard fennel infused tomato sauce. Rice pilaf and naan not included in analysis.

✓✓ CALORIES: Excellent Choice (230) ✓✓ CHOLESTEROL: Excellent Choice (65 mg)
✓✓ FAT: Excellent Choice (12 g)♥ ✓✓ SODIUM: Excellent Choice (170 mg)**
EXCHANGES: 3 Meat, ¼ Veg, ¾ Fat
PROTEIN: 25 g, CARBOHYDRATE: 3 g, FIBER: 1 g

EGGPLANT BHARTHA (½ ORDER) - SPECIAL REQUEST 🍎

Charbroiled eggplant cooked with tomatoes and onion. Request no ghee.

✓✓ CALORIES: Excellent Choice (220) ✓✓ CHOLESTEROL: Excellent Choice (0 mg)
✓✓ FAT: Excellent Choice (15 g)♥ ✓ SODIUM: Good Choice (350 mg)**
EXCHANGES: 3¾ Veg, 2¾ Fat
PROTEIN: 3 g, CARBOHYDRATE: 23 g, FIBER: 3 g

🍎 at least 2 fruit/vegetable servings for entrees

Ruby's Diner with 14 Orange County locations to serve you!

The Original, #1 Balboa Pier	(949) 675-7829
2305 E. Coast Hwy., Corona del Mar	(949) 673-7829
3333 Bear St., Costa Mesa	(714) 662-7829
1301 S. Harbor Blvd., Fullerton	(714) 871-7829
Huntington Beach Pier, Huntington Beach	(714) 969-7829
4602 Barranca Pkwy., Irvine	(949) 552-7829
30622 S. Coast Hwy., Laguna Beach	(949) 497-7829
24155 Laguna Hills Mall, Laguna Hills	(949) 588-7829
27000 Mission Viejo Mall, Mission Viejo	(949) 481-7829
22411 Antonio Pkwy. #C170, R. Santa Margarita	(949) 713-7829
31781 Camino Capistrano, San Juan Capistrano	(949) 496-7829
Seal Beach Municipal Pier, Seal Beach	(562) 431-7829
13102 Newport Ave., Tustin	(714) 838-7829
21450 Yorba Linda Blvd., Yorba Linda	(714) 779-7829

For locations outside Orange County, call 1-800 HEY RUBY or visit our website at www.rubys.com.

Ruby's Diner is the authentic 1940's diner! Step back in time to 40's memorabilia, gleaming red and white interiors and friendly, courteous service. Ruby's offers items to please every palate, including a variety of salads, sandwiches, and home style breakfasts. Swing into Ruby's today and experience great food and great service with a 40's flair. $

ROAST TURKEY BREAST SANDWICH – SPECIAL REQUEST

With lettuce and cranberry sauce on a soft RubyRoll. Just like Thanksgiving!
Request no margarine or mayonnaise.

✓ CALORIES: Good Choice (600) ✓ CHOLESTEROL: Good Choice (120 mg)
✓✓ FAT: Excellent Choice (7 g) SODIUM: Moderate (610 mg)**
EXCHANGES: 6¼ Meat, 3¾ Bread, 1½ Fruit, 1¼ Fat
PROTEIN: 52 g, CARBOHYDRATE: 80 g, FIBER: 3 g

CHICKEN RUBYBURGER – SPECIAL REQUEST

With a tender boneless, skinless chicken breast. Request no margarine or mayonnaise.

✓ CALORIES: Good Choice (485) ✓ CHOLESTEROL: Good Choice (130 mg)
✓✓ FAT: Excellent Choice (10 g) SODIUM: Moderate (950 mg)**
EXCHANGES: 6¾ Meat, 2½ Bread, ¾ Fat
PROTEIN: 55 g, CARBOHYDRATE: 41 g, FIBER: 1 g

TURKEY RUBYBURGER – SPECIAL REQUEST

With a full ⅓ lb. of lean ground turkey. Request no margarine or Ruby sauce.

✓ CALORIES: Good Choice (490) ✓ CHOLESTEROL: Good Choice (145 mg)
✓ FAT: Good Choice (19 g)♥ ✓ SODIUM: Good Choice (485 mg)**
EXCHANGES: 4 Meat, 2¾ Bread, 1½ Fat
PROTEIN: 35 g, CARBOHYDRATE: 43 g, FIBER: 1 g

VEGGIE RUBYBURGER – SPECIAL REQUEST

With a tasty vegetable, rice, oats and wheat Garden Burger patty. Request no margarine or mayonnaise.

✓ CALORIES: Good Choice (500) ✓✓ CHOLESTEROL: Excellent Choice (5 mg)
✓✓ FAT: Excellent Choice (9 g)♥ SODIUM: High (1085 mg)
EXCHANGES: ¼ Meat, 5½ Bread, ¾ Veg, 1¼ Fat
PROTEIN: 19 g, CARBOHYDRATE: 85 g, FIBER: 8 g

VEGGIE SOFT TACOS – SPECIAL REQUEST

Two whole wheat tortillas filled with fresh lettuce, cheese, vegetarian black beans, olives and salsa.
Dressing not included in analysis. Request less cheese (½ oz.) and salsa as dressing.

✓ CALORIES: Good Choice (495) ✓✓ CHOLESTEROL: Excellent Choice (15 mg)
✓ FAT: Good Choice (16 g) SODIUM: High (1375 mg)
EXCHANGES: ½ Meat, 3¾ Bread, 1¼ Veg, 3¼ Fat
PROTEIN: 13 g, CARBOHYDRATE: 66 g, FIBER: 8 g

♥ Primarily unsaturated fat
** If you request no added salt

Winner of San Diego's Best Pizza Award 1989 – 2000 and 2002. Serving gourmet woodfired pizza, heaping salads, fresh pastas, and specialty entrees in a lovely garden atmosphere, Sammy's is known for its imaginative combinations, generous portions, reasonable prices, and exemplary service. Local favorites include Garlic Chicken and New York Style pizzas, Shrimp Angel Hair Pasta and Grilled Chicken Salad. Come enjoy the best! $

Sammy's Woodfired Pizza

18315 Brookhurst Street, Fountain Valley, CA 92708 (714) 593-5800

HEALTHY DINING VEGETARIAN PIZZA (½ PIZZA)

Grilled eggplant, onions, bell peppers, fontina, garlic, zucchini and Roma tomatoes with fat-free mozzarella. Analysis is for ½ of a pizza.

CALORIES: Moderate (885) — ✓✓ CHOLESTEROL: Excellent Choice (20 mg)
✓ FAT: Good Choice (21 g)♥ — SODIUM: High (2110 mg)
EXCHANGES: 2¾ Meat, 7¾ Bread, 1¼ Veg, 3½ Fat
PROTEIN: 38 g, CARBOHYDRATE: 130 g, FIBER: 4 g

HEALTHY DINING TOMATO ANGEL HAIR PASTA

Roma tomatoes, fresh basil and garlic.

✓ CALORIES: Good Choice (650) — ✓✓ CHOLESTEROL: Excellent Choice (15 mg)
✓ FAT: Good Choice (18 g)♥ — ✓✓ SODIUM: Excellent Choice (65 mg)**
EXCHANGES: 5¾ Bread, 2 Veg, 2¾ Fat
PROTEIN: 22 g, CARBOHYDRATE: 105 g, FIBER: 3 g

HEALTHY DINING GRILLED VEGETABLE PENNE

Seasonal grilled vegetables with spinach, olive oil, balsamic vinegar and Romano cheese.

✓ CALORIES: Good Choice (610) — ✓✓ CHOLESTEROL: Excellent Choice (30 mg)
✓ FAT: Good Choice (21 g)♥ — SODIUM: Moderate (685 mg)**
EXCHANGES: 1 Meat, 4¼ Bread, 2 Veg, 3½ Fat
PROTEIN: 24 g, CARBOHYDRATE: 84 g, FIBER: 3 g

HEALTHY DINING CHINESE CHICKEN SALAD

Individual size salad with Chinese greens, bell peppers, sesame seeds, cilantro, scallions, Mandarin oranges and fat-free Oriental dressing.

✓ CALORIES: Good Choice (480) — ✓ CHOLESTEROL: Good Choice (85 mg)
✓✓ FAT: Excellent Choice (13 g) — SODIUM: High (2455 mg)
EXCHANGES: 4½ Meat (extra lean), ½ Bread, 3½ Veg, ¾ Fruit, ¾ Fat
PROTEIN: 42 g, CARBOHYDRATE: 49 g, FIBER: 1 g

HEALTHY DINING CHOPPED CHICKEN SALAD

Individual size salad with chicken breast, lettuce, tomatoes, olives, fat-free mozzarella, basil and fat-free dressing.

✓✓ CALORIES: Excellent Choice (395) — ✓ CHOLESTEROL: Good Choice (90 mg)
✓✓ FAT: Excellent Choice (11 g) — SODIUM: High (3130 mg)
EXCHANGES: 6¾ Meat (extra lean), 1¼ Veg, ¼ Fruit, 1¼ Fat
PROTEIN: 52 g, CARBOHYDRATE: 20 g, FIBER: 1 g

(apple symbol) at least 2 fruit/vegetable servings
** If you request no added salt

SANTA MONICA SEAFOOD

After 60 years in the seafood business, Santa Monica Seafood takes enormous pride in being regarded as Southern California's #1 seafood retailer. Santa Monica Seafood offers oceans of fresh seafood daily, over 30 varieties from all over the world. This guarantees our customers will get the best and freshest of the catch. Santa Monica Seafood also offers fresh produce, fine wines, imported beers, fresh pasta, imported and domestic cheeses, gourmet condiments and fresh bread. Santa Monica Seafood's concern for quality and service to their customers makes visiting this store a truly pleasant experience. $

Santa Monica Seafood

154 East 17th St., Costa Mesa, CA 92627 (949) 574-8862
1700 North Main St., Orange, CA 92865 (714) 921-2632
1205 Colorado Ave., Santa Monica, CA 90404 (310) 393-5244
Visit us on the web at www.santamonicaseafood.com

HAWAIIAN TUNA POKI

Fresh Hawaiian tuna marinated and served with sesame seeds, daikon sprouts and green onions.

✓✓ CALORIES: Excellent Choice (290) ✓✓ CHOLESTEROL: Excellent Choice (75 mg)
✓✓ FAT: Excellent Choice (10 g)♥ SODIUM: Moderate (655 mg)**
EXCHANGES: 5½ Meat (extra lean), 1 Veg, 1¼ Fat
PROTEIN: 42 g, CARBOHYDRATE: 6 g, FIBER: 2 g

GRILLED ALASKAN HALIBUT – SPECIAL REQUEST 🍎

with basil marinated tomatoes and a light herb salad. *Request half portion of marinated tomatoes (3½ oz).*

✓✓ CALORIES: Excellent Choice (370) ✓✓ CHOLESTEROL: Excellent Choice (65 mg)
✓ FAT: Good Choice (18 g)♥ ✓✓ SODIUM: Excellent Choice (235 mg)**
EXCHANGES: 4 Meat (extra lean), 1 Veg, 2¾ Fat
PROTEIN: 43 g, CARBOHYDRATE: 7 g, FIBER: 2 g

SUSHI ROLL COMBINATION

Includes tuna roll, cucumber roll, salmon roll and California roll.

✓✓ CALORIES: Excellent Choice (405) ✓✓ CHOLESTEROL: Excellent Choice (55 mg)
✓✓ FAT: Excellent Choice (5 g)♥ ✓✓ SODIUM: Excellent Choice (125 mg)**
EXCHANGES: 2 Meat (extra lean), 4¼ Bread, ½ Veg, ½ Fat
PROTEIN: 22 g, CARBOHYDRATE: 63 g, FIBER: 4 g

CEVICHE *(8 oz.)*†

Fresh fish, onion, tomato and carrots, marinated in lime juice and spices.

✓✓ CALORIES: Excellent Choice (105) ✓✓ CHOLESTEROL: Excellent Choice (20 mg)
✓✓ FAT: Excellent Choice (1 g)♥ SODIUM: Moderate (245 mg)
EXCHANGES: 1½ Meat (extra lean), ¼ Veg, ¼ Fruit
PROTEIN: 17 g, CARBOHYDRATE: 8 g, FIBER: 1 g

MANHATTAN CHOWDER *(8 oz.)* † 🍎

Clams with lots of vegetables and spices!

✓✓ CALORIES: Excellent Choice (70) ✓✓ CHOLESTEROL: Excellent Choice (10 mg)
✓✓ FAT: Excellent Choice (1 g)♥ SODIUM: High (700 mg)
EXCHANGES: ¾ Meat (extra lean), 1 Veg
PROTEIN: 7 g, CARBOHYDRATE: 11 g, FIBER: 2 g

🍎 at least 2 fruit/vegetable servings, 1 for side dishes
† Side dish guidelines are ⅓ of entrée guidelines

Souplantation is the biggest, the best, the PREMIER, salad experience restaurant. All of our soups, chilis, muffins, and prepared salads are made from scratch. We serve fresh, healthful and wholesome food, which is perfect for everyday family dining. At Souplantation, there's LOTS TO FEEL GOOD ABOUT! Complete nutrition information available at www.souplantation.com. $

Souplantation Locations:

Brea: 555 Pointe Dr. Bldg. #2	(714) 990-4773	Garden Grove: 5939 W. Chapman Ave.	(714) 895-1314
Costa Mesa: 1555 Adams Ave.	(714) 556-1903	Irvine: 2825 Main St.	(949) 474-8682
Fountain Valley: 11179 Talbert	(714) 434-1814	Laguna Niguel: 23870 Aliso Creek Rd.	(949) 831-6055
Fullerton: 1901 W. Malvern Ave.	(714) 446-0566	Tustin: 13681 Newport Ave. #1	(714) 730-5443

Foothill Ranch/Lake Forest: 26572 Towne Centre Dr. (949) 472-1044

FRESH TOSSED SALADS (1 CUP)†

California Cobb, Won Ton Chicken Happiness, Strawberry Fields with Caramelized Walnuts, Watercress & Orange.

✓ CALORIES: Good Choice (130 to 180) ✓✓ CHOLESTEROL: Excellent Choice (10 to 25 mg)
✓ FAT: Good Choice (4 to 8 g), some♥ SODIUM: Strawberry Fields (75 mg), others (190-220)
PROTEIN: 3 to 6 g, CARBOHYDRATE: 4 to 15 g, FIBER: 2 to 3 g

SIGNATURE PREPARED SALADS (½ CUP)†

Carrot Raisin, German Potato, Southern Dill Potato, Summer Barley with Black Beans, Mandarin Noodle with Broccoli, Mandarin Shells with Almonds, Marinated Summer Vegetables, Moroccan Marinated Vegetable, Oriental Ginger Slaw, Spicy Southwestern Pasta.

✓✓ CALORIES: Excellent Choice (70 to 130) ✓✓ CHOLESTEROL: Excellent Choice (0 to 5 mg)
✓✓ FAT: Excellent Choice (3 g) ♥ SODIUM: Carrot Raisin 80 mg; others 280 to 380 mg
PROTEIN: 2 to 5 g, CARBOHYDRATE: 8 to 21 g, Fiber: 2 to 4 g

SOUPS & CHILI (1 CUP)†

Soups: Big Chunk Chicken Noodle, French Onion, Garden Fresh Veg., Hungarian Veg., Living on the Veg., Old Fashioned Veg., Spicy 4 Bean Minestrone, Sweet Tomato Onion, Tomato Parmesan & Veg., Veg. Medley, Vegetarian, Veg. Lentils & Brown Rice, Veggie Jackson. Chilis: 3 Bean Turkey, Deep Kettle House, Santa Fe Black Bean.

✓ CALORIES: Good Choice (80 to 160, House Ch. 230) ✓✓ CHOLESTEROL: Excellent Choice (0 to 20 mg)
✓✓ FAT: Excellent Choice (1 to 3 g), some ♥ SODIUM: High (460 to 990 mg)
PROTEIN: 2 to 15 g, CARBOHYDRATE: 11 to 26 g, Fiber: 1 to 7 g

FRESH BAKED MUFFINS & BREADS †

Muffins: Apple Cinnamon Bran, Cranberry Orange Bran, Fruit Medley Bran, Buttermilk Corn Bread; Breads (1 piece): Big Hearth Focaccia, Garlic Parmesan Focaccia, Sourdough Bread.

✓✓ CALORIES: Excellent Choice (80 to 150) ✓✓ CHOLESTEROL: Excellent Choice (0 to 10 mg)
✓✓ FAT: Excellent Choice (½ to 3 g) ♥ SODIUM: Muffins and Focaccia (110-170 mg)
Corn Bread, Sourdough (240-270 mg)
PROTEIN: 2 to 9 g, CARBOHYDRATE: 15 to 27 g, FIBER: 0 to 2 g

DESSERTS & YOGURT BAR (½ CUP)†

Banana Royale, Butterscotch Pudding, Nutty Waldorf Salad, Apple Medley, Ghirardelli Chocolate Frozen Yogurt, Tapioca or Rice Pudding.

✓✓ CALORIES: Excellent Choice (70 to 140) ✓✓ CHOLESTEROL: Excellent Choice (0 to 20 mg)
✓✓ FAT: Excellent Choice (0 to 4 g) SODIUM: (5 to 80 mg); Tapioca (160 mg)
PROTEIN: 1 to 4 g, CARBOHYDRATE: 12 to 24 g, Fiber: 0 to 3 g

Nutrition information supplied by Souplantation.

† Side dish guidelines are ⅓ of entree guidelines

the sundried tomato
cafe and catering company

The Sundried Tomato staff is pleased to welcome you to our cafe. We have had a café and catering business for over ten years and are very excited to share our creative California cuisine with you. Some of our favorite things in life are brie, fresh herbs, rack of lamb, and a big red. The best is sharing with family and friends, which is what we hope you are about to do. So let your server guide you through a culinary experience, sample our food and our wines, and share in our enthusiasm. $$-$$$

The Sundried Tomato

Laguna Beach: 361 Forest Avenue (949) 494-3312
San Juan Capistrano: 31781 Camino Capistrano (949) 661-1167

PAN SEARED SALMON 🍎

Pan seared salmon topped with cucumber and sesame laced salsa over pan seared vegetables. Rice not included in analysis.

✓ CALORIES: Good Choice (460) ✓ CHOLESTEROL: Good Choice (125 mg)
✓FAT: Good Choice (25 g)♥ ✓ SODIUM: Good Choice (445 mg)**
EXCHANGES: 6 Meat, 1¾ Veg, 2 Fat
PROTEIN: 50 g, CARBOHYDRATE: 9 g, FIBER: 5 g

TERIYAKI CHICKEN BREAST SANDWICH

Teriyaki chicken with provolone cheese garnished with fresh fruit and served with salad of the day (salad not included in analysis).

✓ CALORIES: Good Choice (655) ✓ CHOLESTEROL: Good Choice (115 mg)
✓✓ FAT: Excellent Choice (15 g) ✓✓ SODIUM: High (4880 mg)
EXCHANGES: 6 Meat, 3⅓ Bread, ¼ Fruit, 1 Other Carbs, 1¼ Fat
PROTEIN: 55 g, CARBOHYDRATE: 74 g, FIBER: 3 g

CAJUN CHICKEN BREAST SANDWICH

Cajun chicken sandwich with pears, pasilla pepper, goat cheese and aoli sauce, garnished with fresh fruit and served with salad of the day (salad not included in analysis).

✓ CALORIES: Good Choice (660) ✓ CHOLESTEROL: Good Choice (125 mg)
✓ FAT: Good Choice (20 g) SODIUM: Moderate (950 mg)**
EXCHANGES: 6½ Meat, 3½ Bread, ½ Fruit, 2½ Fat
PROTEIN: 56 g, CARBOHYDRATE: 63 g, FIBER: 5 g

ZITI PASTA

Roma tomatoes, capers, basil and garlic tossed with olive oil over ziti pasta.

✓ CALORIES: Good Choice (565) ✓✓ CHOLESTEROL: Excellent Choice (0 mg)
✓ FAT: Good Choice (16 g)♥ SODIUM: High (1095 mg)
EXCHANGES: 5 Bread, ½ Veg, ¼ Other Carbs, 2¾ Fat
PROTEIN: 15 g, CARBOHYDRATE: 88 g, FIBER: 5 g

♥ Primarily unsaturated
** If you request no added salt

Susan's Healthy Gourmet
fresh · delicious · delivered

Susan's Healthy Gourmet is a one-of-a-kind service that provides delicious, fresh meals for the home that free you of shopping, cooking and clean up. Award winning bakery goods made from scratch and extensive a la carte selections supplement a complete weekly menu of low-fat, low-sodium, and low-cholesterol items offered in three daily calorie levels. All meals are prepared for pick-up or delivery every Monday and Friday. $

Susan's Healthy Gourmet - Meals for the Home and Office

For information & to order call: (949) 833-2929, 1-888-EZ-MEALS (396-3257)
17851 Sky Park Circle, Suite G, Irvine, CA 92614 www.susanshealthygourmet.com

MOM'S POT ROAST ♁

An old-fashioned supper served with garlic mashed potatoes, gravy, green beans and fresh corn.

✓✓ CALORIES: Excellent Choice (370) ✓✓ CHOLESTEROL: Excellent Choice (55 mg)
✓✓ FAT: Excellent Choice (6 g) ✓ SODIUM: Good Choice (370 mg)
EXCHANGES: 3 Meat, 1½ Bread, 2¾ Veg, ¾ Fat
PROTEIN: 31 g, CARBOHYDRATE: 51 g, FIBER: 7 g

TRADITIONAL TURKEY DINNER ♁

Roasted turkey with gravy, herb stuffing, roasted sweet potatoes, cranberry sauce, acorn squash and cabbage.

✓✓ CALORIES: Excellent Choice (400) ✓✓ CHOLESTEROL: Excellent Choice (70 mg)
✓✓ FAT: Excellent Choice (4 g) ✓✓ SODIUM: Excellent Choice (285 mg)
EXCHANGES: 3¾ Meat (extra lean), ½ Bread, 3 Veg, ¾ Fruit
PROTEIN: 32 g, CARBOHYDRATE: 58 g, FIBER: 6 g

SALMON WITH RED PEPPER PESTO ♁

Citrus pineapple marinated salmon with roasted red-pepper pesto on a bed of angel hair pasta. Served with veggies.

✓✓ CALORIES: Excellent Choice (350) ✓✓ CHOLESTEROL: Excellent Choice (50 mg)
✓ FAT: Good Choice (16 g)♥ ✓ SODIUM: Good Choice (340 mg)
EXCHANGES: 2½ Meat, 1 Bread, 2½ Veg, 1½ Fat
PROTEIN: 26 g, CARBOHYDRATE: 29 g, FIBER: 6 g

HONEY THYME PORK ♁

Roasted pork loin glazed with honey, garlic, dijon and thyme and served with roasted lavender potatoes, cabbage, and pecan carrots.

✓ CALORIES: Good Choice (475) ✓✓ CHOLESTEROL: Excellent Choice (65 mg)
✓✓ FAT: Excellent Choice (10 g) ✓✓ SODIUM: Excellent Choice (200 mg)
EXCHANGES: 3 Very Lean Meat, 1¼ Bread, 1¼ Other Carbs, 2½ Veg, 1 Fat
PROTEIN: 29 g, CARBOHYDRATE: 69 g, FIBER: 7 g

BLUEBERRY ORANGE CHICKEN SALAD ♁

Leafy greens mixed with fresh blueberries, orange slices and blue cheese, topped with a grilled chicken breast and served with blueberry vinaigrette and a fresh pear muffin.

✓✓ CALORIES: Excellent Choice (440) ✓ CHOLESTEROL: Good Choice (110 mg)
✓✓ FAT: Excellent Choice (10 g) ✓ SODIUM: Good Choice (380 mg)
EXCHANGES: 5½ Meat, 2 Bread, 1¼ Fruit, ½ Veg, 1¼ Fat
PROTEIN: 45 g, CARBOHYDRATE: 44 g, FIBER: 5 g

SPINACH POLENTA TART DINNER ♁

A creamy polenta tart filled with fresh spinach and mushrooms, topped with tomato slices, served with steamed cauliflower and broccoli and rice pudding.

✓✓ CALORIES: Excellent Choice (380) ✓✓ CHOLESTEROL: Excellent Choice (20 mg)
✓✓ FAT: Excellent Choice (9 g) ✓ SODIUM: Good Choice (420 mg)
EXCHANGES: ½ Meat, 1¾ Bread, 3¾ Veg, ¼ Milk, ¾ Fat
PROTEIN: 21 g, CARBOHYDRATE: 61 g, FIBER: 11 g

Nutrition information provided by Susan's Healthy Gourmet.

♥ Primarily unsaturated fat
♁ at least 2 fruit/vegetable servings

Want lower-fat choices? Try it "Fresco Style." When you voice that choice, we'll know to swap in our freshly-prepared Fiesta Salsa – a zesty mix of diced tomatoes, onions and cilantro – for any sauce or cheese. Fiesta Salsa packs in lots of flavor, but adds only five calories per serving and no fat. Fifteen of our items have under 10 grams of fat when prepared this way. All of our food is made-to-order, with only the finest ingredients: USDA-choice Carne Asada steak, grilled marinated all-white-meat chicken and 100% real cheeses. And no microwaves or pre-made tacos. Never. Not once! You know you're getting real food, that's really good. That's what you get when you "Think Outside The Bun." If you want to see more lower-fat alternatives and full nutritional breakdowns, check out our interactive substitution calculator online at www.TACOBELL.com $

Taco Bell – with 80 locations in Orange County.

GRILLED STEAK SOFT TACO – "FRESCO STYLE"

Chicken soft taco also recommended (with similar nutrition values).

✓✓ CALORIES: Excellent Choice (170) ✓✓ CHOLESTEROL: Excellent Choice (15 mg)
✓✓ FAT: Excellent Choice (5 g) ✓ SODIUM: Good Choice (560 mg)
PROTEIN: 11 g, CARBOHYDRATE: 21 g, FIBER: 2 g

BEAN BURRITO (VEGETARIAN) – "FRESCO STYLE"

✓✓ CALORIES: Excellent Choice (350) ✓✓ CHOLESTEROL: Excellent Choice (0 mg)
✓✓ FAT: Excellent Choice (8 g) SODIUM: High (1220 mg)
PROTEIN: 13 g, CARBOHYDRATE: 56 g, FIBER: 9 g

BURRITO SUPREME® – CHICKEN – "FRESCO STYLE"

Steak version also available.

✓✓ CALORIES: Excellent Choice (350) ✓✓ CHOLESTEROL: Excellent Choice (25 mg)
✓✓ FAT: Excellent Choice (8 g) SODIUM: High (1270 mg)
PROTEIN: 19 g, CARBOHYDRATE: 50 g, FIBER: 6 g

FIESTA BURRITO – CHICKEN – "FRESCO STYLE"

✓✓ CALORIES: Excellent Choice (350) ✓✓ CHOLESTEROL: Excellent Choice (25 mg)
✓✓ FAT: Excellent Choice (9 g) SODIUM: High (1100 mg)
PROTEIN: 16 g, CARBOHYDRATE: 49 g, FIBER: 4 g

TOSTADA (VEGETARIAN) – "FRESCO STYLE"

✓✓ CALORIES: Excellent Choice (200) ✓✓ CHOLESTEROL: Excellent Choice (0 mg)
✓✓ FAT: Excellent Choice (6 g) SODIUM: Moderate (670 mg)
PROTEIN: 8 g, CARBOHYDRATE: 30 g, FIBER: 8 g

ENCHIRITO® – BEEF – "FRESCO STYLE"

Chicken and steak versions also available (with similar nutrition values).

✓✓ CALORIES: Excellent Choice (270) ✓✓ CHOLESTEROL: Excellent Choice (20 mg)
✓✓ FAT: Excellent Choice (9 g) SODIUM: High (1300 mg)
PROTEIN: 13 g, CARBOHYDRATE: 35 g, FIBER: 7 g

Nutrition information supplied by Taco Bell.
Substitution of ingredients may alter nutritional values
Product data is based on current formulations as of January 2004.

"REAL MEXICAN FOOD"

The Taco Company is an upscale fast food Mexican Restaurant. However, unlike most fast food restaurants, everything at The Taco Company is prepared on the premises and made fresh from scratch. While waiting for your order, you can watch homemade tortillas being made. A drive through is provided for patrons in a hurry. Catering and service to private parties is provided, as well as local lunch deliveries, and orders by fax. The Taco Company is located between Katella and Collins off the 55 freeway. We are open every day from 11 am to 9 pm. Our fax number is (714) 289-9167. $

The Taco Company

1009 N. Tustin Ave., Orange, CA 92667 (714) 289-8006

POLLO ASADO TACO

Charbroiled chicken with a soft shell. Analysis is for two tacos.

✓✓ CALORIES: Excellent Choice (215) ✓✓ CHOLESTEROL: Excellent Choice (45 mg)
✓✓ FAT: Excellent Choice (3 g) ✓✓ SODIUM: Excellent Choice (125 mg)**
EXCHANGES: 2¼ Meat (extra lean), 1½ Bread, ¼ Veg, ¼ Fat
PROTEIN: 20 g, CARBOHYDRATE: 26 g

CAMARON TACO

Charbroiled shrimp with a soft shell. Analysis is for two tacos.

✓✓ CALORIES: Excellent Choice (200) ✓ CHOLESTEROL: Good Choice (85 mg)
✓✓ FAT: Excellent Choice (2 g)♥ ✓✓ SODIUM: Excellent Choice (190 mg)**
EXCHANGES: 1¼ Meat (extra lean), 1½ Bread, 1½ Veg, ¼ Fat
PROTEIN: 14 g, CARBOHYDRATE: 33 g

VEGETARIAN TACO

with pinto beans, lettuce, tomato and zucchini. Analysis is for two tacos.

✓✓ CALORIES: Excellent Choice (230) ✓✓ CHOLESTEROL: Excellent Choice (0 mg)
✓✓ FAT: Excellent Choice (5 g) ✓✓ SODIUM: Excellent Choice (195 mg)**
EXCHANGES: ¼ Meat, 2½ Bread, ½ Veg, 1 Fat
PROTEIN: 8 g, CARBOHYDRATE: 40 g

POLLO ASADO BURRITO

Charbroiled chicken and rice.

✓ CALORIES: Good Choice (570) ✓ CHOLESTEROL: Good Choice (110 mg)
✓✓ FAT: Excellent Choice (11 g) SODIUM: Moderate (840 mg)**
EXCHANGES: 5¾ Meat (extra lean), 4¼ Bread, ¼ Veg, 1¼ Fat
PROTEIN: 47 g, CARBOHYDRATE: 66 g

VEGETARIAN TOSTADA

with pinto or black beans. Analysis does not include fried tortilla shell.

✓✓ CALORIES: Excellent Choice (225) ✓✓ CHOLESTEROL: Excellent Choice (5 mg)
✓✓ FAT: Excellent Choice (6 g) ✓✓ SODIUM: Excellent Choice (275 mg)**
EXCHANGES: ¾ Meat, 1¾ Bread, ½ Veg, 1 Fat
PROTEIN: 12 g, CARBOHYDRATE: 32 g

♥ Primarily unsaturated fat
** If you request no added salt

Thai Specialty 2

RESTAURANT

Join us at Thai Specialty 2 for tempting Thai dishes made to order using only fresh ingredients. We carefully prepare every dish from scratch and offer an extensive menu of authentic Thai specialties, from mild to hot. Our friendly staff looks forward to your visit. $

Thai Specialty 2 13572 Newport Ave., Tustin, CA 92780 (714) 731-1711

Analyses below are for ½ order since dishes are usually shared.

APPLE SALAD (½ ORDER) ♁

Green apple and ground chicken, mixed with spicy dressing and cashew nuts.
Analysis does not include fried chili peppers.

✓✓ CALORIES: Excellent Choice (195) ✓✓ CHOLESTEROL: Excellent Choice (35 mg)
✓✓ FAT: Excellent Choice (4 g) SODIUM: High (2155 mg)
EXCHANGES: 2¼ Meat (extra lean), 1¼ Veg, ¾ Fruit, ½ Other Carb, ½ Fat
PROTEIN: 16 g, CARBOHYDRATE: 26 g, FIBER: 4 g

VEGETARIAN EGGPLANT LOVER (½ ORDER) ♁

Tofu sautéed with eggplant, chili, basil, and soy sauce.

✓✓ CALORIES: Excellent Choice (175) ✓✓ CHOLESTEROL: Excellent Choice (10 mg)
✓✓ FAT: Excellent Choice (11 g)♥ ✓✓ SODIUM: Excellent Choice (300 mg)**
EXCHANGES: 1 Meat, 2 Veg, ¼ Other Carb, 1½ Fat
PROTEIN: 10 g, CARBOHYDRATE: 16 g, FIBER: 4 g

SCALLOP AND SHRIMP IN THE POT (½ ORDER)

Scallops and shrimp sautéed with special sauce, onions and glass noodles.

✓✓ CALORIES: Excellent Choice (335) ✓ CHOLESTEROL: Good Choice (105 mg)
✓ FAT: Good Choice (17 g)♥ SODIUM: Moderate (670 mg)**
EXCHANGES: 3¾ Meat (extra lean), ½ Bread, 1¼ Veg, ½ Other Carb, 2¾ Fat
PROTEIN: 28 g, CARBOHYDRATE: 22 g, FIBER: 3 g

SPICY GARLIC CHICKEN (½ ORDER)

Stir-fried chicken with garlic and black pepper.

✓✓ CALORIES: Excellent Choice (310) ✓✓ CHOLESTEROL: Excellent Choice (75 mg)
✓ FAT: Good Choice (17 g) SODIUM: Moderate (805 mg)**
EXCHANGES: 4 Meat (extra lean), ½ Veg, ½ Other Carb, 3 Fat
PROTEIN: 29 g, CARBOHYDRATE: 10 g, FIBER: 1 g

CHICKEN NOODLE (½ ORDER)

Pan-fried flat noodles with chicken, eggs, bean sprouts and crushed peanuts.

✓✓ CALORIES: Excellent Choice (375) ✓ CHOLESTEROL: Good Choice (145 mg)
✓ FAT: Good Choice (20 g) SODIUM: Moderate (810 mg)**
EXCHANGES: 1¾ Meat, 1½ Bread, ½ Veg, ½ Other Carb, 3¼ Fat
PROTEIN: 18 g, CARBOHYDRATE: 33 g, FIBER: 2 g

CHICKEN LARB (½ ORDER)

Chicken cooked with green onion, cilantro, and chili, seasoned with lime juice.

✓✓ CALORIES: Excellent Choice (185) ✓✓ CHOLESTEROL: Excellent Choice (75 mg)
✓✓ FAT: Excellent Choice (3 g) SODIUM: High (2155 mg)
EXCHANGES: 4 Meat (extra lean), ¾ Veg, ¼ Fruit, ¼ Fat
PROTEIN: 30 g, CARBOHYDRATE: 8 g, FIBER: 1 g

GREEN PAPAYA SALAD (½ ORDER) *mixed with dried shrimp, tomatoes, chili and lime.* ♁
CAL: 100, FAT: 1 g♥, CHOL: 5, SOD: 2100 mg; EXCH: ¼ Meat, ½ Veg, ¾ Fr, ½ other c, PROT: 3 g, CARB: 23 g, FIB: 3 g

♁ at least 2 fruit/vegetable servings for entrees, 1 for side dishes

Vie de France – where you go for fine French cuisine the casual way. We serve authentic French breads and pastries from baguettes to sweet-filled croissants baked daily on the premises. Our lunch and dinner menus offer hearty meals and exquisite desserts. Carryout and catering services also available. $

Vie de France

3333 Bristol Ave. #1420
South Coast Plaza, Costa Mesa, CA 92626
(714) 557-1734

SEARED SALMON NICOISE – SPECIAL REQUEST

Salmon on a mound of green beans, tomato wedges, red bliss potatoes, hard cooked egg, black olives and red onions over mixed greens, splashed with fat-free dressing. Request fat-free vinaigrette.

✓ CALORIES: Good Choice (500) | CHOLESTEROL: High (305 mg)
✓ FAT: Good Choice (18 g) | ✓ SODIUM: Good Choice (355 mg)**
EXCHANGES: 5¼ Meat, 1½ Bread, 2¼ Veg, ¼ Fruit, ¾ Fat
PROTEIN: 45 g, CARBOHYDRATE: 40 g, FIBER: 7 g

SEARED AHI TUNA NICOISE – SPECIAL REQUEST

Ahi tuna on a mound of green beans, tomato wedges, red bliss potatoes, hard cooked egg, black olives and red onions over mixed greens, splashed with fat-free dressing. Request fat-free vinaigrette.

✓ CALORIES: Good Choice (590) | CHOLESTEROL: High (310 mg)
✓✓ FAT: Excellent Choice (9 g) | SODIUM: Moderate (990 mg)**
EXCHANGES: 8 Meat, 1½ Bread, 2¼ Veg, 1¾ Fruit, ¾ Fat
PROTEIN: 63 g, CARBOHYDRATE: 60 g, FIBER: 7 g

TOMATO BASIL & ROASTED VEGETABLE PASTA – SPECIAL REQUEST

Fettuccine pasta in homemade tomato basil sauce, topped with oven-roasted vegetables. Request no butter. Garlic bread not included in analysis.

✓ CALORIES: Good Choice (560) | ✓✓ CHOLESTEROL: Excellent Choice (<1 mg)
✓✓ FAT: Excellent Choice (14 g)♥ | SODIUM: High (1300 mg)
EXCHANGES: 5 Bread, 2¼ Veg, 2½ Fat
PROTEIN: 15 g, CARBOHYDRATE: 92 g, FIBER: 8 g

CHICKEN CREOLE PASTA – SPECIAL REQUEST

Chicken breast meat in a spicy blend of peppers, onions, tomatoes and Cajun seasonings with penne pasta. Request less butter (¼ oz). Garlic bread not included in analysis.

✓ CALORIES: Good Choice (750) | ✓ CHOLESTEROL: Good Choice (135 mg)
✓ FAT: Good Choice (21 g) | SODIUM: High (1105 mg)
EXCHANGES: 5 Meat (extra lean), 4¾ Bread, 2 Veg, 2¾ Fat
PROTEIN: 52 g, CARBOHYDRATE: 87 g, FIBER: 7 g

FRENCH DIP

Tender slices of warm roast beef heaped on a freshly baked French baguette, served au jus, garnished with lettuce and tomato, and served with orzo salad.

✓ CALORIES: Good Choice (640) | ✓ CHOLESTEROL: Good Choice (80 mg)
✓✓ FAT: Excellent Choice (15 g) | SODIUM: High (3660 mg)
EXCHANGES: 5½ Meat (extra lean), 2¼ Bread, ½ Veg, 2 Fat
PROTEIN: 49 g, CARBOHYDRATE: 77 g, FIBER: 5 g

at least 2 fruit/vegetable servings

Wahoo's Fish Taco serves a unique menu featuring Mexican dishes with a Brazilian twist in a beach-casual atmosphere. Known for our charbroiled fish tacos and Banzai burritos, we also serve chicken, steak, pork shrimp, and veggie dishes. All ingredients are prepared fresh daily. $

Wahoo's Fish Taco Orange County Locations:

Aliso Viejo: 26741 Aliso Creek Rd. #D (949) 389-9399
Costa Mesa: 1862 Placentia Ave. (949) 631-3433
3000 Bristol Ave. (714) 435-0130
Fashion Island: 1091 Newport Ctr. Dr. (949) 760-0290
Foothill Ranch Coming soon!
Fullerton: 444 N. Harbor Blvd. #100 (714) 525-4110
Huntington Beach: 120 Main St. (714) 536-2050
Irvine: 2967 Michelson #F (949) 253-9532
Irvine Spectrum: 81 Fortune Dr. #151 (949) 753-0251
Laguna Beach: 1133 S. Coast Hwy (949) 497-0033
Lake Forest: 23600 Rockfield #2D½ (949) 830-7386
S. Coast Plaza: 3333 Bear St. #211 (714) 549-0565
Tustin: 13791 Newport Ave. #4 (714) 544-1154
Yorba Linda: 23042 East Park Dr. (714) 921-3051
San Clemente: 641 Camino de Los Mares #A100 (949) 487-6995
Visit www.wahoos.com for other locations.

CHARBROILED FISH TACO

✓✓ CALORIES: Excellent Choice (235)
✓✓ FAT: Excellent Choice (4 g)
✓✓ CHOLESTEROL: Excellent Choice (55 mg)
✓ SODIUM: Good Choice (325 mg)**
EXCHANGES: 2 Meat, 1¾ Bread, ½ Veg, ½ Fat
PROTEIN: 16 g, CARBOHYDRATE: 28 g, FIBER: 3 g

CHARBROILED CHICKEN TACO

✓✓ CALORIES: Excellent Choice (260)
✓✓ FAT: Excellent Choice (6 g)
✓✓ CHOLESTEROL: Excellent Choice (50 mg)
✓ SODIUM: Good Choice (305 mg)**
EXCHANGES: 2½ Meat, 1¾ Bread, ½ Veg, ½ Fat
PROTEIN: 20 g, CARBOHYDRATE: 28 g, FIBER: 3 g

½ RICE & ½ BEAN COMBO BOWL

✓✓ CALORIES: Excellent Choice (390)
✓✓ FAT: Excellent Choice (3 g)
✓✓ CHOLESTEROL: Excellent Choice (0 mg)
SODIUM: High (1005 mg)
EXCHANGES: ¾ Meat, 4¾ Bread, ¼ Veg, ½ Fat
PROTEIN: 16 g, CARBOHYDRATE: 74 g, FIBER: 13 g

CHARBROILED CHICKEN BURRITO

✓ CALORIES: Good Choice (540)
✓ FAT: Good Choice (17 g)
✓ CHOLESTEROL: Good Choice (110 mg)
SODIUM: High (1080 mg)
EXCHANGES: 5½ Meat, 3 Bread, ¾ Veg, 2¼ Fat
PROTEIN: 46 g, CARBOHYDRATE: 49 g, FIBER: 3 g

VEGETARIAN BURRITO

✓ CALORIES: Good Choice (600)
✓✓ FAT: Excellent Choice (14 g)
✓✓ CHOLESTEROL: Excellent Choice (15 mg)
SODIUM: High (1460 mg)
EXCHANGES: 1 Meat, 6 Bread, 1 Veg, 2¼ Fat
PROTEIN: 21 g, CARBOHYDRATE: 98 g, FIBER: 12 g

CHARBROILED FISH BURRITO

✓ CALORIES: Good Choice (480)
✓✓ FAT: Excellent Choice (14 g)
✓ CHOLESTEROL: Good Choice (120 mg)
SODIUM: High (1125 mg)
EXCHANGES: 4¼ Meat, 3 Bread, 1 Veg, 2¼ Fat
PROTEIN: 38 g, CARBOHYDRATE: 50 g, FIBER: 4 g

♥ Primarily unsaturated fat
** If you request no added salt

Walt's Wharf is located on Main Street in what Sunset Magazine describes as "The Last of America's Small Towns." We offer the freshest seafood cooked over a red oak fire, lean Limousin beef, fresh homemade pastas and specially grown vegetables, all served in a comfortable, friendly neighborhood building built in the early 1930s. Walt Babcock, retired dentist and winery owner, has found a way to "take the guilt out of eating a juicy steak" by serving Limousin beef from Nebraska. $$

Walt's Wharf

201 Main Street, Seal Beach, CA 90740 (562) 598-4433

ROASTED CHICKEN PASTA

with portabello mushrooms, garlic, tomatoes and basil.

✓ CALORIES: Good Choice (595)
FAT: Moderate (26 g)
✓ CHOLESTEROL: Good Choice (100 mg)
✓ SODIUM: Good Choice (325 mg)**

EXCHANGES: 4¾ Meat, 2 Bread, 1¾ Veg, 3¼ Fat
PROTEIN: 43 g, CARBOHYDRATE: 43 g, FIBER: 4 g

OAK GRILLED SWORDFISH

Swordfish marinated in lemongrass, soy ginger and garlic, served with sautéed Asian vegetables. Analysis includes plain baked potato.

✓ CALORIES: Good Choice (630)
✓✓ FAT: Excellent Choice (12 g)♥
✓ CHOLESTEROL: Good Choice (80 mg)
✓✓ SODIUM: Excellent Choice (300 mg)**

EXCHANGES: 4½ Meat, 4 Bread, 1¾ Veg, ¾ Fat
PROTEIN: 49 g, CARBOHYDRATE: 81 g, FIBER: 11 g

HAWAIIAN AHI SALAD – SPECIAL REQUEST

Blackened ahi sashimi served on organic baby field greens, with fresh papaya and cilantro salsa and oak roasted red peppers. Request dressing on the side (not included in analysis).

✓✓ CALORIES: Excellent Choice (295)
✓✓ FAT: Excellent Choice (12 g)♥
✓✓ CHOLESTEROL: Excellent Choice (60 mg)
✓✓ SODIUM: Excellent Choice (130 mg)**

EXCHANGES: 3¾ Meat (extra lean), 2½ Veg, ¼ Fruit, 2 Fat
PROTEIN: 30 g, CARBOHYDRATE: 18 g, FIBER: 4 g

OAK GRILLED VEGETABLE PLATTER

with artichoke, zucchini, crookneck squash, Bermuda onion, eggplant, and red & green peppers. Aioli not included in analysis.

✓✓ CALORIES: Excellent Choice (275)
✓✓ FAT: Excellent Choice (13 g)
✓✓ CHOLESTEROL: Excellent Choice (35 mg)
✓✓ SODIUM: Excellent Choice (270 mg)**

EXCHANGES: 6¾ Veg, ¼ Fruit, 2½ Fat
PROTEIN: 10 g, CARBOHYDRATE: 39 g, FIBER: 16 g

SPAGHETTINI POMODORO WITH JUMBO PRAWNS – SPECIAL REQUEST

Fresh roma tomatoes and basil sautéed in olive oil & garlic with five jumbo prawns. Request less oil (¼ Tbs).

✓ CALORIES: Good Choice (585)
✓✓ FAT: Excellent Choice (11 g)♥
CHOLESTEROL: Moderate (295 mg)
SODIUM: Moderate (820 mg)**

EXCHANGES: 2½ Meat (extra lean), 4 Bread, 4¾ Veg, 2 Fat
PROTEIN: 37 g, CARBOHYDRATE: 85 g, FIBER: 7 g

GRILLED LEAN LIMOUSIN FILET MIGNON

over tobacco onions with roasted shallot demiglace and fresh green beans with tomatoes and basil. Analysis includes plain baked potato.

✓ CALORIES: Good Choice (695)
✓✓ FAT: Excellent Choice (14 g)
✓ CHOLESTEROL: Good Choice (150 mg)
✓✓ SODIUM: Excellent Choice (220 mg)**

EXCHANGES: 5¼ Meat (extra lean), 4 Bread, 2¼ Veg, 1 Fat
PROTEIN: 54 g, CARBOHYDRATE: 98 g, FIBER: 11 g

♥ Primarily unsaturated fat
** If you request no added salt

Whole Foods Markets are dedicated to supplying the finest, most natural, wholesome foods available, including an ever-increasing selection of organically grown ingredients. Our savory salads, delectable dressings, steamy soups, enticing entrees and many of our delicious baked goods are prepared in our own kitchen, using time honored recipes with no artificial flavors, artificial colors, artificial sweeteners or preservatives. $

Whole Foods Market

14945 Holt Avenue, Tustin, CA 92680 (714) 731-3400

TUSTIN CHICKEN *(½ lb. serving)*

✓✓ CALORIES: Excellent Choice (320) ✓ CHOLESTEROL: Good Choice (115 mg)
✓✓ FAT: Excellent Choice (10 g) ✓ SODIUM: Good Choice (425 mg)
EXCHANGES: 6 Meat (extra lean), ¾ Veg, 1 Fat
PROTEIN: 44 g, CARBOHYDRATE: 10 g, FIBER: 2 g

EDAMAME TOFU SALAD *(½ lb. serving)*

✓✓ CALORIES: Excellent Choice (350) ✓✓ CHOLESTEROL: Excellent Choice (0 mg)
✓ FAT: Good Choice (19 g)♥ SODIUM: Moderate (850 mg)
EXCHANGES: 3½ Meat, ¾ Bread, ½ Veg, ¼ Fruit, 1½ Fat
PROTEIN: 28 g, CARBOHYDRATE: 23 g, FIBER: 10 g

CRANBERRY KASHI *(½ lb. serving)*

✓✓ CALORIES: Excellent Choice (275) ✓✓ CHOLESTEROL: Excellent Choice (0 mg)
✓✓ FAT: Excellent Choice (4 g)♥ ✓✓ SODIUM: Excellent Choice (20 mg)
EXCHANGES: 2¼ Bread, ¼ Veg, 1¼ Fruit, ¾ Fat
PROTEIN: 7 g, CARBOHYDRATE: 54 g, FIBER: 9 g

BALSAMIC GRILLED VEGETABLES *(½ lb. serving)*

✓✓ CALORIES: Excellent Choice (105) ✓✓ CHOLESTEROL: Excellent Choice (0 mg)
✓✓ FAT: Excellent Choice (6 g)♥ ✓✓ SODIUM: Excellent Choice (255 mg)
EXCHANGES: 2 Veg, 1 Fat
PROTEIN: 2 g, CARBOHYDRATE: 12 g, FIBER: 4 g

LEMON CAPELLINI SALAD *(½ lb. serving)*

✓✓ CALORIES: Excellent Choice (285) ✓✓ CHOLESTEROL: Excellent Choice (0 mg)
✓✓ FAT: Excellent Choice (12 g)♥ ✓✓ SODIUM: Excellent Choice (245 mg)
EXCHANGES: 2 Bread, ¾ Veg, 2¼ Fat
PROTEIN: 6 g, CARBOHYDRATE: 39 g, FIBER: 3 g

at least 2 fruit/vegetable servings

Known for the world's largest selection of draft beer and remembered for the excellent food, Yard House offers an eclectic menu of American Fusion cuisine including salads, seafood, pizza, and burgers. Friendly, attentive service in a casual and relaxed atmosphere contribute to Yard House being the perfect destination for family gatherings, business luncheons and time spent with friends. Kids Klub menu available daily. Visit us at YardHouse.com. $$

Yard House
1875 Newport Blvd., Costa Mesa (949) 642-0090
71 Fortune Drive, Irvine (949) 753-9373

MOO SHU CHICKEN

Filled with chicken and chili cream cheese with apple ginger plum sauce.
Analysis is for 1 order (2 egg rolls and 2 oz. apple ginger plum sauce).

✓ CALORIES: Good Choice (540) — CHOLESTEROL: Moderate (155 mg)
✓ FAT: Good Choice (22 g) — SODIUM: Moderate (950 mg)**
EXCHANGES: 6½ Meat, 1 Bread, 1 Veg, 1 Fruit, 2¾ Fat
PROTEIN: 50 g, CARBOHYDRATE: 36 g, FIBER: 2 g

SPICY TUNA DYNAMITE ROLL (½ ORDER)

Layered with cucumber, edamame, crushed avocados, wasabi soy and sesame oil.
Analysis is for ½ order, assuming it is shared by two people.

✓✓ CALORIES: Excellent Choice (315) — ✓✓ CHOLESTEROL: Excellent Choice (20 mg)
✓ FAT: Good Choice (19 g)♥ — SODIUM: High (1120 mg)
EXCHANGES: 1¾ Meat, 3 Veg, ¼ Fruit, 3¼ Fat
PROTEIN: 18 g, CARBOHYDRATE: 19 g, FIBER: 4 g

BBQ CHICKEN SALAD – SPECIAL REQUEST

Marinated BBQ chicken with pinto beans, tomatoes, corn, greens, and cheese.
Request no fried onions or tortilla strips and dressing on the side (dressing not included in analysis).

✓ CALORIES: Good Choice (710) — CHOLESTEROL: Moderate (155 mg)
✓ FAT: Good Choice (23 g) — SODIUM: High (1410 mg)
EXCHANGES: 7¾ Meat (extra lean), 2¾ Bread, 2¼ Veg, ¼ Fruit, 2¾ Fat
PROTEIN: 64 g, CARBOHYDRATE: 64 g, FIBER: 11 g

MISO GLAZED SEA BASS – SPECIAL REQUEST

with bok choy and edamame atop Jasmine rice. Request less oil (½ oz.) and no butter. Jasmine rice not included in analysis; rice adds 305 calories, 5 mg sodium, 6 g protein, 67 g carbs, 1 g fiber.

✓ CALORIES: Good Choice (665) — ✓ CHOLESTEROL: Good Choice (95 mg)
✓ FAT: Good Choice (23 g)♥ — SODIUM: High (1920 mg)
EXCHANGES: 5 Meat (extra lean), ¼ Bread, 3 Veg, 2¾ Fruit, 3 Fat
PROTEIN: 53 g, CARBOHYDRATE: 59 g, FIBER: 5 g

MARGHERITA PIZZA (½ PIZZA) – SPECIAL REQUEST

Oven roasted roma tomatoes and garlic with mozzarella and fresh basil.
Request less cheese (2 oz). Pizza has 8 slices; analysis is for 4 slices.

✓ CALORIES: Good Choice (545) — ✓✓ CHOLESTEROL: Excellent Choice (35 mg)
✓ FAT: Good Choice (22 g) — SODIUM: High (1315 mg)
EXCHANGES: 1½ Meat, 3¼ Bread, 1 Veg, 3 Fat
PROTEIN: 21 g, CARBOHYDRATE: 66 g, FIBER: 3 g

AHI CRUNCHY SALAD – SPECIAL REQUEST

Seared ahi and mixed greens, tossed in a soy vinaigrette.
Request fried wontons on the side (not included in analysis) and half portion of dressing (1½ oz).

✓✓ CALORIES: Excellent Choice (355) — ✓✓ CHOLESTEROL: Excellent Choice (50 mg)
✓ FAT: Good Choice (18 g)♥ — SODIUM: High (1325 mg)
EXCHANGES: 3½ Meat (extra lean), ¼ Bread, 2¼ Veg, ¼ Fruit, 3 Fat
PROTEIN: 31 g, CARBOHYDRATE: 20 g, FIBER: 7 g

at least 2 fruit/vegetable servings

Offering a unique blend of culinary craftsmanship, health-conscious philosophy and superior quality, Z Pizza remains in a league of its own. Z Pizza began using only Montana winter wheat flour and award-winning low fat mozzarella from Wisconsin. Nearly 20 years later, our premium ingredients also include certified organic tomato sauce and reduced-fat and additive-free meats. Z's fire-baked pizza, calzones, sandwiches, salads and gourmet pasta have never tasted better! $

Z Pizza

Orange County locations in Aliso Viejo, Belmont Shore, Corona Del Mar, Crystal Cove, Huntington Beach, Laguna Beach, Lake Forest, Newport Beach, San Clemente, Seal Beach, & South Coast Metro. For other locations, please visit www.zpizza.com.

Analyses for pizzas below are for ½ of the small size pizza.

TUSCAN MUSHROOM PIZZA (½ OF SMALL 10-INCH PIZZA)

Mushrooms, green onions, oregano, garlic sauce, and feta cheese on whole wheat pizza crust.

✓✓ CALORIES: Excellent Choice (325) ✓✓ CHOLESTEROL: Excellent Choice (15 mg)
✓✓ FAT: Excellent Choice (9 g) ✓ SODIUM: Good Choice (595 mg)
EXCHANGES: ¼ Meat, 2¾ Bread, ½ Veg, 1½ Fat
PROTEIN: 11 g, CARBOHYDRATE: 51 g, FIBER: 4 g

SANTA FE PIZZA (½ OF SMALL 10-INCH PIZZA) – SPECIAL REQUEST

Chicken sausage, red onions, corn, serrano chiles, tomatoes, cilantro, and southwest chipotle pesto. Request non-fat mozzarella cheese.

✓✓ CALORIES: Excellent Choice (440) ✓✓ CHOLESTEROL: Excellent Choice (25 mg)
✓✓ FAT: Excellent Choice (10 g) SODIUM: High (1075 mg)
EXCHANGES: 2 Meat (extra lean), 2¾ Bread, ½ Other Carbs, 1 Veg, 1¼ Fat
PROTEIN: 27 g, CARBOHYDRATE: 60 g, FIBER: 8 g

PROVENCE PIZZA (½ OF SMALL 10-INCH PIZZA) – SPECIAL REQUEST

Artichoke hearts, capers, tomatoes, roasted garlic, basil and marinara. Request non-fat mozzarella cheese.

✓✓ CALORIES: Excellent Choice (425) ✓✓ CHOLESTEROL: Excellent Choice (10 mg)
✓✓ FAT: Excellent Choice (8 g)♥ SODIUM: High (1480 mg)
EXCHANGES: 2¾ Meat, 2¾ Bread, 1¼ Veg, 1¼ Fat
PROTEIN: 28 g, CARBOHYDRATE: 62 g, FIBER: 7 g

THAI PIZZA (½ OF SMALL 10-INCH PIZZA) – SPECIAL REQUEST

Spicy chicken, red onions, cilantro, carrots, bean sprouts, and peanut sauce. Request non-fat mozzarella cheese.

✓✓ CALORIES: Excellent Choice (430) ✓✓ CHOLESTEROL: Excellent Choice (35 mg)
✓✓ FAT: Excellent Choice (6 g) SODIUM: High (1305 mg)
EXCHANGES: 3¾ Meat (extra lean), 2¾ Bread, 1¼ Veg, ¼ Fat
PROTEIN: 36 g, CARBOHYDRATE: 58 g, FIBER: 7 g

YUPPEE VEGGIE SANDWICH

Avocado, mozzarella, lettuce, onions, cucumber, artichoke hearts, and vinaigrette dressing.

✓ CALORIES: Good Choice (460) ✓✓ CHOLESTEROL: Excellent Choice (15 mg)
✓ FAT: Good Choice (24 g) SODIUM: Moderate (665 mg)**
EXCHANGES: 1¼ Meat, 2 Bread, 2¼ Veg, ¼ Fruit, 3¾ Fat
PROTEIN: 19 g, CARBOHYDRATE: 46 g, FIBER: 8 g

Z TUNA SALAD

Tuna over romaine and looseleaf lettuce, with cucumber, tomato, basil, and Oriental non-fat dressing.

✓✓ CALORIES: Excellent Choice (215) ✓✓ CHOLESTEROL: Excellent Choice (25 mg)
✓✓ FAT: Excellent Choice (2 g)♥ SODIUM: Moderate (915 mg)**
EXCHANGES: 2¾ Meat (extra lean), 2 Veg, ¼ Fat
PROTEIN: 25 g, CARBOHYDRATE: 22 g, FIBER: 4 g

♥ Primarily unsaturated fat
** If you request no added salt

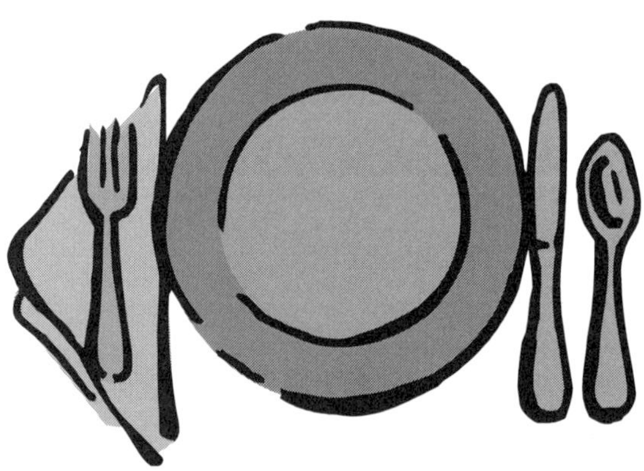

Part III
Chefs' Recipes

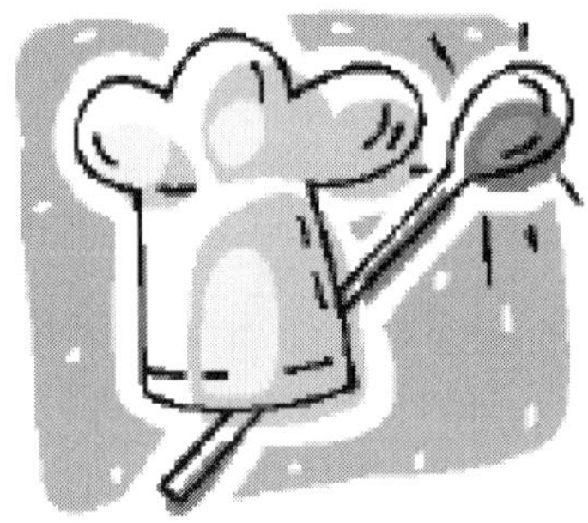

Measure Equivalents:

3 teaspoons (tsp.) = 1 Tablespoon (Tbs.)
16 Tablespoons (Tbs.) = 1 cup
2 Tablespoons (Tbs.) = 1 ounce (oz.) for liquids
1 Tablespoon = ½ ounce

Healthy Dining in Orange County is pleased to present a diverse selection of recipes created by chefs of restaurants participating in this book and other **Healthy Dining** books from Southern California. We are delighted that so many restaurants have elected to participate in this section, sharing some of their culinary "trade secrets."

Types of Recipes

The recipes include a wide range of selections --- varying ethnic and regional origins, combinations of flavors, preparation time required, preparation difficulty, and types of dishes (soups, entrees, salads, desserts, etc.)

The Recipe Index

On pages 116 to 119 you'll find the Recipe Index, first arranged by type of dish, then by the name of the restaurant that submitted the recipe. Many recipes could easily fall into more than one category within the Recipe Index. For example, a seafood salad could be under either the salads or seafood category. We suggest that you scan the entire Recipe Index to identify dishes that may appeal to you.

Nutritional analysis and modification of the recipes

Most recipes represent dishes that appear on the restaurant's menu page in ***Healthy Dining***. We've stated on each recipe page that "This nutritional analysis corresponds to the recipe below. The restaurant version may differ." This notice indicates: (1) The recipe originally submitted to us for nutrition analysis was in bulk quantity and was adjusted to make 2 to 6 servings. In the process, we may have reformulated the recipe slightly so that amounts are expressed in convenient units – for example, ½ cup and not $\frac{7}{12}$ of a cup, or one tomato, not 6 oz. of tomato; (2) We may have substituted more common ingredients; or (3) We may have adjusted the quantities of some ingredients to further improve the nutrition profile.

Unfamiliar ingredients

When an ingredient is included that might be unfamiliar to the "average" cook, we've given some explanation and direction for finding it. If you need further explanation, please call the restaurant, a cooking school, or a specialty market. Or use your creativity and try your own substitutions!

Talk to us!

We wish you enjoyment and satisfaction, challenge and variety in experimenting with the recipes included. We're eager to get your feedback on the recipes included -- please return the questionnaire at the back of your book!

Recipe Index

By Type of Cuisine

Salads

Ahi Salad – *Yard House* 121
Apple-Chicken Salad – *Thai Specialty 2* 122
Chinese Chicken Salad – *J. T. Schmid's Brewhouse & Eatery* 123
Crab Stack – *Roppongi* 124
Fresh Albacore Tuna Salad – *The Health Emporium* 125
Fresh Papaya Salad – *Diho Siam* 126
Grilled Salmon Salad – *Mi Piace* 127
Orange and Jicama Salad – *Melissa's/World Variety Produce, Inc.* 128
Warm Lentil Salad – *Gelson's Market* 129

Fish

Apple Braised Salmon – *Green Parrot Café* 130
Broiled Seabass with Tropical Fruit Salsa – *Bluewater Grill* 131
Carmelized Halibut – *BeachFire Bar & Grill* 132
Charbroiled Fish Taco – *Wahoo's Fish Taco* 133
Chef Mark Tydell's Grilled Pacific Swordfish – *Walt's Wharf* 134
Fresh Sea Bass Taquitos Appetizer – *Ranchos Cocina* 135
Grilled Alaskan Halibut – *Santa Monica Seafood* 136
Salmon Atashi – *Ferdussi Taste of Persia* 137
Sautéed Bluenose Bass – *The Beach House* 138
Seared Blackened Ahi – *McCormick & Schmick's* 139

Other Seafood

Camerones a la Mexicana – *El Callejon* 140
Cioppino – *McKenna's on the Bay* 141
Jumbo Sea Scallops – *G5-Georges on Fifth* 142
Lite Ginger Wine Shrimp – *Café Chin Chin* 143
Lobster Tacos – *Pacific Coast Grill* 144
Pasta Angelica with Scallops – *The Fish Market* 145

Recipe Index, continued

Poultry

Chicken Breast a la Provencal – *Pascal* 146
Chicken Marengo – *Susan's Healthy Gourmet* 147
Chicken Vermicelli – *Luciana's Ristorante* 148
Culinary Wrap – *The Culinary Wrap* 149
Karahi Chicken – *Royal Khyber* 150
Lettuce Wraps with Plum Sauce – *Newport Beach Brewing Company* 151
Mushroom Chicken – *Pick Up Stix* 152
Poblano Turkey Chili – *Chili My Soul* 153

Pasta

Capellini al Pomodoro Fresco – *Pane e Vino* 154
Chicken Creole Pasta – *Vie de France* 155
Italian Country Linguini – *Lino's* 156
Linguini alla Trevi – *Il Forno* 157
Pasta Mare e Monti – *Il Moro* 158
Rock Shrimp with Cilantro – *Pizza Nova* 159
Spaghetti with Mushroom Sauce – *The Old Spaghetti Factory* 160

Vegetables and/or Vegetarian

Aloo Gobi – *Star of India* 161
Cauliflower Enchiladas – *Jimbo's Markets* 162
Neptune Loaf – *The Spot* 163
Vegetable Burrito – *Casa Guadalajara* 164
Vegetable Stir Fry with Tofu Over Rice – *Henry's Marketplace* 165
Whole Earth Casserole – *Angie's Cuisine Italiano* 166

Soups, Sauces & Side Dishes

Clam and Mushroom Miso Soup – *Chaya Venice & Brasserie* 167
Garlic Mashed Potatoes – *Skew's Fresh & Fire Grilled* 168
Shrimp & Lemon Grass Soup – *California Wok* 169
Tomato Bruschetta – *Whole Foods Market* 170

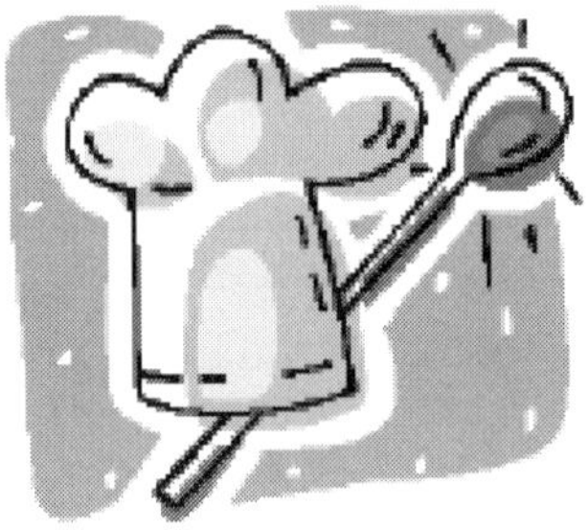

Recipe Index

by Restaurant Name

Angie's Cuisine Italiano – Whole Earth Casserole 166

The Beach House – Sautéed Bluenose Bass 138

BeachFire Bar & Grill – Carmelized Halibut 132

Bluewater Grill – Broiled Seabass with Tropical Fruit Salsa 131

Café Chin Chin – Lite Ginger Wine Shrimp 143

California Wok – Shrimp & Lemon Grass Soup 169

Casa Guadalajara (San Diego) – Vegetable Burrito 164

Chaya Venice & Brasserie (Los Angeles) – Clam and Mushroom Miso Soup 167

Chili My Soul (Los Angeles area) – Poblano Turkey Chili 153

The Culinary Wrap – Culinary Wrap 149

Diho Siam – Fresh Papaya Salad 126

El Callejon (San Diego area) – Camerones a la Mexicana 140

Ferdussi Taste of Persia – Salmon Atashi 137

The Fish Market – Pasta Angelica with Scallops 145

Gelson's Market – Warm Lentil Salad 129

G5-Georges on Fifth (San Diego) – Jumbo Sea Scallops 142

Green Parrot Café – Apple Braised Salmon 130

The Health Emporium – Fresh Albacore Tuna Salad 125

Henry's Marketplace – Vegetable Stir Fry with Tofu Over Rice 165

Il Forno (Los Angeles) – Linguini alla Trevi 157

Il Moro (Los Angeles) – Pasta Mare e Monti 158

Jimbo's Markets (San Diego area) – Cauliflower Enchiladas 162

J. T. Schmid's Brewhouse & Eatery – Chinese Chicken Salad 123

Recipe Index, continued

Lino's (San Diego) – Italian Country Linguini 156

Luciana's Ristorante – Chicken Vermicelli 148

McCormick & Schmick's – Seared Blackened Ahi 139

McKenna's on the Bay – Cioppino 141

Melissa's/World Variety Produce, Inc. – Orange and Jicama Salad 128

Mi Piace (Los Angeles area) – Grilled Salmon Salad 127

Newport Beach Brewing Company – Lettuce Wraps with Plum Sauce 151

The Old Spaghetti Factory – Spaghetti with Mushroom Sauce 160

Pacific Coast Grill (San Diego area) – Lobster Tacos 144

Pane e Vino – Capellini al Pomodoro Fresco 154

Pascal – Chicken Breast a la Provencal 146

Pick Up Stix – Mushroom Chicken 152

Pizza Nova (San Diego) – Rock Shrimp with Cilantro 159

Ranchos Cocina (San Diego) – Fresh Sea Bass Taquitos Appetizer 135

Roppongi (San Diego) – Crab Stack 124

Royal Khyber – Karahi Chicken 150

Santa Monica Seafood – Alaskan Halibut 136

Skew's Fresh & Fire Grilled (Los Angeles) – Garlic Mashed Potatoes 168

The Spot (Los Angeles area) – Neptune Loaf 163

Star of India (San Diego) – Aloo Gobi 161

Susan's Healthy Gourmet – Chicken Marengo 147

Thai Specialty 2 – Apple-Chicken Salad 122

Vie de France – Chicken Creole Pasta 155

Wahoo's Fish Taco – Charbroiled Fish Taco 133

Walt's Wharf – Chef Mark Tydell's Grilled Pacific Swordfish 134

Whole Foods Market – Tomato Bruschetta 170

Yard House – Ahi Salad 121

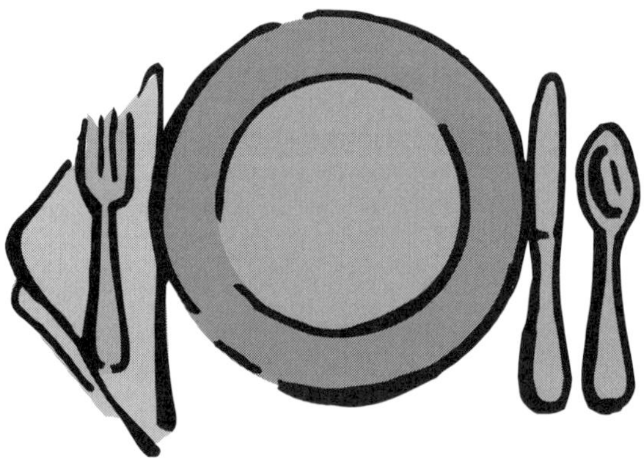

AHI SALAD ♁

Nutrition Information per serving

✓✓ CALORIES: Excellent Choice (340) ✓✓ CHOLESTEROL: Excellent Choice (50 mg)
✓✓ FAT: Excellent Choice (14 g)♥ SODIUM: High (1400 mg)
EXCHANGES: 3½ Meat (extra lean), 2¼ Veg, ½ Fruit, 2¼ Fat
PROTEIN: 33 g, CARBOHYDRATE: 21 g, FIBER: 5 g

This nutrition analysis corresponds to the recipe below. The restaurant version may differ.

Ingredients (4 servings):

Soy Vinaigrette

¼ cup soy sauce
¼ cup rice vinegar
1 Tbs. dijon mustard
2 Tbs. sugar
¼ tsp. salt
¼ tsp. pepper
½ yellow onion, chopped
¼ cup salad oil
¼ cup sesame oil

Salad

3 cups cilantro, chopped
1½ cups green cabbage, shredded
1½ cups red cabbage, shredded
1 cup julienned carrots
1¼ cups bean sprouts
1 cup broccoli slaw
1 lb. fresh ahi tuna
4 tsp. Cajun seasoning
2 tsp. olive oil
6 cups baby lettuce greens
about 40 stems of radish sprouts
1 tsp. sesame seeds

Directions:

Soy Vinaigrette: Combine all ingredients except oils into blender. Blend while slowly adding oils to emulsify the dressing.
Asian Slaw: Combine first 6 salad ingredients and toss until thoroughly combined.
Ahi: Coat ahi with Cajun seasoning. Heat oil in cast iron pan to almost smoking point. Place ahi in pan and allow blackening on all sides. Remove from pan and cut into slices.
Salad: Add baby greens to Asian Slaw and ½ cup Soy Vinaigrette and toss. Mound lettuce mix in bowls creating as much height as possible. Top with radish sprouts and arrange ahi on top. Drizzle another 1 Tbs. Soy Vinaigrette per plate over the ahi and salads. Reserve the remaining Vinaigrette Dressing for another use. Finish the salads by garnishing with sesame seeds.
Note: The restaurant recommends adding fried wonton strips (not included in analysis) to add crunch to the salad.

Recipe supplied by:

Yard House

1875 Newport Blvd., Costa Mesa (949) 642-0090
71 Fortune Drive, Irvine (949) 753-9373

♁ at least 2 fruit/vegetable servings

APPLE-CHICKEN SALAD

Nutrition Information per Serving:

✓✓ CALORIES: Excellent Choice (195) ✓✓ CHOLESTEROL: Excellent Choice (35 mg)
✓✓ FAT: Excellent Choice (4 g) SODIUM: Moderate (765 mg)
EXCHANGES: 2¼ Meat (extra lean), 1¼ Veg, ¾ Fruit, ½ Other Carb, ½ Fat
PROTEIN: 16 g, CARBOHYDRATE: 26 g, FIBER: 4 g

This nutrition analysis corresponds to the recipe below. The restaurant version may differ.

Ingredients (4 servings):

6 oz. chicken breast
2 Tbs. fish sauce
2 Tbs. lime juice
2 Tbs. sugar
2 green apples, peeled, cored & diced
2 carrots, shredded
1 cup sliced red onion
2 Tbs. chopped green onion
6 Tbs. (⅜ cup) chopped cilantro
2 Tbs. cashews, dry roasted & salted

Directions:

1. Grill chicken breast or sauté with non-stick spray. Cool and shred the chicken.
2. Mix fish sauce, lime juice and sugar together.
3. Mix apples, carrots, onions, cilantro and shredded chicken together.
4. Pour fish sauce mixture over apple mixture and stir gently.
5. Garnish with cashews and serve.

Recipe supplied by:

Thai Specialty 2
13572 Newport Ave.
Tustin, CA 92780
(714) 731-1711

at least 2 fruit/vegetable servings

Chinese Chicken Salad

Nutrition Information per Serving:

✓ Calories: Good Choice (510) ✓ Cholesterol: Good Choice (130 mg)
✓ Fat: Good Choice (19 g) ✓ Sodium: Good Choice (470 mg)
Exchanges: 7 Meat, ¼ Bread, 1½ Veg, ¾ Fruit, 2½ Fat
Protein: 54 g, Carbohydrate: 30 g, Fiber: 5 g

This nutrition analysis corresponds to the recipe below. The restaurant version may differ.

Ingredients (2 servings):

Wasabi Vinaigrette
1 Tbs. rice vinegar
½ Tbs. honey
¾ Tbs. hoisin sauce
⅛ oz. (about 1 tsp.) wasabi powder
¼ Tbs. garlic, chopped fine
¼ Tbs. ginger, chopped fine
1 Tbs. canola oil
¼ Tbs. sesame oil

2 chicken breasts, skinless (6 oz. each)
⅓ red bell pepper, julienned
⅓ yellow bell pepper, julienned
⅓ green bell pepper, julienned
⅓ cup red onion, julienned
2 Tbs. peanuts, unsalted
2 Mandarin oranges, sectioned
1 oz. (about ⅔ cup) bean sprouts
4 cups spring lettuce
½ carrot, shredded

Directions:

1. For Wasabi Vinaigrette, puree all ingredients except canola oil and sesame oil in a food processor. Just before serving, mix in oils.
2. Grill chicken breasts. Cool and slice into 1-inch slices.
3. Toast peanuts in oven until slightly browned.
4. Place greens on two plates or large bowls.
5. Add bell peppers, onions, peanuts, Mandarin orange segments, bean sprouts and shredded carrots.
6. Top salads with chicken strips and drizzle dressing over salads.

Recipe supplied by:

J T Schmid's Brewhouse & Eatery
2610 E. Katella Avenue
Anaheim, CA 92806
(714) 634-9200

at least 2 fruit/vegetable servings

POLYNESIAN DUNGENESS CRAB STACK ♁

Mango, pea shoots, cucumber, tomato, avocado & peanuts served with spicy ginger lime dressing.

Nutrition Information per Serving:

✓✓ CALORIES: Excellent Choice (280) ✓✓ CHOLESTEROL: Excellent Choice (45 mg)
✓✓ FAT: Excellent Choice (10 g)♥ SODIUM: Moderate (780 mg)
EXCHANGES: 2 Meat (extra lean), 1 Bread, ¾ Veg, ¼ Fruit, 1¾ Fat
PROTEIN: 18 g, CARBOHYDRATE: 33 g

This nutrition analysis corresponds to the recipe below. The restaurant version may differ.
♥Primarily unsaturated fat

Ingredients (4 servings)#:

Crab Stack:

1 cup pea shoots, cut in 2" pieces
1 cup mango, diced in ½" pieces
1 cup cucumber, seeded & sliced
1 cup red onion, thinly sliced
1 cup roma tomatoes, seeded & sliced
½ avocado, diced in ½" pieces
8 oz. Dungeness crab meat, squeeze dry
¼ cup peanuts, ground & toasted
1½ Tbs. cilantro leaves
ginger lime dressing

Ginger Lime Dressing:

½ tsp. garlic, minced
1 Tbs. chile paste
2 Tbs. ginger root, minced
3 Tbs. fish sauce
3 Tbs. lime juice
¼ cup + 1 Tbs. water
¼ cup + 1 Tbs. sugar

For the most effective presentation, the restaurant suggests using a tubular mold that is open at both ends (1 per person) for preparation.

Directions:

1. Combine ingredients of ginger lime dressing in a medium-sized bowl and set aside.
2. Place the four tubular molds on the serving plates. Beginning with pea shoots and ending with crabmeat, place each ingredient in turn into the four tubular molds. Pack firmly. If you're not using molds, stack ingredients on the plates.
3. Garnish with peanuts and cilantro leaves, and drizzle with dressing.
4. Take off the mold by pressing down on the stack and lifting the tube at the same time.

Recipe supplied by:

ROPPONGI RESTAURANT · BAR · CAFE ™

Roppongi Restaurant, Bar & Cafe
875 Prospect Street
La Jolla, CA 92037
(858) 551-5252

♁ at least 2 fruit/vegetable servings

FRESH ALBACORE TUNA SALAD

Nutrition Information per Serving:

✓✓ CALORIES: Excellent Choice (205)
✓✓ CHOLESTEROL: Excellent Choice (50 mg)
✓✓ FAT: Excellent Choice (10 g)♥
✓✓ SODIUM: Excellent Choice (225 mg)

EXCHANGES: 3 Meat, ¼ Veg, ¼ Fruit, 1¾ Fat
PROTEIN: 22 g, CARBOHYDRATE: 6 g, FIBER: <1 g

This nutrition analysis corresponds to the recipe below. The restaurant version may differ.
♥ primarily unsaturated fat

Ingredients (5 servings):

8 oz. (1 cup) apple juice
2 cups water
3 cloves garlic, chopped
½ bunch fresh dill, chopped
½ celery stalk, cut
½ carrot, cut
½ onion, cut
1 lb. fresh albacore tuna
¼ bunch green onions, minced
¼ cup (2 oz.) red onions, minced
½ lemon, freshly squeezed
¼ cup organic mayonnaise
¼ cup non-fat yogurt, plain
¼ tsp. sea salt

Directions:

1. Combine apple juice, water, garlic, dill, celery, carrot, and onion & simmer for 10 minutes.
2. Add tuna, cooking gently until cooked through. Remove tuna, cool and flake.
3. Combine tuna with remaining ingredients.
4. Divide into five portions and serve as a sandwich, on top of a salad, or as a snack on crackers.

Recipe supplied by:

The Health Emporium
3347 East Pacific Coast Hwy.
Corona del Mar, CA 92625
(949) 673-2244

FRESH PAPAYA SALAD

Papaya with chilies, carrots, green beans, tomatoes and peanuts with Thai spicy-lime dressing.

Nutrition Information per Serving:

✓✓ CALORIES: Excellent Choice (255) ✓✓ CHOLESTEROL: Excellent Choice (0 mg)
✓✓ FAT: Excellent Choice (7 g)♥ SODIUM: High (1160 mg)
EXCHANGES: 1 Meat (extra lean), ½ Bread, 2¼ Veg, 1 Fruit, 1¼ Fat
PROTEIN: 12 g, CARBOHYDRATE: 40 g, FIBER: 8 g

This nutrition analysis corresponds to the recipe below. The restaurant version may differ.
** sodium may be reduced by reducing quantity of fish sauce

Ingredients (2 servings):

2 cups papaya, peeled & grated
2 Thai chilies, seeded, chopped & crushed
½ carrot, shredded
½ Tbs. minced fresh garlic
¼ cup green beans, cut to 1 inch long pieces
1 Tbs. dried shrimp
2 Tbs. peanuts, roasted & unsalted
2 Tbs. fish sauce
3 Tbs. lime juice
1 Tbs. sugar
2 large lettuce leaves
⅛ head cabbage, shredded
1 tomato, cut into wedges

Directions:

1. Prepare papaya and vegetables.
2. Blanch green beans. Reserve a few pieces for garnish.
3. Grind or crush ½ of the peanuts. Leave the other peanuts whole.
4. For Thai dressing, mix crushed chilies, ground peanuts, fish sauce, lime juice and sugar.
5. Mix all other ingredients together except lettuce, cabbage, tomato and the green beans reserved for garnish. Add Thai dressing and mix gently.
6. Serve salad by placing a lettuce leaf on each plate. Spread cabbage on top, then papaya mixture. Arrange tomato wedges on top, and garnish with remaining green beans.

Recipe supplied by:

DIHO SIAM Restaurant THAI/CHINESE

Diho Siam Restaurant
Costa Mesa: 1835 Newport Blvd. (949) 645-3259
Lake Forest: 23600 Rockfield, Suite 2L (949) 859-4192
Mission Viejo: 27001 La Paz, Suite 100 (949) 597-1550

THAI DISHES: Fountain Valley: 10065 Garfield Ave. (at Brookhurst) (714) 962-1312

at least 1 fruit/vegetable servings for side dishes

GRILLED SALMON SALAD

with Star Anise dressing, Asian spicy mix, cucumber, tomatoes and onion.

Nutrition Information per Serving:

✓✓ CALORIES: Excellent Choice (300) ✓✓ CHOLESTEROL: Excellent (60 mg)
✓ FAT: Good Choice (18 g) ✓✓ SODIUM: Excellent Choice (60 mg)
EXCHANGES: 3½ Meat, 1Veg, 3 Fat
PROTEIN: 25 g, CARBOHYDRATE: 11 g, FIBER: 3 g

This nutrition analysis corresponds to the recipe below. The restaurant version may differ.

Ingredients (4 servings):

Star Anise Dressing:
¾ tsp. star anise
¾ tsp. honey
¾ Tbs. white wine vinegar
1 tsp. balsamic apple cider
¼ tsp. sugar
2 Tbs. olive oil
salt and pepper to taste (not included in analysis)

Salmon Salad:
1 Tbs. olive oil
1 lb. Salmon, cut into 4 pieces
12 oz. Asian spicy lettuce mix
1 cucumber, sliced
1 small onion, diced
2 medium organic tomatoes, peeled and sliced
1 tsp. chives, diced
½ tsp. balsamic vinegar

Directions:

1. Combine all dressing ingredients and allow to sit for several hours in the refrigerator to allow flavors to mix.
2. Heat sauté pan. Add olive oil.
3. Grill salmon until done.
4. Toss Asian lettuce mix with cucumber, onion, tomato and chives.
5. Toss with star anise dressing.
6. Drizzle with balsamic vinegar.

Recipe supplied by:

Mi Piace
25 E. Colorado Blvd., Old Town Pasadena
(626) 795-3131
801 N. San Fernando Rd., Burbank
(818) 843-1111
4799 Commons Way, Calabasas
(818) 591-8822

at least 2 fruit/vegetable servings

ORANGE AND JICAMA SALAD

Nutrition Information per Serving:†

✓✓ CALORIES: Excellent Choice (65)
✓✓ FAT: Excellent Choice (<1 g)♥
✓✓ CHOLESTEROL: Excellent Choice (0 mg)
✓✓ SODIUM: Excellent Choice (50 mg)
EXCHANGES: 1 Veg, ¾ Fat
PROTEIN: 1 g, CARBOHYDRATE: 16 g, FIBER: 5 g

† Side dish guidelines are ⅓ of entrée guidelines
♥ primarily unsaturated fat

Ingredients (6 servings):

3 organic oranges, cut into ⅛ inch slices
1 medium jicama (about ¾ pound)
1 cup strawberry (or other flavor) papayas, peeled, seeded & cut into ¼ inch cubes
¼ cup diced red onion
2 Tbs. fresh lime juice
pinch sea salt
⅛ tsp. cayenne pepper or to taste
½ cup chopped fresh cilantro

Directions:

1. Peel the jicama, including the fibrous layer just beneath the skin. Slice into ¼ inch pieces, then dice into ⅛ inch pieces.
2. Combine all ingredients in a large bowl and mix thoroughly.
3. Allow to chill 2 hours before serving.

Recipe supplied by:

www.melissas.com

Melissa's
Melissa's/World Variety Produce, Inc.
P.O. Box 21127
Los Angeles, CA 90021
(800) 588-0151

at least 1 fruit/vegetable servings for side dishes

WARM LENTIL SALAD

Nutrition Information per Serving:

✓✓ CALORIES: Excellent Choice (190) ✓✓ CHOLESTEROL: Excellent Choice (0 mg)
✓✓ FAT: Excellent Choice (3½ g)♥ ✓✓ SODIUM: Excellent Choice (145 mg)
PROTEIN: 12 g, CARBOHYDRATE: 30 g, FIBER: 14 g

This nutrition analysis corresponds to the recipe below. The restaurant version may differ.
Nutrition information provided by Gelson's ♥ primarily unsaturated fat

Ingredients (5 servings):

3 cups water
1 cup lentils, picked over and rinsed
1 carrot, diced
¾ tsp. dried thyme
¼ tsp. salt
½ tsp. pepper
2 Tbs. red wine vinegar
1 Tbs. white wine vinegar
1 Tbs. olive oil
2 tsp. Dijon mustard
3 cups cluster tomatoes (about 4 medium tomatoes), diced
½ yellow bell pepper, diced
2 Tbs. green onions, thinly sliced

Directions:

1. Bring water to a boil and add lentils, carrot, thyme, salt and pepper. Cover, reduce heat to low and let simmer until tender, about 25 minutes.
2. Drain lentil mix and transfer to a large bowl. Toss with red and white vinegars, olive oil, Dijon mustard, tomatoes, bell pepper and green onions.
3. Serve warm, or to serve cold, chill cooked lentils and toss with cold ingredients before serving.

Recipe supplied by:

GELSON'S THE Super MARKET

Gelson's Orange County locations:

Irvine: 5521 Alton Parkway, Irvine, CA 92618 (949) 551-6093
Dana Point: 24 Monarch Bay Plaza, Dana Pt., CA 92629 (949) 488-8147
Newport Beach: 1660 San Miguel Dr., Newport Beach, CA 92660 (949) 644-8660

at least 1 fruit/vegetable servings for side dishes

Apple Braised Salmon

with fine herbs, served over spinach.

Nutrition Information per Serving:

✓✓ Calories: Excellent Choice (390) ✓ Cholesterol: Good Choice (90 mg)
✓ Fat: Good Choice (17 g)♥ ✓✓ Sodium: Excellent Choice (195 mg)
Exchanges: 4¼ Meat, 2 Veg, ½ Fruit, 1¼ Fat
Protein: 38 g, Carbohydrate: 18 g, Fiber: 6 g

This nutrition analysis corresponds to the recipe below. The restaurant version may differ.
♥ primarily unsaturated fat

Ingredients (4 servings):

1½ lbs. salmon
1½ Tbs. vegetable oil
1 cup dry white wine or Riesling
1 cup apple juice
4 shallots, chopped
1 celery stalk, matchstick
1 carrot, matchstick
½ lb. (about 12) asparagus stalks
2 roma tomatoes, seeded and diced
1 oz. (about ½ cup) fresh herbs of your choice (parsley, tarragon, chives, etc.)
1 lb. fresh spinach

Directions:

1. Sauté presentation side of salmon in oil until golden. Pour off oil.
2. Turn salmon and add white wine and apple juice. Bring to a simmer, then cook for approximately one minute.
3. Place salmon and apple juice sauce in 400° oven and bake until salmon is just done.
4. Blanch shallots, celery, carrot and asparagus until almost done.
5. Wilt spinach (steam or microwave 30 to 60 seconds) and place evenly on four dinner plates. Place salmon on top of spinach.
6. Place apple juice sauce in sauté pan, and reduce for two minutes. Add blanched vegetables and then reduce heat. Add tomato and herbs. Continue to reduce to your liking (a thin broth or reduce further for a thicker sauce).
7. Spoon sauce and vegetables over salmon and serve.

Recipe supplied by:

Green Parrot Café
2035 North Main Street
Santa Ana, CA 92706
(714) 550-6040

at least 2 fruit/vegetable servings

BROILED SEABASS WITH TROPICAL FRUIT SALSA

Nutrition Information per Serving:

✓✓ CALORIES: Excellent Choice (340) ✓ CHOLESTEROL: Good Choice (115 mg)
✓✓ FAT: Excellent Choice (6 g)♥ ✓✓ SODIUM: Excellent Choice (270 mg)
EXCHANGES: 5½ Meat (extra lean), ¼ Veg, ¾ Fruit
PROTEIN: 55 g, CARBOHYDRATE: 15 g

This nutrition analysis corresponds to the recipe below. The restaurant version may differ.
♥Primarily unsaturated fat

Ingredients (6 servings):

½ cup red onion, diced
1 cup mango, chopped
1 cup papaya, chopped
1-2 jalapenos, seeded, diced
juice of ½ fresh lime
juice of ½ fresh orange
⅓ cup rice vinegar (or use seasoned rice vinegar which has higher sodium)
1 Tbs. fresh cilantro, chopped
¼ tsp. white pepper
½ tsp. salt (optional, not included in analysis)

6 seabass steaks, 8 oz. each

Directions:

1. Combine all ingredients except fish in bowl. Chill for 30 minutes.
2. Barbecue or broil seabass steaks.
3. Serve salsa on top of fish steaks.

Recipe supplied by:

BLUEWATER GRILL
SEAFOOD RESTAURANT
& OYSTER BAR

Bluewater Grill
630 Lido Park Drive
Newport Beach, CA 92663 (949) 675 3474
1621 W. Sunflower Avenue
Santa Ana, CA 92704 (714) 546-3474

Carmelized Halibut

Served with seasonal mixed vegetables.

Nutrition Information per Serving:

✓ Calories: Good Choice (550)
✓ Cholesterol: Good Choice (130 mg)
✓ Fat: Good Choice (25 g)
✓✓ Sodium: Excellent Choice (155 mg)
Exchanges: 5¾ Meat (extra lean), ¼ Bread, 1 Veg, 1¼ Other Carbs, 4¾ Fat
Protein: 49 g, Carbohydrate: 31 g, Fiber: 2 g

This nutrition analysis corresponds to the recipe below. The restaurant version may differ.

Ingredients (4 servings):

Carmelized Shallot Sauce

1 shallot, minced
¾ tsp. white wine
⅜ cup brown sugar
⅜ cup butter

Halibut & Vegetables

4 halibut steaks, 7 oz. each
3 large carrots, julienned
2 zucchini, julienned
½ red onion, sliced

Directions:

Carmelized Shallot Sauce:

1. Sauté shallots in ½ Tbs. butter. Add white wine and half of remaining butter and let butter melt.
2. Whisk in the brown sugar. Add remaining butter and stir until completely mixed. Keep warm until served.

Halibut and Vegetables:

1. Grill halibut or sauté with non-stick spray.
2. Steam vegetables lightly and arrange on plates beside halibut.
3. Drizzle Carmelized Shallot Sauce over halibut and enjoy!

Recipe supplied by:

BeachFire
204 Avenida Del Mar Suite D
San Clemente, CA 92672
(949) 366-3232

CHARBROILED FISH TACO

Nutrition Information per Serving:

✓✓ CALORIES: Excellent Choice (225) ✓✓ CHOLESTEROL: Excellent Choice (50 mg)
✓✓ FAT: Excellent Choice (4 g) ✓ SODIUM: Good Choice (340 mg)
EXCHANGES: 1¼ Meat, 1¾ Bread, ¼ Veg, ½ Fat
PROTEIN: 15 g, CARBOHYDRATE: 27 g, Fiber: 3g

This nutrition analysis corresponds to the recipe below. The restaurant version may differ.

Ingredients (4 servings):

½ lb. fresh mahi mahi fillets (¾-1 inch thick)
pinch of garlic salt
8 corn tortillas
1 oz. shredded cheese (Jack and/or cheddar)
2 oz. cabbage, shredded
4 oz. salsa
2 limes, quartered
cilantro (optional)

Directions:

1. Season fish with pinch of garlic salt.
2. Grill each side over medium heat until done. Divide into 4 portions.
3. Heat tortillas in pan and keep warm.
4. Fill tortillas with fish and top with cheese, cabbage, and salsa. In the restaurant the tacos are made using a double layer of corn tortillas. Alternatively, you can divide the filling evenly between all 8 tortillas to make 2 tacos per serving that contain less filling per taco.
5. Garnish with lime and cilantro.

Recipe supplied by:

Wahoo's Fish Taco locations:

Aliso Viejo, Costa Mesa, Fashion Island, Foothill Ranch (coming soon), Fullerton, Huntington Beach, Irvine, Irvine Spectrum, Laguna Beach, Lake Forest, San Clemente, South Coast Plaza, Tustin, and Yorba Linda.

Visit www.wahoos.com for a list of all Southern California locations!

Chef Mark Tydell's Grilled Pacific Swordfish

Nutrition Information per Serving:

✓✓ CALORIES: Excellent Choice (250)
✓✓ FAT: Excellent Choice (9 g)♥
✓✓ CHOLESTEROL: Excellent Choice (65 mg)
✓✓ SODIUM: Excellent Choice (260 mg)

EXCHANGES: 3¾ Meat, 1 Veg, ¼ Fat

PROTEIN: 36 g, CARBOHYDRATE: 5 g, FIBER: 3 g

This nutrition analysis corresponds to the recipe below. The restaurant version may differ.

♥ primarily unsaturated fat

Ingredients (4 servings):

Marinade:

½ cup low sodium soy sauce
½ cup extra virgin olive oil
20 turns fresh cracked pepper
2 stalks lemongrass, thinly sliced
2 tsp. fresh grated ginger
2 tsp. fresh diced garlic
⅓ cup lemon juice

Swordfish Meal:

1½ lb. swordfish steak
4 cups steamed vegetables (a mix of Asian vegetables is a good choice)

Directions:

1. Mix all marinade ingredients in a saucepan and bring to a boil for 1 minute. Cool.
2. Pour the cooled mixture over the swordfish steaks and marinate for at least 4 hours in the refrigerator. Drain and discard the marinade.
3. Divide swordfish into portions for 4 people. Grill the swordfish for approximately 4 or 5 minutes on each side, depending on the thickness.
4. Arrange swordfish and vegetables on plates and garnish if desired.

Recipe supplied by:

Walt's Wharf

201 Main Street
Seal Beach, CA 90740
(562) 598-4433

FRESH SEABASS TAQUITOS APPETIZER

Nutrition Information per Serving†:

✓✓ CALORIES: Excellent Choice (130) ✓✓ CHOLESTEROL: Excellent Choice (25 mg)
✓✓ FAT: Excellent Choice (2 g)♥ ✓✓ SODIUM: Excellent Choice (50 mg)
EXCHANGES: 1¾ Meat, 1 Bread, ½ Veg
PROTEIN: 13 g, CARBOHYDRATE: 16 g, FIBER: 2 g

This nutrition analysis corresponds to the recipe below. The restaurant version may differ.
♥ primarily unsaturated fat † Side dish guidelines are ⅓ of entree guidelines

Ingredients (4 servings):

1 cup shredded cabbage
1 Tbs. non-fat yogurt
juice from ¼ lemon
½ cup chopped tomato
2 Tbs. chopped onion
2 Tbs. chopped cilantro
⅛ tsp. Mexican seasoning
cooking spray*
8 oz. seabass
4 corn tortillas (6-inch) or 8 mini tortillas

Directions:

1. In a medium bowl, combine cabbage, yogurt, lemon juice, tomato, onion, cilantro and seasoning.
2. Spray a non-stick pan with cooking spray* and cook seabass about 1 minute on each side, or until done. Cut into slices.
3. Heat tortillas and roll with vegetable mix and fish.

*or use 1 Tbs. olive oil for cooking (adds 30 calories and 3 grams fat per serving).

Recipe supplied by:

Ranchos Cocina

Mexican & Vegetarian Cuisine

1830 Sunset Cliffs Blvd. #H, Ocean Beach (619) 226-7619
4705 Point Loma Ave., Ocean Beach (619) 224-9815
3910 30th St., San Diego (619) 574-1288

GRILLED ALASKAN HALIBUT

with basil marinated tomatoes and a light herb salad.

Nutrition Information per Serving:

✓✓ CALORIES: Excellent Choice (390) ✓✓ CHOLESTEROL: Excellent Choice (65 mg)
✓ FAT: Good Choice (19 g)♥ ✓ SODIUM: Good Choice (350 mg)
EXCHANGES: 4 Meat, 1½ Veg, 2¾ Fat
PROTEIN: 43 g, CARBOHYDRATE: 11 g, FIBER: 2 g

This nutrition analysis corresponds to the recipe below. The restaurant version may differ.
♥ primarily unsaturated fat

Ingredients (4 servings):

Basil Marinated Tomatoes

2 cups vine ripe cherry tomatoes, halved
¼ cup fresh basil, julienned
1 Tbs. shallots, finely diced
½ tsp. fresh garlic, minced
¼ cup red pepper puree
¼ cup extra virgin olive oil
pinch sea salt or kosher salt
fresh ground black pepper to taste
juice of 1 lemon

Herb Salad

½ bunch flat parsley, leaves only
¼ bunch fresh chives, cut 1½ inch long
¼ bunch fresh baby dill, small sprigs
¼ cup fresh basil, small leaves only
¼ cup fresh mint, small leaves only
1 baby fennel, shaved very thin

Halibut

4 halibut filets, 7 oz. each

Directions:

1. Core and cut the tomatoes and combine with other ingredients in first column in a stainless steel bowl. Cover with plastic wrap and hold in a warm place for several hours to extract juices from the tomatoes. Adjust seasoning if desired.
2. Prepare the salad ingredients and store in a bowl with a damp cloth.
3. Season the halibut with salt and pepper if desired (salt and pepper not included in analysis). Grill halibut filets or sauté in pan with ½ tsp. olive oil for approx. 4 to 5 minutes on each side.
4. To serve, place ½ cup Basil Marinated Tomatoes (with the juices) in the bottom of each of four large bowls. Rest the cooked halibut filets on top of the tomato mixture. Lightly dress the herb salad with a few drops of lemon juice and fresh ground black pepper, and arrange on top of the halibut and tomato mixtures.

Recipe supplied by:

SANTA MONICA SEAFOOD

Santa Monica Seafood

154 East 17th St., Costa Mesa, CA 92627 (949) 574-8862
424 South Main St., Suite F., Orange, CA 92868 (714) 456-0234
1205 Colorado Ave., Santa Monica, CA 90404 (310) 393-5244
Visit us on the web at www.smseafood.com

at least 2 fruit/vegetable servings

Salmon Atashi

With crushed tomato sauce and fresh pepper.

Nutrition Information per Serving:

✓✓ Calories: Excellent Choice (360) ✓ Cholesterol: Good Choice (90 mg)
✓ Fat: Good Choice (18 g)♥ ✓ Sodium: Good Choice (405 mg)
Exchanges: 4¼ Meat, 2¼ Veg, 1¼ Fat
Protein: 37 g, Carbohydrate: 13 g, Fiber: 5 g

This nutrition analysis corresponds to the recipe below. The restaurant version may differ.

Ingredients (4 servings):

1½ lbs. salmon
1½ lbs. fresh tomato
2 Tbs. olive oil
½ tsp. salt
2 tsp. black pepper
8 basil leaves, chopped
4 cups steamed vegetables (e.g. broccoli, carrots, cauliflower)

Directions:

1. Grill or bake salmon.
2. Puree or finely chop tomatoes
3. Heat oil in sauté pan. Add tomatoes. Sauté until tomatoes are hot. Lower heat and simmer several minutes. Add salt, pepper, and basil leaves.
4. Steam vegetables, mix with sauce in sauté pan, and heat through.
5. Place mixture over salmon and serve.

Recipe supplied by:

FERDUSSI
TASTE OF PERSIA

Ferdussi Taste of Persia
3605 S. Bristol St., Santa Ana, CA 92704
at MacArthur Blvd., one block north of South Coast Plaza
(714) 545-9096

SAUTÉED BLUENOSE BASS
(OR OTHER WHITE FISH)

with garlic, red onion, tomatoes, artichoke hearts, mushrooms, basil and wine.

Nutrition Information per Serving:

✓✓ CALORIES: Excellent Choice (380)
✓ CHOLESTEROL: Good Choice (80 mg)
✓✓ FAT: Excellent Choice (10 g)♥
✓✓ SODIUM: Excellent Choice (290 mg)

EXCHANGES: 5¾ Meat (extra lean), 3¼ Veg, 1 Fat
PROTEIN: 44 g, CARBOHYDRATE: 21 g, Fiber: 9 g

This nutrition analysis corresponds to the recipe below. The restaurant version may differ.
♥primarily unsaturated fat

Ingredients (4 servings):

4 tsp. olive oil
8 cloves fresh garlic, crushed
8 slices red onion
4 bluenose bass filets, 7 oz. each, or other type of white fish
4 roma tomatoes, diced
4 artichoke hearts, quartered
16 mushrooms, sliced
12 leaves of fresh basil
1 cup chardonnay wine
⅛ tsp. pepper
⅛ tsp. salt
1 bunch asparagus, steamed

Directions:

1. Heat oil in pan. Sauté the garlic, onions and mushrooms.
2. Add fish and one half of the wine, and cook fish on one side.
3. Flip fish and add remaining ingredients.
4. Cook for 4 minutes or until the fish is done.
5. Serve with steamed asparagus on the side.

Recipe supplied by:

The Beach House

619 Sleepy Hollow Lane, Laguna Beach, CA 92651 (949) 494-9707
25001 Dana Drive, Dana Point, CA 92629 (949) 496-7310

at least 2 fruit/vegetable servings

SEARED BLACKENED AHI

Served rare with Cajun spices, pickled ginger and wasabi.

Nutrition Information per Serving:

✓✓ CALORIES: Excellent Choice (175)
✓✓ CHOLESTEROL: Excellent Choice (50 mg)
✓✓ FAT: Excellent Choice (2 g)♥
SODIUM: High (1680 mg)
EXCHANGES: 3½ Meat, ¼ Veg, ¾ Fruit
PROTEIN: 31 g, CARBOHYDRATE: 9 g, FIBER: 1 g

This nutrition analysis corresponds to the recipe below. The restaurant version may differ.
♥Primarily unsaturated fat

Ingredients (4 servings):

1 Tbs. paprika
1¼ tsp. onion powder
1¼ tsp. garlic powder
¼ Tbs. white pepper
¼ Tbs. black pepper
1¼ Tbs. thyme
½ Tbs. oregano
1¼ tsp. cayenne pepper
½ tsp. salt
1 lb. ahi tuna, sashimi quality
cooking spray
4 tsp. ginger root, grated
1 oz. pickled ginger
1 oz. wasabi
½ cup soy sauce, reduced sodium

Directions:

1. Combine dry seasonings (first 9 ingredients) and mix thoroughly.
2. Coat both sides of tuna with seasoning mix, shaking off excess.
3. Heat a cast-iron skillet over high heat with exhaust fan on.
4. Spray tuna with nonstick spray and place in super-hot pan.
5. Sear fish about 1 minute on all sides. Do not overcook. Fish should be rare or medium-rare.
6. Slice thinly and fan on plate.
7. Serve with soy sauce mixed with grated ginger in a small bowl, pickled ginger and wasabi.

Recipe supplied by:

McCORMICK&SCHMICK'S SEAFOOD RESTAURANT

McCormick & Schmick's Seafood Restaurant

2000 Main Street, Irvine, CA 92614 (949) 756-0505

Camarones a la Mexicana

Giant shrimp in a tomato sauce.

Nutrition Information per Serving:

✓✓ Calories: Excellent Choice (245) Cholesterol: Moderate (295 mg)
✓✓ Fat: Excellent Choice (7 g)♥ ✓ Sodium: Good Choice (360 mg)
Exchanges: 4½ Meat (extra lean), 1½ Veg, 1 Fat
Protein: 34 g, Carbohydrate: 13 g, Fiber: 2 g

This nutrition analysis corresponds to the recipe below. The restaurant version may differ.
♥ Primarily unsaturated fat

Ingredients (6 servings):

2 Tbs. olive oil
¾ cup onion, chopped
3 cloves garlic, minced
2 lbs. tomatoes, peeled, seeded, and chopped
½ Tbs. pepper
2 bay leaves
5½ Tbs. thyme
salt to taste (not included in analysis)
1–2 Tbs. juice from chilies gueros (below)
2 lbs. shrimp (16–20/lb size)
2 Tbs. buttermilk
3 Tbs. parsley, chopped
chiles gueros (or other chiles) to taste for garnish (not included in analysis)

Directions:

1. Heat oil in large pan. Add onions and garlic and cook for about 2 minutes until golden and transparent.
2. Add tomatoes and cook over medium heat for about 5 minutes, constantly stirring.
3. Add pepper, laurel, thyme, chile juice and salt to taste (salt not included in analysis).
4. Cover and cook on low for about 5 minutes.
5. Coat another pan with non-stick cooking spray and heat over medium heat. Add shrimp and cook for two minutes.
6. Add the shrimp to the sauce and cook for about 3-4 minutes or until heated through and shrimp is completely cooked. Add buttermilk and stir.
7. To serve, divide shrimp & sauce mixture into 6 equal portions. Place each serving on a warm dish and sprinkle with parsley. If desired, garnish with chiles gueros.

Recipe supplied by:

El Callejon Restaurant

345 South Coast Highway 101
Encinitas, CA 92024
(760) 634-2793
www.el-callejon.com

at least 2 fruit/vegetable servings

CIOPPINO ⍥

Nutrition Information per Serving:

✓ CALORIES: Good Choice (590) CHOLESTEROL: Moderate (205 mg)
✓ FAT: Good Choice (20 g)♥ SODIUM: High (1515 mg)
EXCHANGES: 6¾ Meat, 2 Veg, 2½ Fat
PROTEIN: 64 g, CARBOHYDRATE: 39 g, FIBER: 8 g

This nutrition analysis corresponds to the recipe below. The restaurant version may differ.
♥ primarily unsaturated fat

Ingredients (2 servings):

Base

½ Tbs. olive oil
16 cloves garlic, minced
¼ small onion, chopped
⅔ cup mushrooms, sliced
¼ green bell pepper, chopped
1 medium to large tomato, diced
½ cup tomato sauce
3 Tbs. clam juice
⅓ cup red wine
½ Tbs. oregano
½ tsp. black pepper
⅓ tsp. salt

Cioppino

3 oz. prawns (about 4 medium 21/25)
4 oz. dungeness crab
8 mussels
8 small clams
8 oz. assorted fish
1 Tbs. olive oil
¼ cup white wine
2 tsp. minced garlic
2 tsp. minced shallots

Directions:

Base:
1. In a saucepan, heat the oil, add garlic, onion, mushrooms, and bell pepper. Cook until soft.
2. Add tomatoes, tomato sauce, clam juice, wine, and flavorings, cover and simmer for 45 minutes.

Cioppino:
1. Cook the seafood and fish.
3. Sauté garlic and shallots in olive oil. Add white wine and reduce.
4. Add the base (above), heat and serve.

Recipe supplied by:

McKenna's on the Bay
190 Marina Drive
Long Beach, CA 90803
(562) 342-9411

⍥ at least 2 fruit/vegetable servings

JUMBO SEA SCALLOPS

Pan seared scallops with watercress, new potatoes, sun dried tomatoes & green goddess dressing.

Nutrition Information per Serving:

✓ CALORIES: Good Choice (660) — CHOLESTEROL: Moderate (165 mg)
✓ FAT: Good Choice (20 g)♥ — SODIUM: High (1300 mg)
EXCHANGES: 2¾ Meat, 3 Bread, 4½ Veg, 3 Fat
PROTEIN: 44 g, CARBOHYDRATE: 86 g, FIBER: 9 g

This nutrition analysis corresponds to the recipe below. The restaurant version may differ.
♥ primarily unsaturated fat

Ingredients (4 servings):

1¼ lb. scallops
2 eggs
4 Tbs. flour
2 Tbs. oil
½ cup panko (Japanese) breadcrumbs
4 new potatoes (8 oz.)
½ bunch raw watercress (approx. 2 cups)
1 medium large tomato, diced
4 oz. sun dried tomatoes, diced

Green Goddess Dressing
½ bunch watercress
2 to 3 leaves fresh basil
2 Tbs. lemon juice
¼ tsp. salt
1½ cups olive oil
pepper to taste

Directions:

Scallops: Whip eggs. Dip scallops in flour, then egg, then breadcrumbs. Add oil to sauté pan and heat. Sauté scallops for 3 minutes on each side.

New Potatoes: Steam or boil.

Dressing: Place all ingredients in blender except the oil. Blend ingredients together, adding a little oil at a time until all oil is mixed in.

Assembling the dish:

1. Clean the watercress and place in the center of each of four plates.
2. Top watercress with diced tomato.
3. Slice the potatoes into "coins." Place each cooked scallop on a potato "coin" and arrange around the plate. Sprinkle sun dried tomatoes on top of scallops.
4. Drizzle 1 Tbs. dressing over each dish. Save remaining dressing for future use.

Recipe supplied by:

G5–Georges on Fifth
835 Fifth Ave, San Diego, CA 92101
(619) 702-0444

at least 2 fruit/vegetable servings

LITE GINGER WINE SHRIMP

Classic light sauce with shrimp, ginger, snow peas, water chestnuts, carrots and Chinese wine.

Nutrition Information per Serving:

✓✓ CALORIES: Excellent Choice (435) CHOLESTEROL: Moderate (290 mg)
✓✓ FAT: Excellent Choice (2 g)♥ SODIUM: Moderate (685 mg)
EXCHANGES: 4½ Meat (extra lean), 1 Bread, 5½ Veg
PROTEIN: 35 g, CARBOHYDRATE: 67 g, FIBER: 13 g

This nutrition analysis corresponds to the recipe below. The restaurant version may differ.
** Sodium can be reduced by using less salt in the White Ginger Sauce.

Ingredients (2 servings):

Shrimp Mixture

1¼ Tbs. corn starch
1 egg white
10 oz. shrimp
4 oz. (about 1 cup) snow peas
3 carrots, thinly sliced and blanched
6 oz. water chestnuts
2 Tbs. thinly sliced fresh ginger
1 Tbs. corn starch
¼ cup rice wine

White Ginger Sauce

1 cup hot water
½ green onion, sliced
1 tsp. thinly sliced ginger
1 Tbs. sugar
½ Tbs. rice wine
½ tsp. salt
¼ tsp. chicken powder
pinch minced garlic
pinch white pepper

Directions:

1. Whip egg white and mix in corn starch.
2. Marinate shrimp in egg white mixture for at least 2 hours in the refrigerator.
3. For White Ginger Sauce, mix all ingredients into the hot water and allow to stand for 30 to 40 minutes. Strain mixture.
4. Put marinated shrimp into boiling water for approximately 60 seconds. Add vegetables to water for another 15 seconds. Strain shrimp and vegetables. Discard remaining egg white marinade mixture.
5. Mix 1 Tbs. corn starch with 1 Tbs. water.
6. Put ginger into wok, add White Ginger Sauce and heat quickly to boiling.
7. Add shrimp and vegetables.
8. Add corn starch mixture and stir until mixture thickens. Add wine and stir another 10 seconds to finish cooking. Transfer to platter to serve.

Recipe supplied by:

CAFÉ Chin Chin
ASIAN FAST CASUAL

Café Chin Chin
Lakewood Mall: Candlewood Restaurant Row (562) 616-7171
Tustin Market Place: 2945 El Camino Real (714) 689-3131

Lobster Tacos

with roasted corn salsa, black beans and tortillas. Analysis includes 2 tacos per person.

Nutrition Information per Serving (2 tacos):

✓✓ Calories: Excellent Choice (355) ✓✓ Cholesterol: Excellent Choice (60 mg)
✓✓ Fat: Excellent Choice (4 g)♥ Sodium: High (1255 mg)
Exchanges: 2 Meat (extra lean), 3 Bread, ½ Veg, ½ Fat
Protein: 28 g, Carbohydrate: 53 g, Fiber: 10 g

This nutrition analysis corresponds to the recipe below. The restaurant version may differ.
♥ primarily unsaturated fat

Ingredients (4 servings):

½ Tbs. oil
2 tsp garlic, crushed
4 tsp shallots, minced
12 oz. lobster meat
1 cup salsa
4 oz. corn (about 2 ears)
¼ cup cilantro, chopped
1 cup tomatoes, diced
1½ cups cooked black beans
8 corn tortillas

Directions:

1. Roast corn (either on the cob on the BBQ and then remove from cob, or boil/steam corn and then briefly broil in oven).
2. In a hot sauté pan, sauté garlic and shallots in oil. Add lobster and cook for about 1 minute.
3. Add salsa, roasted corn, and cilantro. Sauté until lobster meat is cooked, but still tender (overcooked lobster can be very tough).
4. Heat black beans. Warm tortillas. Spoon black beans, lobster, and tomatoes into corn tortillas. If you'd like, you can use 2 tortillas for each taco (only one tortilla per taco included in analysis).

Recipe supplied by:

Pacific Coast Grill

Pacific Coast Grill
437 South Highway 101
Solana Beach, CA 92075
(858) 794-4632

PASTA ANGELICA WITH SCALLOPS

Angel hair pasta tossed with scallops, pesto, garlic and tomatoes.

Nutrition Information per Serving:

✓ CALORIES Good Choice (610) ✓✓ CHOLESTEROL: Excellent Choice (40 mg)
✓ FAT: Good Choice (17 g)♥ ✓ SODIUM: Good Choice (540 mg)
EXCHANGES: 2¾ Meat (extra lean), 4¼ Bread, 2¼ Veg, 3 Fat
PROTEIN: 33 g, CARBOHYDRATE: 80 g, FIBER: 5 g

This nutrition analysis corresponds to the recipe below. The restaurant version may differ.
♥primarily unsaturated fat

Ingredients (4 servings):

12 oz. angel hair pasta (dry weight)
2 Tbs. olive oil
2 – 8 Tbs. Garlic, pureed or minced
1 lb. (2 cups) scallops (or rock shrimp)
½ cup red wine vinegar
2 cups stewed tomatoes, pureed, or tomato sauce
¼ cup pesto sauce
2 Tbs. fresh chopped parsley

Directions:

1. Cook pasta according to instructions. Drain.
2. Place oil, garlic, 1 Tbs. of the parsley, and scallops in a sauté pan. Sauté on medium heat for several minutes.
3. Add red wine vinegar and reduce for approximately one minute.
4. Add tomato puree and pesto. Mix well.
5. Add pasta and stir to distribute sauce completely.
6. Garnish with parsley. Serve and enjoy!

Recipe supplied by:

The Fish Market
85 Fortune Drive #329
Irvine, CA 92615
(949) 727-FISH (3474)

at least 2 fruit/vegetable servings

CHICKEN BREAST A LA PROVENCAL

Roasted breast of chicken served with olives, sweet garlic and tomatoes and garnished with steamed asparagus.

Nutrition Information per Serving:

✓ CALORIES: Good Choice (530) | CHOLESTEROL: Moderate (180 mg)
✓ FAT: Good Choice (19 g) | SODIUM: Moderate (840 mg)
EXCHANGES: 9 Meat (extra lean), 1½ Veg, ¼ Other Carbs, 2¾ Fat
PROTEIN: 69 g, CARBOHYDRATE: 18 g, FIBER: 5 g

This nutrition analysis corresponds to the recipe below. The restaurant version may differ.

Ingredients (4 servings):

4 chicken breast filets, 8 oz. each
1 Tbs. extra virgin olive oil
16 garlic cloves, blanched in milk for 3 min.
2 medium tomatoes, diced
8 oz. pitted black olives, halved
4 oz. (¼ cup) dry Chardonnay
10 oz. chicken stock or bouillon
1 tsp. olive oil
salt & pepper (optional)
1 lb. asparagus, steamed
fresh herbs of your choice (garnish)

Directions:

1. Season chicken with salt and pepper if desired (not included in analysis).
2. Sauté the chicken in olive oil until golden color. Remove any fat from the pan.
3. Add tomatoes, garlic, olives and fresh herbs into the pan with the chicken breasts.
4. Add wine and chicken stock.
5. Heat oven to 400° and braise chicken for about 12 minutes. Remove chicken from pan.
6. Reduce the sauce to ⅓ (over medium heat on stove top). Add olive oil to sauce.
7. Place warm chicken onto plates and pour hot sauce over.
8. Garnish with asparagus and fresh herbs.

Recipe supplied by:

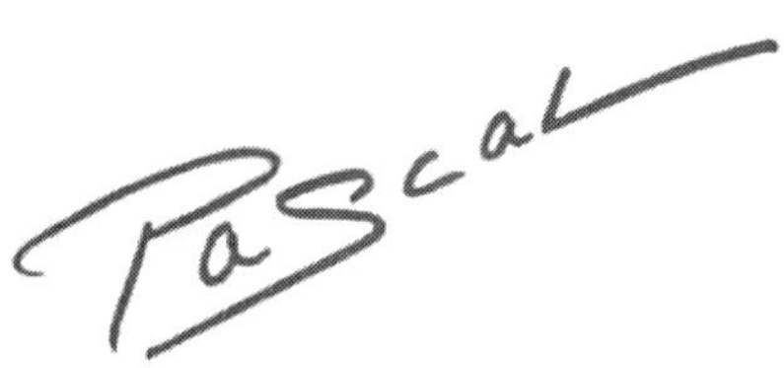

Pascal Restaurant/Epicerie & Wine
1000 Bristol Street
Newport Beach, CA 92660
(949) 752-0107/ (949) 261-9041

at least 2 fruit/vegetable servings

CHICKEN MARENGO

Delicious tomato and mushroom sauce served over chicken breasts and brown rice.

Nutrition Information per Serving:

✓✓ CALORIES: Excellent Choice (345) ✓ CHOLESTEROL: Good Choice (100 mg)
✓✓ FAT: Excellent Choice (3 g) ✓✓ SODIUM: Excellent Choice (170 mg)
PROTEIN: 44 g, CARBOHYDRATE: 31 g, FIBER: 3 g

This nutrition analysis corresponds to the recipe below. The restaurant version may differ.
Nutrition information supplied by Susan's Healthy Gourmet.

Ingredients (4 servings):

4 chicken breasts, 6 oz. each, skinless
Pam cooking spray
2 Tbs. cooking sherry
1½ cups chicken stock
1½ cups fresh mushrooms
2 Tbs. flour
2 Tbs. water
1 Tbs. tomato paste
1 bay leaf
2 Tbs. chives
⅛ tsp. black pepper
3 roma tomatoes, chopped in large chunks
2 cups cooked brown rice

Directions:

1. Sear chicken breasts in skillet sprayed with Pam. Remove from heat and place in shallow baking dish.
2. Pour sherry over chicken and cover with aluminum foil. Bake until tender, 20 to 30 minutes or until temperature is 165°.
3. Add ¼ cup chicken broth to skillet and sauté mushrooms until tender. Remove and save.
4. Combine flour and water, stirring until smooth. Add to skillet with remaining chicken broth, heat and stir until thickened.
5. Add tomato paste, bay leaf, chives and pepper. Simmer 15 minutes. Remove bay leaf.
6. Add mushrooms and chopped tomatoes and simmer another 5 minutes.
7. Pour over chicken breasts and brown rice.

Recipe supplied by:

SUSAN'S Healthy Gourmet
fresh · delicious · delivered

Susan's Healthy Gourmet
(949) 833-2929, 1-888-EZ-MEALS (396-3257)
www.susanshealthygourmet.com
Conveniently located pick-up locations throughout Orange County.

CHICKEN VERMICELLI ♁

Glass noodles with chicken breast, asparagus, carrots and red onion.

Nutrition Information per Serving:

✓ CALORIES: Good Choice (525) ✓ CHOLESTEROL: Good Choice (100 mg)
✓✓ FAT: Excellent Choice (9 g) ✓✓ SODIUM: Excellent Choice (120 mg)
EXCHANGES: 5 Meat (extra lean), 3¾ Bread, 2¼ Veg, 1 Fat
PROTEIN: 39 g, CARBOHYDRATE: 69 g, FIBER: 5 g

This nutrition analysis corresponds to the recipe below. The restaurant version may differ.

Ingredients (2 servings):

4 cups soaked vermicelli (glass noodles)
2 tsp. olive oil
½ lb. chicken breasts, skinless
2 tsp. olive oil
½ red onion, sliced
2 carrots, sliced
4 to 6 stalks asparagus, sliced
¼ cup white wine
¼ cup chicken stock, low sodium
Salt & pepper to taste
(not included in analysis)

Directions:

1. Soak vermicelli in hot water according to package instructions. Rinse and drain.
2. Grill or sauté chicken breast with olive oil until almost done and then slice.
3. Sauté red onions and carrots in olive oil in large hot pan for about one minute.
4. Add asparagus & chicken and sauté for one additional minute or until vegetables are done.
5. Add wine and chicken stock, bring to boil to reduce alcohol.
6. Mix in vermicelli, season with salt & pepper (optional), and serve immediately.

Recipe supplied by:

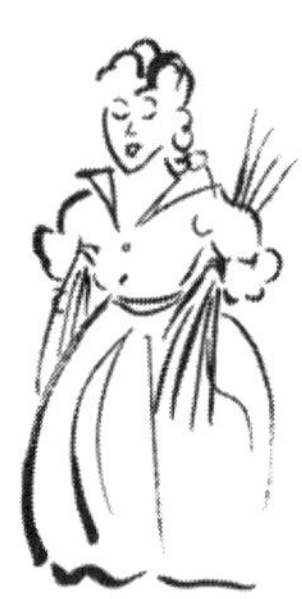

Luciana's Ristorante
24312 Del Prado (PCH)
Dana Point, CA 92629
(949) 661-6500

♁ at least 2 fruit/vegetable servings

CULINARY WRAP

Chicken, lettuce, tomatoes, red onion, avocado, Jack cheese & creamy vinaigrette.

Nutrition Information per Serving:

✓✓ CALORIES: Excellent Choice (435) ✓✓ CHOLESTEROL: Excellent Choice (75 mg)
✓✓ FAT: Excellent Choice (13 g) SODIUM: Moderate (750 mg)
EXCHANGES: 3¾ Meat, 2¼ Bread, ¾ Veg, ½ Fruit, 1½ Fat
PROTEIN: 35 g, CARBOHYDRATE: 47 g, FIBER: 7 g

This nutrition analysis corresponds to the recipe below. The restaurant version may differ.

Ingredients (4 servings):

2 chicken breasts, 6 oz. each
1 clove garlic, crushed or minced
pinch salt and pepper (optional)
4 cups romaine lettuce, broken or cut
1 medium tomato, diced
¾ cup chopped red onion
½ avocado, sliced or chopped
6 Tbs. creamy Italian dressing
2 oz. grated Jack cheese
4 tortilla/wrappers or
4 pita bread, cut in half

Directions:

1. Season chicken with garlic, salt and pepper (optional, not included in analysis). Grill about 15 minutes until done and cut into ¾ inch squares.
2. Toss the lettuce, tomatoes, red onions, chicken, avocado and Italian dressing. Add Jack cheese and toss lightly.
3. Warm each tortilla, wrapper, or pita for 30 seconds.
4. Fill each wrapper with ¼ of mixture (or each pita slice with 1/8 of mixture), cut in half, and serve.

Recipe supplied by:

The Culinary Wrap

Brea (Brea Union Plaza):
2435 E. Imperial Hwy., Suite E (714) 672-9727

Costa Mesa (Hillgren Square):
250 E. 17th St., Suite D (949) 548-4403

Cal State Long Beach on campus (49ER Shops):
6049 E. 7th St. (562) 494-9727

KARAHI CHICKEN

Chicken breast with a light Karahi sauce of garlic, tomatoes, olive oil and herbs.

Nutrition Information per Serving:

✓✓ CALORIES: Excellent Choice (355) ✓ CHOLESTEROL: Good Choice (130 mg)
✓✓ FAT: Excellent Choice (10 g) ✓✓ SODIUM: Excellent Choice (140 mg)
EXCHANGES: 6¾ Meat, 2¼ Veg, ¾ Fat
PROTEIN: 51 g, CARBOHYDRATE: 15 g, FIBER: 3 g

This nutrition analysis corresponds to the recipe below. The restaurant version may differ.

Ingredients (4 servings):

1½ lbs. chicken breast, skinless
2 lbs. tomatoes
4 red chilies
½ Tbs. coriander seeds
1 Tbs. extra virgin olive oil
1 Tbs. garlic paste
4 green chilies, deseeded & chopped
2 Tbs. chopped ginger
1 cup fresh chopped cilantro
1 tsp. dry fenugreek
1 tsp. garam masala (Indian spice available in many specialty stores)

Directions:

1. Clean chicken and cut each breast into 1 to 1½ inch pieces.
2. Wash tomatoes, then remove skin, chop and coarsely puree.
3. Remove stems from the chilies. Wash, slit, deseed and chop.
4. Pound the red chilies and coriander seeds with a pestle.
5. Heat oil in a Karahi (Indian wok). Add garlic paste and sauté over medium heat until light brown.
6. Add the pounded seeds, stir for 30 seconds and then add the tomatoes.
7. Bring to a boil, add green chilies, ¾ of the ginger and a third of the chopped cilantro. Reduce heat and simmer for 4 to 5 minutes.
8. Add chicken and bring to a boil. Simmer, stirring occasionally, until the gravy becomes thick and the chicken is tender.
9. Sprinkle garam masala and fenugreek into the mixture, and stir for one minute. Adjust seasoning, if desired.
10. Serve and garnish with remaining ginger and cilantro. Serve with Indian bread of your choice (not included in analysis).

Recipe supplied by:

Royal Khyber
FINE INDIAN CUISINE

Royal Khyber
South Coast Village Plaza
1621 W. Sunflower Ave., Santa Ana
(714) 436-1010

LETTUCE WRAPS WITH PLUM SAUCE 🍎

Nutrition Information per Serving:

✓ CALORIES: Good Choice (495) ✓ CHOLESTEROL: Good Choice (130 mg)
✓✓ FAT: Excellent Choice (10 g) SODIUM: Moderate (865 mg)
EXCHANGES: 6¾ Meat (extra lean), ½ Bread, 6¼ Veg, ¼ Fruit, ½ Fat
PROTEIN: 58 g, CARBOHYDRATE: 47 g, FIBER: 12 g

This nutrition analysis corresponds to the recipe below. The restaurant version may differ.

Ingredients (2 servings):

Plum Sauce

¼ cup plum sauce (commercially bottled)
2 Tbs. hoisin sauce
1 tsp. sesame oil
pinch crushed red pepper
¼ tsp. ginger
1 Tbs. soy sauce
1 tsp. orange juice
1 green onion, sliced

Lettuce Wraps

2 chicken breasts, 6 oz. each
1 head of lettuce
2 cups shredded carrots
2 cups bean sprouts
1 cucumber, sliced into thin strips

Directions:

1. For the plum sauce, combine all ingredients and blend well.
2. Grill chicken and slice into thin strips.
3. Remove the larger leaves from the head of lettuce (about ½ of the head) for this recipe. Discard smaller leaves or save for another use.
4. Place lettuce leaves, chicken strips, carrots, sprouts and cucumber in sections on plates.
5. Serve sauce on the side. Each person can prepare his/her own wraps and dip in sauce or spread sauce within the lettuce wraps.

Recipe supplied by:

Newport Beach Brewing Co.
2920 Newport Blvd.
Newport Beach
(949) 675-8449

Mushroom Chicken

Nutrition Information per Serving:

✓✓ Calories: Excellent Choice (175) ✓✓ Cholesterol: Excellent Choice (60 mg)
✓✓ Fat: Excellent Choice (2 g) ✓✓ Sodium: Excellent Choice (145 mg)
Exchanges: 3¼ Meat (extra lean), ½ Bread, 1¼ Veg
Protein: 26 g, Carbohydrate: 12 g, Fiber: 2 g

This nutrition analysis corresponds to the recipe below. The restaurant version may differ.

Ingredients (2 servings):

7 oz. white meat chicken, diced
2 oz. cut carrots (½ cup)
2 oz. cut zucchini (½ cup)
6 oz. sliced mushrooms (2 cups)
1 green onion, chopped
2 Tbs. white cooking wine
⅜ cup chicken broth (no salt added)
pinch each, garlic & ginger
dash white pepper
1 Tbs. corn starch
1 Tbs. water
drop sesame oil

Directions:

1. Blanch or steam chicken, carrots, zucchini, and mushrooms, and set aside.
2. In sauté pan, combine green onion, wine, broth, garlic, ginger and pepper and heat until almost boiling.
3. Mix cornstarch with water.
4. Add chicken-vegetable mix and cornstarch mix to sauté pan and cook 1 to 2 minutes until cornstarch is thickened.
5. Add drop of sesame oil for flavor.

Recipe supplied by:

Pick Up Stix

with 23 Orange County locations.
Please visit www.pickupstix.com
for the location nearest you.

at least 2 fruit/vegetable servings

Poblano Turkey Chili

The creative blending of mild poblano and pasilla peppers enriches the character of this healthy, substantive chili reminiscent of Mexican mole. Analysis for 8oz. (cup) serving.

Nutrition Information per Serving:

✓✓ Calories: Excellent Choice (215) ✓ Cholesterol: Good Choice (95 mg)
✓✓ Fat: Excellent Choice (4 g) ✓ Sodium: Good Choice (410 mg)
Exchanges: 5 Meat, 1¼ Veg, ½ Fat
Protein: 36 g, Carbohydrate: 9 g, Fiber: 2 g

This nutrition analysis corresponds to the recipe below. The restaurant version may differ.

Ingredients (12 servings):

2 Tbs. vegetable oil
2 large yellow onions, coarsely chopped
3 lbs. ground white meat turkey (no skin)
4 Tbs. ground Pasilla chili powder
2 whole poblano chile peppers, seeded & coarsely chopped
4 cloves garlic, minced
1 Tbs. ground cumin
1 can (28 oz.) chopped tomatoes with liquid
1 tsp each salt and pepper

Directions:

For best results, use heavy sauce pan or dutch oven with lid.

1. Sauté the chopped onions in vegetable oil until slightly softened (excess oil will be removed later in process).
2. Add ground turkey and Poblano chile and continue to cook with onions while stirring frequently until turkey is "crumbly".
3. Cover with water and bring to a low boil.
4. Add Pasilla chile powder, garlic, salt and pepper.
5. Reduce heat to simmer, partially cover with lid and continue to simmer for about one hour.
6. Skim any residual fat from surface, stir and continue to cook for 10 minutes*.
7. Serve with fresh scallions and cilantro.

* For a slightly "thicker chili, after defatting, add 3 Tbs. corn masa flour or 2 Tbs. cornstarch diluted with warm water. Masa flour or cornstarch not included in analysis.

Recipe supplied by:

Chili My Soul

4928 Balboa Blvd.
Encino, CA 91316
(818) 981-SOUL (7685)

Capellini al Pomodoro Fresco

Nutrition Information per Serving:

✓ Calories: Good Choice (475)
✓✓ Cholesterol: Excellent Choice (0 mg)
✓ Fat: Good Choice (16 g)♥
✓✓ Sodium: Excellent Choice (20 mg)

Exchanges: 4 Bread, 1¼ Veg, 2¾ Fat

Protein: 12 g, Carbohydrate: 71 g, Fiber: 4 g

This nutrition analysis corresponds to the recipe below. The restaurant version may differ.

♥ primarily unsaturated fat

Ingredients (4 servings):

12 oz. capellini pasta (dry weight)
1 lb. fresh ripe Roma tomatoes
¼ cup olive oil
4 cloves garlic, thinly sliced
½ cup chopped fresh basil leaves
⅛ tsp. pepper
salt to taste (not included in analysis)
grated parmesan or romano cheese (optional, not included in analysis)

Directions:

1. Remove skins from tomatoes by piercing with a paring knife on the tip and then putting in boiling water for 15 to 20 seconds. Drain, peel and dice the tomatoes and set aside.
2. Cook the pasta according to package instructions.
3. While pasta is cooking, sauté the garlic, tomatoes, and basil over medium heat until almost cooked. Add salt to taste (optional, not included in analysis) & pepper.
4. When the pasta is cooked "al dente," rinse, drain and place back in cooking pan.
5. Add the tomato mix, toss well, and serve.
6. Sprinkle with grated cheese (optional, not included in analysis).

Recipe supplied by:

Pane e Vino

240 S. Brea Blvd., Brea, CA 92821
(714) 256-7779 www.panevino.biz

CHICKEN CREOLE PASTA

Chicken breast meat in a spicy blend of peppers, onions, tomatoes, Cajun seasonings & penne pasta.

Nutrition Information per Serving:

✓ CALORIES: Good Choice (610) CHOLESTEROL: Moderate (165 mg)
✓ FAT: Good Choice (17 g) ✓ SODIUM: Good Choice (450 mg)
EXCHANGES: 6¾ Meat (extra lean), 2½ Bread, 2½ Veg, 1¾ Fat
PROTEIN: 60 g, CARBOHYDRATE: 56 g, FIBER: 6 g

This nutrition analysis corresponds to the recipe below. The restaurant version may differ.

Ingredients (4 servings):

Creole Sauce

2 Tbs. butter
½ Tbs. minced garlic
2 cups chopped yellow onions
2 green bell peppers, chopped
2 red bell peppers, chopped
1 Tbs. Cajun spice or to taste
pinch cayenne pepper
1 cup low-sodium chicken broth
½ cup diced tomatoes

Entrée

1½ lbs. chicken breast, skinless
8 oz. penne pasta (dry weight)
1 Tbs. butter
6 oz. mushrooms (2½ cups), sliced
½ cup low-sodium chicken broth
2 tsp. chopped parsley for garnish

Directions:

Creole Sauce:

1. Melt butter in stockpot or kettle. Add garlic, onions and green and red bell peppers. Stir occasionally until onions are translucent.
2. Add Cajun spice and cayenne pepper and stir well.
3. Add chicken broth and diced tomatoes and stir well.
4. Cook over medium heat until volume is reduced by half. Sauce will thicken during this time (approx. 15 to 20 minutes). Remove from stove and cool.

Entrée:

1. Cook chicken until almost done. Slice into ½ inch slices.
2. Cook pasta according to package instructions. Drain well.
3. Melt butter in a sauté pan. Add mushrooms and chicken and cook until mushrooms lose their raw appearance.
4. Add Creole Sauce and chicken broth. Add pasta and toss well to coat.
5. Cook until all ingredients are hot. Place on plates or pasta bowls with a twisting motion to mound ingredients in the center of the plate/bowl. Garnish with parsley.

Recipe supplied by:

Vie de France
3333 Bristol Ave. #1420 South Coast Plaza
Costa Mesa, CA 92626
(714) 557-1734

at least 2 fruit/vegetable servings

ITALIAN COUNTRY LINGUINI

Nutrition Information per Serving:

✓✓ CALORIES: Excellent Choice (340) ✓✓ CHOLESTEROL: Excellent Choice (5 mg)
✓✓ FAT: Excellent Choice (6 g) SODIUM: Moderate (685 mg)
EXCHANGES: ½ Meat, 3 Bread, 1¾ Veg, ¾ Fat
PROTEIN: 12 g, CARBOHYDRATE: 55 g, FIBER: 5

This nutrition analysis corresponds to the recipe below. The restaurant version may differ.

Ingredients (4 servings):

8 oz. linguini (dry weight)
1 Tbs. olive oil
4 Tbs. garlic, minced
4 tomatoes, chopped
1½ oz. lean ham, chopped into bite-size pieces
1¼ cup mushrooms, chopped
½ tsp. salt
2 tsp. black pepper
¾ cup chicken broth
½ cup white wine
2 Tbs. oregano
4 orange slices, twisted (garnish)
2 Tbs. green onion, finely chopped (garnish)

Directions:

1. Cook pasta according to package directions until al dente.
2. Heat a separate sauté pan over medium heat. Add olive oil, minced garlic, tomatoes, ham, mushrooms, chicken broth and white wine.
3. Cook until mushrooms are tender and alcohol has evaporated.
4. Season with salt, pepper and oregano.
5. Toss pasta with sauce and portion onto 4 dishes.
6. Garnish each dish with an orange twist and green onion.

Recipe supplied by:

Lino's Italian Restaurant

Lino's
Bazaar del Mundo Old Town
San Diego State Historic Park
2754 Calhoun Street
(619) 299-7124

at least 2 fruit/vegetable servings

LINGUINE ALLA TREVI

Linguine pasta with eggplant, basil, garlic, fresh tomatoes and extra virgin olive oil.

Nutrition Information per Serving:

✓✓ CALORIES: Excellent Choice (390)
✓✓ FAT: Excellent Choice (7 g)
✓✓ CHOLESTEROL: Excellent Choice (0 mg)
✓✓ SODIUM: Excellent Choice (15 mg)**

EXCHANGES: 5½ Bread, ¾ Veg, 1 Fat
PROTEIN: 15 g, CARBOHYDRATE: 91 g, FIBER: 6 g

This nutrition analysis corresponds to the recipe below. The restaurant version may differ.

Ingredients (4 servings):

1 large eggplant
12 oz. pasta, dry weight
4 tsp. olive oil
3 medium tomatoes, chopped
4 cloves garlic, minced
16 fresh basil leaves, chopped
½ tsp. pepper
salt to taste (not included in analysis)

Directions:

1. Chop eggplant. Spread out eggplant pieces on a cookie sheet and bake at 350° until soft (10 – 15 minutes).
2. Boil water and cook pasta as directed on package.
3. Add oil to sauté pan, and sauté eggplant, tomato, garlic, basil, salt and pepper.
4. Drain pasta and add to tomato/eggplant mix. Sauté until hot.

Recipe supplied by:

il Forno

2901 Ocean Park Blvd., Santa Monica 90405 (310) 450-1241

Pasta Mare e Monti

Pasta with Italian porcini mushrooms, shrimp, garlic, white wine & light tomato sauce.

Nutrition Information per Serving:

✓ CALORIES: Good Choice (500)
✓✓ FAT: Excellent Choice (10)*
CHOLESTEROL: Moderate (220 mg)
SODIUM: High (1560 mg)**
EXCHANGES: 3½ Meat (extra lean), 2½ Bread, ¼ Veg, 1¼ Fat
PROTEIN: 38 g, CARBOHYDRATE: 62 g

This nutrition analysis corresponds to the recipe below. The restaurant version may differ.

* Primarily unsaturated fat

** Sodium may be reduced by using low-sodium marinara sauce

Ingredients (4 servings):

8 oz. dry pasta
2 Tbs. olive oil
4 tsp. garlic, minced
4 oz. dried porcini mushrooms, thinly sliced
10 oz. white shrimp
¾ cup white wine
3½ cups marinara sauce
4 tsp. parsley
1 tsp. black pepper
1 tsp. red pepper

Directions:

1. Cook pasta al dente and set aside.
2. Rehydrate porcini mushrooms in water for a few minutes.
3. Heat olive oil in a saucepan.
4. Add garlic, shrimp and mushrooms and sauté.
5. Add white wine to shrimp mix and allow to fully evaporate (approx. 2 min.).
6. Add tomato sauce, parsley, pepper (and salt to taste if desired - not included in analysis above).
7. Simmer 10 to 20 minutes.
8. Drain pasta and add to sauce. Sauté together until heated.

Recipe supplied by:

IL MORO
RISTORANTE • CAFE

Il Moro
11400 W. Olympic Blvd.
Los Angeles, CA 90064
(310) 575-3530

ROCK SHRIMP WITH CILANTRO

Linguine and shrimp with feta cheese, garlic, cilantro and tomatoes..

Nutrition Information per Serving:

✓ CALORIES: Good Choice (455)   CHOLESTEROL: Moderate (235 mg)
✓✓ FAT: Excellent Choice (9 g)   ✓ SODIUM: Good Choice (505 mg)
EXCHANGES: 2½ Meat (extra lean), 3¼ Bread, ½ Veg, 1 Fat
PROTEIN: 30 g, CARBOHYDRATE: 58 g, FIBER: 3 g

This nutrition analysis corresponds to the recipe below. The restaurant version may differ.

Ingredients (4 servings):

14 oz. fresh linguini pasta with egg
nonstick cooking spray
¼ cup red onion, chopped
3 cloves garlic, minced
10 oz. rock shrimp
6 oz. (¾ cup) white wine
¼ cup feta cheese
¼ cup cilantro, chopped, divided
½ cup tomato, diced
salt and pepper to taste
(not included in analysis)

Directions:

1. Cook pasta according to instructions.
2. Coat pan with cooking spray.
3. Sauté onions, garlic and shrimp.
4. Add white wine and heat until most of the liquid has evaporated.
5. Add feta cheese, 3 Tbs. of the cilantro, tomatoes and pasta.
6. Simmer for a few minutes.
7. Garnish with remaining cilantro. Serve immediately.

Recipe supplied by:

Pizza Nova
Hillcrest: 3955 Fifth Ave. (619) 296-6682
Point Loma: 5120 North Harbor Dr. (619) 226-0268
Solana Beach: 945 Lomas Santa Fe Dr. (858) 259-0666

Spaghetti with Mushroom Sauce 🍎

Fresh tender mushrooms, swimming in authentic Italian tomato sauce.

Nutrition Information per Serving:

✓✓ Calories: Excellent Choice (440) ✓✓ Cholesterol: Excellent Choice (0 mg)
✓✓ Fat: Excellent Choice (4 g)♥ ✓ Sodium: Good Choice (580 mg)
Exchanges: 2¼ Veg, 5¼ Bread, ½ Fat,
Protein: 12 g, Carbohydrate: 91 g, Fiber: 5 g

This nutrition analysis corresponds to the recipe below. The restaurant version may differ.
♥ primarily unsaturated fat

Ingredients (6 servings):

1 Tbs. vegetable oil, divided
⅓ cup onion, chopped fine
3 cloves garlic, minced
1 28 oz. can diced tomatoes in juice
6 oz tomato puree
1 tsp. salt
¾ Tbs. sugar
1 pinch black pepper
½ Tbs. crushed oregano
½ Tbs. fresh parsley (chopped fine)
1 Tbs. red wine
⅓ cup water
½ Tbs. corn starch
½ lb. large mushrooms, sliced
16 oz. Spaghetti, uncooked

Directions:

1. Place a large saucepan on stove over medium heat.
2. Add the ½ Tablespoon oil, onions and garlic. Cook the garlic and onions until tender; stir frequently. (add a little water to prevent scorching if needed).
3. Add the diced tomatoes and tomato puree. Mix thoroughly.
4. Add spices, parsley, and wine. Mix thoroughly.
5. Bring all ingredients to a boil. Simmer for 30 minutes.
6. While sauce simmers, cook pasta according to package directions.
7. Mix cornstarch with water and stir into sauce and continue simmering.
8. In a separate sauté pan, heat the remaining ½ tablespoon oil.
9. Add mushrooms and sauté until they start to "sweat".
10. Stir the mushrooms into the sauce.
11. Portion spaghetti into dishes. Spoon sauce over pasta.

Recipe supplied by:

the old spaghetti factory

The Old Spaghetti Factory

Newport Beach: 2110 Newport Blvd. (949) 675-8654
Fullerton: 110 East Santa Fe Ave. (714) 526-6801
Riverside: 3191 Mission Inn Ave. (909) 784-4417
Rancho Cucamonga: 11896 Foothill Blvd. (909) 980-3585

🍎 at least 2 fruit/vegetable servings

Aloo Gobi

Cauliflower and potatoes cooked with herbs and spices.

Nutrition Information per Serving:

✓✓ Calories: Excellent Choice (160) ✓✓ Cholesterol: Excellent Choice (0 mg)
✓✓ Fat: Excellent Choice (8 g)♥ ✓✓ Sodium: Excellent Choice (65 mg)
Exchanges: ¼ Bread, 2¾ Veg, 1¼ Fat
Protein: 6 g, Carbohydrate: 21 g, Fiber 8 g

This nutrition analysis corresponds to the recipe below. The restaurant version may differ.
♥ primarily unsaturated fat

Ingredients (4 servings):

1 medium (20 oz.) cauliflower
2 medium potatoes
2 Tbs. soybean oil
½ tsp. cumin seeds
1 large onions, chopped
1 tsp. garlic, minced
½ tsp. ginger, minced
¼ to 1 green chili, minced, or ⅛ to ½ tsp. chili powder
½ tsp. turmeric powder
½ tsp. dhania (coriander) powder
½ tsp. red pepper (optional, to taste)
½ tsp. garam masala spices
2 large tomatoes, chopped
½ Tbs. coriander (cilantro), chopped

Directions:

1. Break cauliflower into florettes. Chop potatoes in medium sized chunks.
2. Simmer in boiling water for 3-5 minutes. Drain and set aside.
3. Heat soybean oil in a pan, add cumin seeds, allow to sputter.
4. Add onions, garlic, ginger, and green chili; sauté until cooked.
5. Add turmeric powder, dhania powder, red pepper, and masala spices; sauté for 2 to 3 minutes, stirring continuously.
6. Add tomatoes, potatoes and cauliflower; cook until liquid thickens, stirring occasionally to avoid burning.
7. Add salt to taste (salt not included in analysis).
8. Garnish with coriander.

Recipe supplied by:

Star of India
Pacific Beach: 1820 Garnet Ave. (858) 459-3355
Del Mar: 3860 Valley Center Drive (858) 792-1111
Downtown: 423 F Street (619) 234-8000

at least 2 fruit/vegetable servings

CAULIFLOWER ENCHILADAS

Nutrition Information per Serving:

✓✓ CALORIES: Excellent Choice (315) ✓✓ CHOLESTEROL: Excellent Choice (45 mg)
✓ FAT: Good Choice (16 g) SODIUM: Moderate (955 mg)
EXCHANGES: 1¼ Meat, 1¼ Bread, ¾ Veg, ¼ Milk, 2¼ Fat
PROTEIN: 13 g, CARBOHYDRATE: 28 g, FIBER: 4 g

This nutrition analysis corresponds to the recipe below. The restaurant version may differ.

Ingredients (6 servings):

2½ cups organic cauliflower, coarsely chopped
8 oz. jack cheese
6 oz. light sour cream
4 oz. can green chilies
⅓ cup organic onion, chopped
½ tsp. organic cumin, ground
¼ tsp. salt
20 oz. can green enchilada sauce
12 mini-corn tortillas 4" diameter (or 8 tortillas 6" diameter)
2 Tbs. black olives, diced
3 Tbs. fresh organic parsley

Directions:

1. Filling: Steam the cauliflower and chop it finely. In a large bowl, combine and mix well the cauliflower, 2 oz. of the cheese, sour cream, 3 oz. of the chilies, onion, cumin and salt.
2. Ladle a layer of enchilada sauce in a 9x9" baking pan. Dip 4 tortillas in the sauce and layer on the bottom of the pan. Place ½ of the filling over the tortillas and spread evenly.
3. Dip 4 more tortillas in the sauce and layer over the filling mix and then top with remaining cheese. Place remaining filling over cheese and spread evenly.
4. Place remaining tortillas on top. Ladle remaining sauce over tortillas.
5. Cover with foil. Heat at 350 degrees for 40 – 45 minutes. Garnish with olives, parsley, remaining chilies, and serve.

Recipe supplied by:

Jimbo's...Naturally!

Del Mar Heights: 12853 El Camino Real (858) 793-7755
Escondido: 1633 S. Centre City Parkway (760) 489-7755
Carlsbad: 1923 Calle Barcelona, Ste. 149 (760) 334-7755

at least 2 fruit/vegetable servings

NEPTUNE LOAF

Fettucine pasta, veggies, tofu & cheese, smothered in Savory Sauce.

Nutrition Information per Serving:

✓✓ CALORIES: Excellent Choice (250) ✓✓ CHOLESTEROL: Excellent Choice (65 mg)
✓✓ FAT: Excellent Choice (12 g) ✓✓ SODIUM: Excellent Choice (285 mg)**
EXCHANGES: 1½ Meat, 1¼ Bread, ½ Veg, 1½ Fat
PROTEIN: 15 g, CARBOHYDRATE: 22 g

This nutrition analysis corresponds to the recipe below. The restaurant version may differ.

Ingredients (12 servings):

12 oz. whole wheat noodles (dry weight)
½ bell pepper
1½ stalks celery
½ cup chopped onion
2 cups assorted vegetables of your choice
3 cups shredded cheddar cheese
1 lb. tofu, chopped into small cubes
2 eggs
½ tsp. minced garlic
1 Tbs. Bragg liquid aminos
1 tsp. tamari sauce

Directions:

1. Cook noodles as directed on package. Drain and rinse.
2. Steam bell pepper, celery, onion and assorted vegetables for 3 to 5 minutes.
3. Mix 2 cups of cheese and remaining ingredients in a large bowl. Add pasta and vegetables and stir until well combined.
4. Press into a lightly oiled 9x12-inch pan. Sprinkle with remaining cheese and bake 40 to 45 minutes in a 400° oven.

Recipe from: ***Recipes from the Heart*** book by Tonya Beaudet, owner of :

The Spot

Natural Food Restaurant
110 Second Street
Hermosa Beach, CA 90254
(310) 301-7074

at least 2 fruit/vegetable servings

Vegetable Burrito

Fresh colorful garden vegetables in a burrito topped with tomatillo sauce.

Nutrition Information per Serving:

✓✓ Calories: Excellent Choice (440) ✓✓ Cholesterol: Excellent Choice (0 mg)
✓ Fat: Good Choice (17 g)♥ Sodium: High (1845 mg)
Exchanges: ¼ Meat, 2¾ Bread, 4 Veg, ½ Fruit, 3 Fat
Protein: 14 g, Carbohydrate: 65 g, Fiber: 7 g

This nutrition analysis corresponds to the recipe below. The restaurant version may differ.
♥ Primarily unsaturated fat

Ingredients (4 servings):

½ Tbs. vegetable oil
½ bell pepper, chopped
1½ cups fresh mushrooms, chopped
½ cup onions, chopped
½ cup carrots, chopped
1 cup yellow squash, chopped
1 cup zucchini, chopped
1 cup tomatillo sauce
4 flour tortillas, 12 inch diameter

Directions:

1. Heat oil in a large sauté pan over medium-high heat.
2. Add all of the vegetables and sauté until golden brown.
3. Fill each tortilla with ¼ of the cooked vegetables, fold and roll.
4. Place rolled tortilla on each plate and top with tomatillo sauce.

Recipe supplied by:

Casa Guadalajara
Bazaar del Mundo Old Town
San Diego State Historic Park
4105 Taylor Street
(619) 295-5111

at least 2 fruit/vegetable servings

VEGETABLE STIR FRY WITH TOFU OR CHICKEN OVER BROWN RICE

Nutrition Information per Serving:
(Analysis for Tofu version)

✓✓ CALORIES: Excellent Choice (385) ✓✓ CHOLESTEROL: Excellent Choice (0 mg)
✓✓ FAT: Excellent Choice (15 g)♥ ✓✓ SODIUM: Excellent Choice (220 mg)
EXCHANGES: 1¼ Meat, 1½ Bread, 1½ Veg, 1 Fat
PROTEIN: 19 g, CARBOHYDRATE: 44 g, FIBER: 6 g

♥ primarily unsaturated fat

Ingredients (2 servings):

8 oz. Pulmuone extra firm tofu or 6 oz. Foster Farms chicken
1 cup broccoli, chopped
¾ cup snow peas, halved
1 Tbs. freshly grated ginger
2 Tbs. canned water chestnuts or sliced carrots
1 Tbs. Spectrum olive oil or sesame oil
2 tsp. low sodium soy sauce or Bragg aminos
½ cup bok choy, cut in 1 inch pieces
1½ cups cooked brown rice (can be made ahead)

Directions:

1. Chop tofu or chicken into medium-sized cubes.
2. Heat large frying pan or wok and add oil. Add ginger & tofu or chicken. Toss until cooked; set aside.
3. Add broccoli to pan or wok, toss for several minutes.
4. Add the other vegetables. When all vegetables are cooked until crisp and tender, add soy sauce & tofu or chicken, tossing until well-mixed. Season to taste (not included in analysis).
5. Serve over rice.

Recipe supplied by:

Henry's Marketplace

Costa Mesa: 3030 Harbor Blvd. (714) 751-6399
Laguna Niguel: 27271 La Paz Road (949) 349-1999
Mission Viejo: 27765 Santa Margarita Parkway (949) 587-3003
Yorba Linda: 17482 Yorba Linda Blvd. (714) 572-3535
Chino Hills: 3630 Grand Ave. (909) 548-0440
Call (619) 258-2900 for more locations and information.

at least 2 fruit/vegetable servings

WHOLE EARTH CASSEROLE

Spaghetti in marinara with onions, mushrooms, zucchini, green bell pepper, alfalfa sprouts, black olives and tomatoes, covered with cheese and oven baked.

Nutrition Information per Serving:

✓✓ CALORIES: Excellent Choice (395) ✓✓ CHOLESTEROL: Excellent Choice (15 mg)
✓ FAT: Good Choice (17 g) SODIUM: Moderate (805 mg)
EXCHANGES: 1 Meat, 2 Bread, 2 Veg, 2¼ Fat
PROTEIN: 15 g, CARBOHYDRATE: 49 g, FIBER: 5 g

This nutrition analysis corresponds to the recipe below. The restaurant version may differ.

Ingredients (4 servings):

6 oz. dry spaghetti (dry weight)
1 medium white onion, chopped
1 green bell pepper, chopped
1 medium zucchini, chopped
6 oz. fresh mushrooms, sliced
1 medium tomato, chopped
⅓ cup alfalfa sprouts
6 oz. black olives (15-20 large), chopped
26 oz. marinara sauce
4 oz. part skim milk mozzarella cheese

Directions:

1. Cook spaghetti according to directions. Rinse and drain.
2. Spray pan with non-stick spray. Sauté onion, bell pepper, zucchini, mushrooms and tomato. Add alfalfa sprouts and olives.
3. Mix vegetables, marinara sauce, and spaghetti together and place in baking dish.
4. Top with cheese and bake at 350° for 10 to 15 minutes until cheese melts.

Recipe supplied by:

Angie's

Angie's Cuisine Italiano
14425 Newport Ave.
Tustin, CA 92780
(714) 832-3434

at least 2 fruit/vegetable servings

Clam and Mushroom Miso Soup

Nutrition Information per Serving †:

✓ Calories: Good Choice (165) ✓ Cholesterol: Good Choice (35 mg)
✓✓ Fat: Excellent Choice (3 g)* Sodium: High (925 mg)
Exchanges: 2 Meat (extra lean), 1 Bread, ½ Veg, ½ Fat
Protein: 17 g, Carbohydrate: 19 g, Fiber: 1 g

This nutrition analysis corresponds to the recipe below. The restaurant version may differ.
† Side dish guidelines are 1/3 of entrée guidelines

Ingredients (4 servings):

2 lbs. marina clams
2 oz. oyster mushrooms, chopped
2 oz. shiitake mushrooms, chopped
2 oz. white mushrooms, chopped
1½ cups spinach
4 cups water
5 oz. white miso soy pesto (soy bean paste)
2 green onion stems, chopped
½ bunch chives, chopped

Directions:

1. In a medium saucepan add clams, chopped mushrooms, spinach and water.
2. Heat at medium-high heat until clamshells open.
3. Next, add miso soy pesto, stir, and cook for approximately 2½ minutes.
4. To serve – Pour in soup bowls and garnish with chopped green onions and chives.

Recipe supplied by:

CHAYA BRASSERIE
8741 Alden Dr., Los Angeles 90048
(310) 859-883

CHAYA VENICE
110 Navy St., Venice 90291
(310) 396-1179

GARLIC MASHED POTATOES

Nutrition Information per Serving †:

✓ CALORIES: Good Choice (180) ✓✓ CHOLESTEROL: Excellent Choice (0 mg)
✓✓ FAT: Excellent Choice (0 g) ✓ SODIUM: Good Choice (160 mg)
EXCHANGES: 2¼ Bread, ¼ Milk
PROTEIN: 5 g, CARBOHYDRATE: 40 g, Fiber: 4 g

This nutrition analysis corresponds to the recipe below. The restaurant version may differ.
† Side dish guidelines are 1/3 of entrée guidelines

Ingredients (4 servings):

1½ lb red potatoes
8-10 garlic cloves, peeled
½ cup non-fat sour cream
¼ tsp kosher salt
1/3 tsp black pepper

Directions:

1. Clean and peel potatoes. It is okay to leave some of the potato skin on.
2. Boil potatoes and garlic until fork-tender in a large pot.
3. Drain water.
4. Add non-fat sour cream, salt and black pepper to cooked potatoes and garlic.
5. Hand mash ingredients together, creating a smooth and lumpy texture.

Recipe supplied by:

Skew's Fresh and Fire Grilled

300 South Grand Ave., Los Angeles 90036 (213) 613-0300

SHRIMP & LEMON GRASS SOUP ♁

A hot, sour and spicy shrimp soup with lemon grass.

Nutrition Information per Serving†:

✓✓ CALORIES: Excellent Choice (110) CHOLESTEROL: High (110 mg)
✓✓ FAT: Excellent Choice (1 g)♥ SODIUM: High (445 mg)
EXCHANGES: 1¾ Meat, 1¼ Veg
PROTEIN: 15 g, CARBOHYDRATE: 11 g, FIBER: 3 g

This nutrition analysis corresponds to the recipe below. The restaurant version may differ.
† Side dish guidelines are ⅓ of entree guidelines ♥ primarily unsaturated fat

Ingredients (4 servings):

4 to 6 stalks lemon grass, crushed
4 shallots or ½ red onion
6 to 8 Kefir lime leaves
8 cups water
8 oz. shrimp (31/35), peeled & deveined
16 to 20 fresh mushrooms, sliced
2 Thai chiles
2 Tbs. chopped fresh cilantro
4 tsp. fish sauce
4 tsp. lemon juice
2 tsp. chili paste (optional)
½ tsp. sugar (optional)

Directions:

1. In a 6 to 8-quart stainless steel pan, put lemon grass, shallots, kefir lime leaves and cold water and bring to a boil. Simmer at low heat for 15 to 20 minutes.
2. Add sliced mushrooms and continue to boil for another 10 minutes.
3. Add shrimp and bring to a boil again. Then turn off the heat. Add the remaining ingredients and adjust flavor to your taste. Please keep in mind that Thai chili can be very spicy and should be used sparingly.

Recipe supplied by:

CALIFORNIA WOK
Natural Chinese and Thai Cuisine

California Wok
4466 Cerritos Ave.
Los Alamitos, CA 90720
(714) 527-0226

TOMATO BRUSCHETTA

Nutrition Information per Serving:†

✓✓ CALORIES: Excellent Choice (145) ✓✓ CHOLESTEROL: Excellent Choice (0 mg)
✓✓ FAT: Excellent Choice (5 g)♥ SODIUM: Moderate (310 mg)
EXCHANGES: 1 Bread, 1½ Veg, ¾ Fat
PROTEIN: 4 g, CARBOHYDRATE: 24 g, FIBER: 3 g

This nutrition analysis corresponds to the recipe below. The restaurant version may differ.
† Side dish guidelines are 1/3 of entrée guidelines ♥ primarily unsaturated fat

Ingredients (4 servings):

1 lb. plum tomatoes, chopped
2 cloves garlic, minced (1 tsp.)
1 small red onion, minced
2 Tbs. fresh parsley, minced
3 Tbs. fresh basil, chopped
¼ tsp. salt
¼ tsp. black pepper
1 Tbs. olive oil
4 tsp. balsamic vinegar
1 Tbs. red wine vinegar
½ French bread baguette, sliced ¼ inch thick

Directions:

1. Preheat oven to 400° F.
2. Combine tomatoes, garlic onion, parsley, basil, salt, pepper, olive oil, and vinegars in a large mixing bowl to make the bruschetta.
3. Place the baguette slices on a baking pan in a single layer. Bake the slices until just golden and remove from the oven, flip them, and return to the oven until golden.
4. Serve the warm baguette slices topped with the bruschetta.

As seen in:

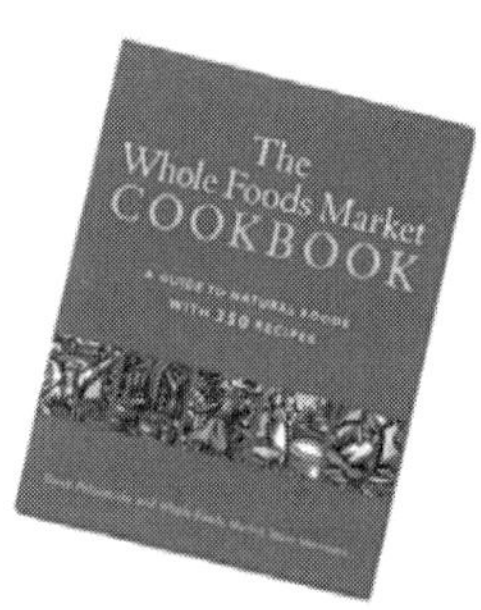

Whole Foods Market
14945 Holt Avenue
Tustin, CA 92680
(714) 731-3400

at least 1 fruit/vegetable serving for side dishes

Part IV
Health Resource Guide

It's probably easier to live a more healthful lifestyle in Southern California than anywhere in the country. The agreeable climate, gentle pace, health-conscious mindset, and accessibility to health-oriented products and services all promote a healthier way of life.

Healthful living includes more than healthy dining. So in the Health Resource Guide that follows, you'll find an array of "tools" to further support your healthful lifestyle. We think you'll find this guide useful, informative and interesting. The **Healthy Dining** team recognizes the Health Resource Guide companies and organizations for their contribution to a healthier community.

Index

1. American Cancer Society 173
2. American Council on Exercise 174
3. American Diabetes Association 175
4. American Heart Association 176
5. California Dietetic Association 177
6. California 5 a Day Campaign 178
7. Henry's Marketplace 179
8. Juvenile Diabetes Research Foundation 180
9. Melissa's/World Variety Produce, Inc. 181
10. Orange County Farmers' Markets 182
11. Orange County Wellness Coalition 183
12. Pediatric Adolescent Diabetes Research Foundation 184

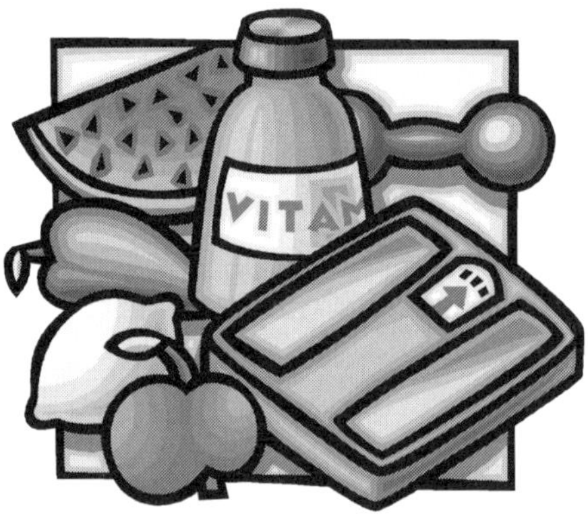
VITA

AMERICAN CANCER SOCIETY

NUTRITION, EXERCISE & CANCER

American Cancer Society®

1.800.ACS.2345
www.cancer.org

Hope.Progress.Answers.

THE BASICS

Poor diet and physical inactivity may be responsible for 1 of 3 cancer deaths. Overweight and obesity have increased dramatically in California. Nearly 60% of Californians were overweight or obese in 2001, compared to 38% in 1984. The number of teenagers who are overweight is about 28%. In general, men are more likely to be overweight than women, though women are more likely to be obese.

The American Cancer Society recommends eating at least five servings of fruits and vegetables each day. Few Californians meet this recommendation. In general, people who eat fast food on a regular basis eat fewer fruits and vegetables. Nearly 1 in 3 teens and 1 in 5 adults eat fast food on a typical day.

Regular physical activity is also strongly recommended. In 2001, only 1 in 3 California adults reported having engaged in physical activity for 30 minutes or more at least five times a week.

NUTRITION & EXERCISE GUIDELINES

- Eat 5 or more servings of fruits/vegetables each day. Choose whole grains instead of processed grains.
- Limit your consumption of red meats, especially those processed and high in fat.
- Adults should engage in at least moderate activity for 30 minutes or more on 5 or more days of the week; Children and teens at least 60 minutes.
- Stay within your healthy weight range. Balance caloric intake with physical activity.
- If you drink alcoholic beverages, limit consumption.
- Public, private and community organizations should work to create social and physical environments that support the adoption and maintenance of healthful nutrition and physical activity behaviors.

Most Californians Don't Eat Enough Fruits & Vegetables

percentage who don't eat the recommended five or more fruits & vegetables a day

Boys & Men

Age	% NOT eating 5-a-day
9-11	78%
12-13	73%
14-15	80%
16-17	78%
18+	70%

Girls & Women

Age	% NOT eating 5-a-day
9-11	80%
12-13	60%
14-15	62%
16-17	66%
18+	65%

Source: Public Health Institute, 2001

1/3 OF CANCERS MAY BE CAUSED BY POOR DIET AND INACTIVITY

Half of Californians are Overweight

Percentage of Overweight Californians is Skyrocketing

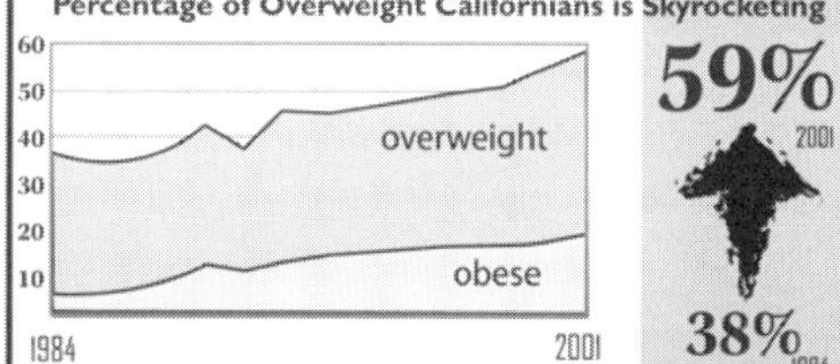

Many Californians are not Physically Active

In 2001, only one out of three California adults reported being engaged in moderate physical activity for 30 minutes or more at least 5 times a week.

Source: American Cancer Society & California Cancer Registry

AMERICAN DIABETES ASSOCIATION

1570 Brookhollow Drive, Suite 120
Santa Ana, CA 92705
(714) 662-7940

10445 Old Placerville Road
Sacramento, CA 95827
1-800-DIABETES

American Diabetes Association®
Cure • Care • Commitment®

The American Diabetes Association is the nation's leading nonprofit health organization providing diabetes research, information and advocacy. The mission of the organization is to "prevent and cure diabetes, and to improve the lives of all people affected by diabetes." To fulfill this mission, the American Diabetes Association funds research, publishes scientific findings, and provides information, education programs and other services to people with diabetes, their families, health care professionals, and the public.

The 1-800-DIABETES program is the cornerstone of the Association's information programs. 1-800-DIABETES is a toll-free help line for people who have questions and concerns about diabetes. Through 1-800-DIABETES, people can request information and literature about diabetes-related topics, including exercise, nutrition and self-management.

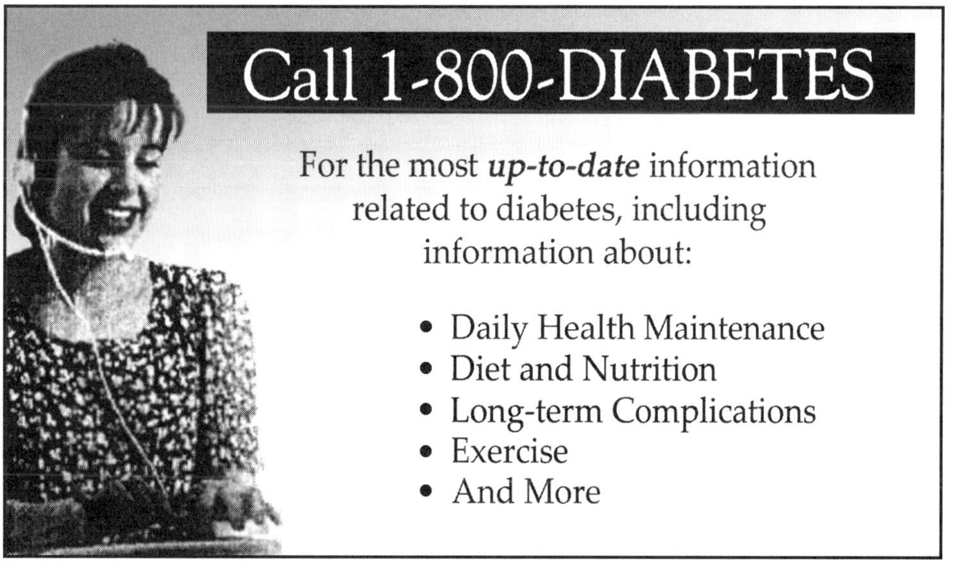

American Heart Association

Western States Affiliate, Orange County
4600 Campus Drive, Irvine, CA 92612
(949) 856-3555

Heart disease is the leading cause of death in America, claiming almost one million lives a year. Stroke is the third leading cause of death and the number one cause of disability. The goal of the American Heart Association is to reduce death, disability and risk of heart disease and stroke by 25% by the year 2010.

The American Heart Association, founded in 1924, is the largest national voluntary organization focused on cardiovascular diseases. Funds are raised through private and corporate donations and used to support research and professional and public education. For more information, call (949) 856-3555 or reach us online at www.americanheart.org.

Food Guide Pyramid

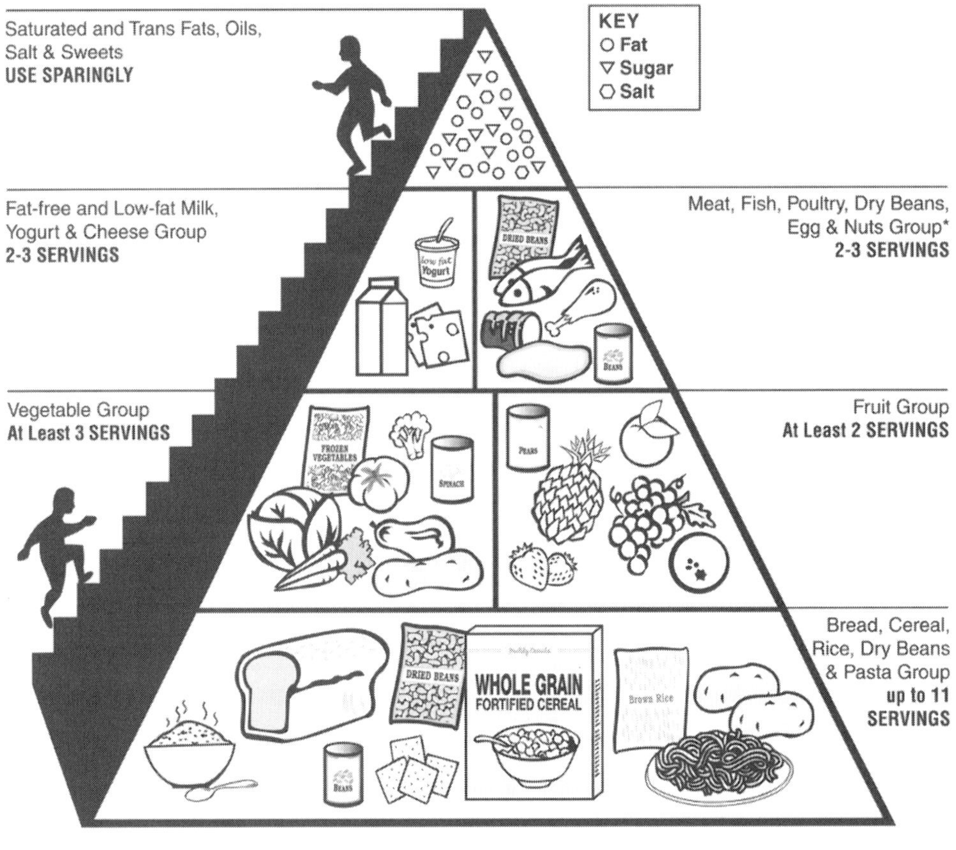

*Substitutes for 1 ounce of meat: 1/2 cup of cooked dry beans, 2 tablespoons of peanut butter, or 1 oz of nuts.
Note: 1 egg yolk has 213 mg of cholesterol. The American Heart Association recommends no more than 300 mg of cholesterol a day.

 12/03 HL-0590

CALIFORNIA DIETETIC ASSOCIATION/ ORANGE DISTRICT

1046 N. Tustin Avenue, Suite O
Orange, CA 92867
(714) 538-5819
www.cdaorangedistrict.org
cda@hotmail.com

CALIFORNIA DIETETIC ASSOCIATION/ ORANGE DISTRICT:

YOUR LINK TO NUTRITION AND HEALTH

- **Think Registered Dietitian as the best source of nutrition information.**
- **For a personalized eating plan, contact a Registered Dietitian.**
- **When too much confusing nutrition information clogs the airways, a Registered Dietitian can give you expert and accurate nutrition information.**
- **To locate a Registered Dietitian in your area:**
    1. **call us at (714) 538-5819**
    2. **visit us on the internet at www.cdaorangedistrict.org**
    3. **email us at cda@hotmail.com**

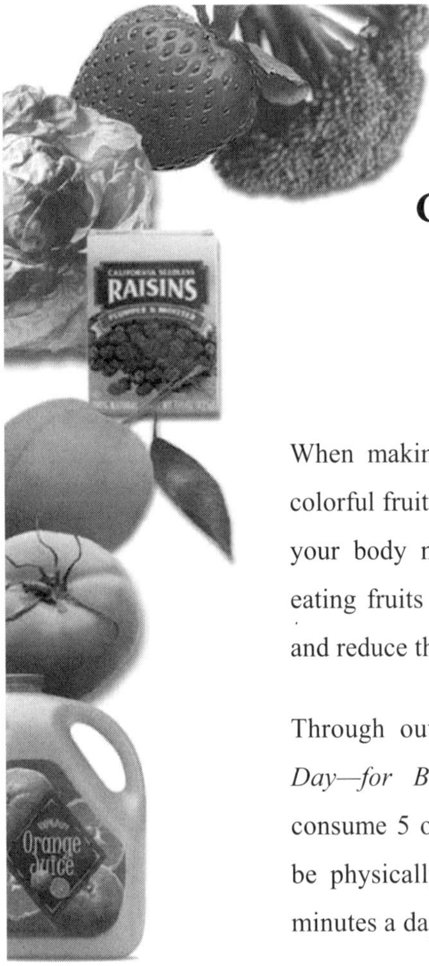

CALIFORNIA 5 a DAY CAMPAIGN

1616 Capitol Ave., Suite 74.516
Sacramento, CA 95814

When making healthy dining decisions, think color! A variety of colorful fruits and vegetables provide the vitamins, minerals and fiber your body needs to maintain good health and high energy. Plus, eating fruits and vegetables can protect against the effects of aging and reduce the risk of cancer and heart disease.

Through outreach and educational activities, the *California 5 a Day—for Better Health! Campaign* empowers Californians to consume 5 or more servings of fruits and vegetables every day and be physically active at least 30 minutes a day for adults and 60 minutes a day for children.

So next time you enjoy a meal out with friends or family, remember to put more color in your life by reaching for nature's answer to better health.

For more information about the *California 5 a Day Campaign*, visit www.ca5aday.com or call 1-888-EAT-FIVE

EAT 5 A DAY for better health AND BE ACTIVE

HENRY'S MARKETPLACE

Costa Mesa: 3030 Harbor Blvd. (714) 751-6399
Laguna Niguel: 27271 La Paz Road (949) 349-1999
Mission Viejo: 27765 Santa Margarita Parkway (949) 587-3003
Yorba Linda: 17482 Yorba Linda Blvd. (714) 572-3535
Chino Hills: 3630 Grand Ave. (909) 548-0440
Call (619) 258-2900 for more locations and information.

Henry's is known for its farm fresh produce at great prices, but did you know that Henry's also carries bulk bin items like healthy cereals, beans and pastas? How about the finest seafood, hormone-free beef and poultry? We also have one of Southern California's largest selections of natural vitamins and supplements, natural cosmetics, plus much more, like...

- Save 10% off retail on all major brands of vitamins and supplements, herbs, natural cosmetics, body care products and books when you purchase $100 or more of these items.
- Seniors 55+ receive 10% off retail on all Henry's brand vitamins and supplements with their Henry's Senior Discount Card.

In a nutshell, Henry's is quality products, great prices, friendly and knowledgeable people -- all for you! Call (619) 258-2900 to find the Henry's Marketplace nearest you.

Trust
Henry's Marketplace
For Life™

JUVENILE DIABETES RESEARCH FOUNDATION INTERNATIONAL

ORANGE COUNTY CHAPTER
(949) 553-0363
www.jdrf.org

The Juvenile Diabetes Research Foundation International (JDRF) is the leading charitable funder and advocate of juvenile (type 1) diabetes research worldwide. JDRF was founded more than 30 years ago by parents of children with juvenile diabetes, with the mission to find a cure for diabetes and its complications through the support of research. To date, the foundation has provided more than $680 million in grants for diabetes research around the world.

JDRF is accessible to people 24 hours per day, seven days per week—particularly those struggling with difficult moments after a diagnosis of juvenile diabetes. Each year, JDRF handles more than 25,000 inquiries by telephone (1-800-533-2873), through its innovative Online Diabetes Support Team accessed through the JDRF website at www.jdrf.org, and through its more than 100 locations worldwide.

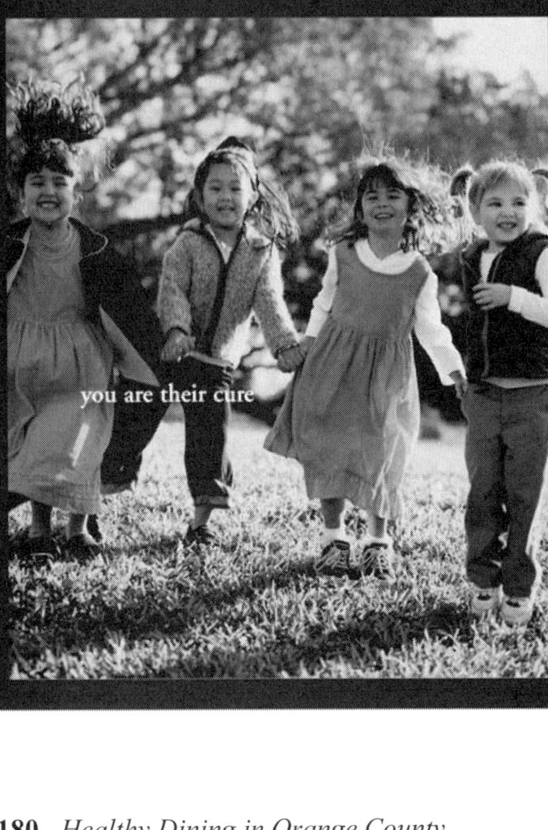

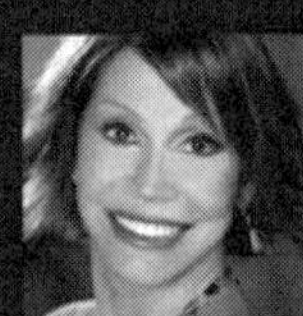

Mary Tyler Moore
International Chairman

These kids and millions more have Juvenile Diabetes, a disease that threatens their lives every day. None of them can outgrow it. But we're closer than ever to a cure. Please, help us make life-saving research possible.

Call 1.800.533.CURE or visit www.jdrf.org.

JDRF Juvenile Diabetes Research Foundation International

dedicated to finding a cure

MELISSA'S

Melissa's/World Variety Produce, Inc.
P.O. Box 21127
Los Angeles, CA 90021
www.melissas.com
(800) 588-0151

Think tasty, creamy, tangy, aromatic, tart, sweet, crunchy and delectable. Established in 1984, Melissa's Produce is currently the largest distributor of specialty produce in the United States, offering the best variety of organic and exotic fruits and vegetables. With over 800 items available at any given time, Melissa's imports and distributes exotic fresh fruits and vegetables from around the globe. Look for Melissa's fresh organic produce and specialty items in the produce department of your local grocery store.

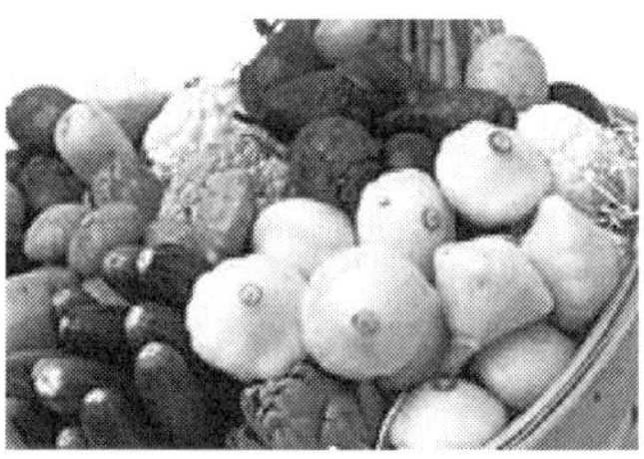

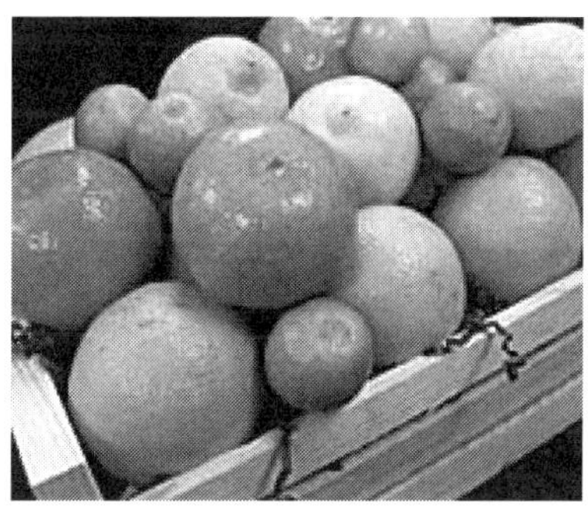

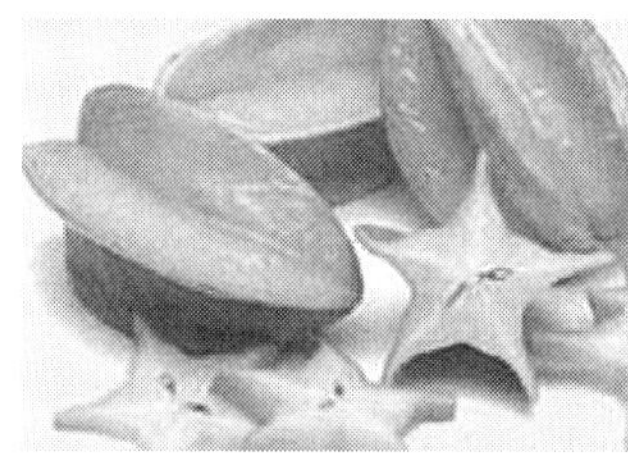

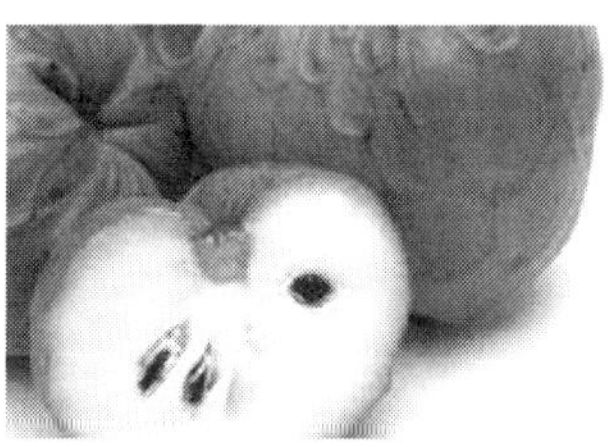

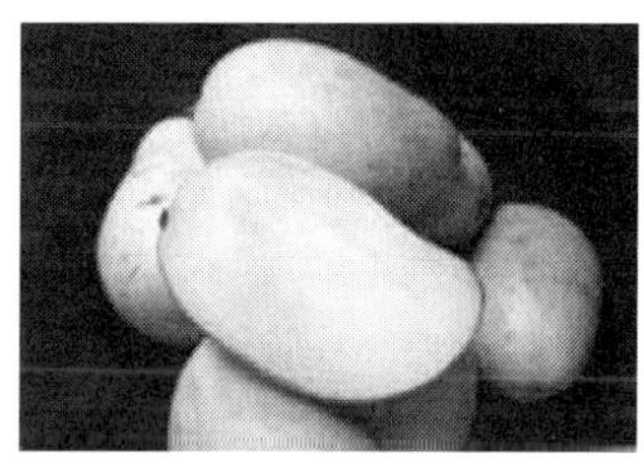

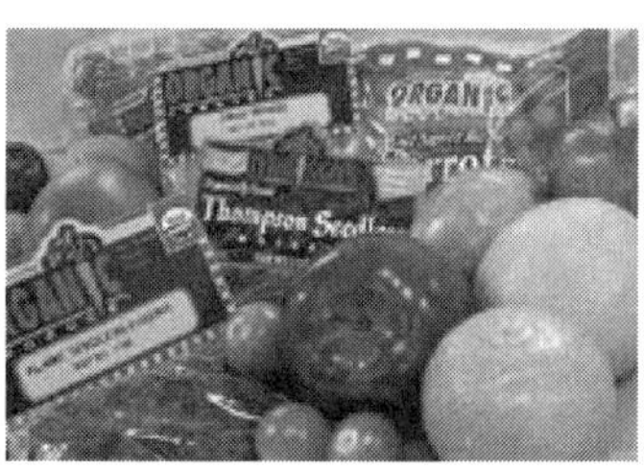

You can also visit us on the web at www.melissas.com, where you can buy healthy and natural organic produce, fresh gourmet food, baked goods, corporate gift baskets, gift certificates, and holiday treats online and have them delivered direct to your door. Also, browse our online cookbook for lots of wonderful free recipes – Asian, Latin, vegetarian, holiday, ethnic and others, or enjoy our magazine, Melissa's in Minutes.

Melissa's is also involved in many community efforts, has sponsored the James Beard Foundation Awards, and is affiliated with the National 5 A Day Partnership and the Produce for Better Health Foundation.

For more information, visit our website www.melissas.com or call (800) 588-0151.

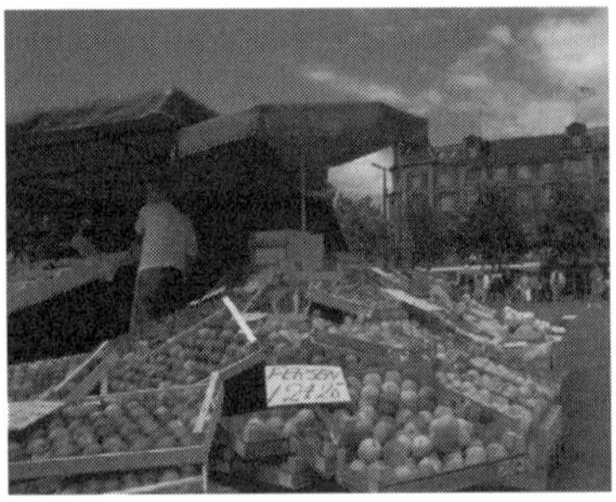

ORANGE COUNTY FARMERS' MARKETS

Farmers markets offer great-tasting fresh produce for your enjoyment and your health! Below is a list of Orange County farmers markets compiled from public websites. For more information, please visit www.ocpfrd.com/ag/ser_farmers_market_certified.asp or www.ams.usda.gov/farmersmarkets/States/California.

Anaheim: Center Street Promenade, Thursday, 9:30 am-1:30 pm (May Sept.) (714) 956-3586

Brea: Birch Street near Brea & Imperial, Tuesday, 4:00 pm- 8:00pm (714) 329-6755

Cerritos: Park Plaza at Towne Center Dr., Saturday, 8:00 am-12 noon (562) 433-3881

Corona Del Mar: Margarite & PCH, Saturday, 9:00 am-1:00 pm (seasonal) (949) 361-0764

Costa Mesa: Orange County Fairgrounds, Thursday, 9:00 am-1:00 pm (714) 573-0374

Dana Point: Community Center, Tuesday, 9:00 am-1:00 pm (714) 573-0374

Diamond Bar: Grand Ave. & Golden Springs Rd., Sat., 9:00 am-2:00 pm (seasonal) (714) 534-3172

Fullerton: Wiltshire & Pomona, Thurs., 4:00 pm-9:00 pm (open air/seasonal May-Nov.) (714) 526-5814

Fullerton: Woodcrest Park, Wednesday, 8:30 am-2:00 pm (714) 871-5304

Huntington Beach: Pier Plaza, Friday, 1:00 pm-6:00 pm (714) 573-0374

Irvine University Center: Campus & Bridge, Saturday, 9:00 am-1:00 pm (714) 573-0374

Laguna Beach: Lumberyard parking lot, City Hall, Saturday, 8:00 am-12 noon (714) 573-0374

Laguna Hills: El Toro & I-5, Friday, 9:00 am-1:00 pm (714) 573-0374

Laguna Niguel: Plaza de La Paz Ctr., Sunday, 9:00 am-1:00 pm (open-air/seasonal) (714) 573-0374

Long Beach: Broadway & the Promenade, Friday, 10:00 am-4:00 pm (562) 433-3881

Long Beach East: Wardlow Rd. & Norwalk Blvd. Saturday, 10:00 am-sellout (562) 433-3881

Long Beach Marina: Marina Dr., south of 2nd St., Sunday, 9:00 am-1:00 pm (562) 433-3881

Los Alamitos : Pine & Florista, Friday, 9:00 am-1:00 pm (open air/seasonal) (714) 573-0374

Old Capistrano: Yorba south of Mission, Wed., 3:00 pm-7:00 pm (3-6 in winter) (858) 272-7054

Orange: Antique Station parking lot, Thurs., 2:00 pm-6:00 pm (open air/seasonal) (714) 744-1821

Rancho Santa Margarita: Dove Canyon & Plano Trabuco, Wed., 9:00 am-1:00 pm (909) 229-3329

San Clemente Village: 200 Avenida Del Mar Dr., Sunday, 9:00 am-1:00 pm (949) 492-6000

Tustin: El Camino & 3d Streets, Wednesday, 9:00 am-1:00 pm (714) 573-0374

Tustin Old Town: El Camino & 3d Streets, Saturday, 9:00 am-1:00 pm (949) 248-1846

Yorba Linda-Old Towne: Lemon & Imperial Hwy, Saturday, 9:00 am-1:00 pm (619) 516-1618

The Orange County Wellness Coalition

Phone: 310-563-1445
www.ocwellness.org

Working to enhance the health status of individuals, both in the community and at the worksite. Providing educational programs, resources and technical assistance.

Vision – The Orange County Wellness Coalition is a professional resource network committed to creating healthy work sites and healthy communities.

Mission – We promote healthy lifestyles and wellness concepts by providing innovative programs, educational resources and networking opportunities for health professionals.

Goals – Through our highly qualified executive board, committee structure and membership networking, we will work to accomplish:

- Build partnerships with leaders.
- Develop a state-of-the art resource network of educational and training materials and speakers.

Join us - Meetings are held the 3rd Thursday of each month (except December and August) from 7:30 a.m. to 9:00 a.m. at Orange Coast Memorial Medical Center – 9920 Talbert Ave., Fountain Valley, CA.

~ Your first meeting is complimentary! ~

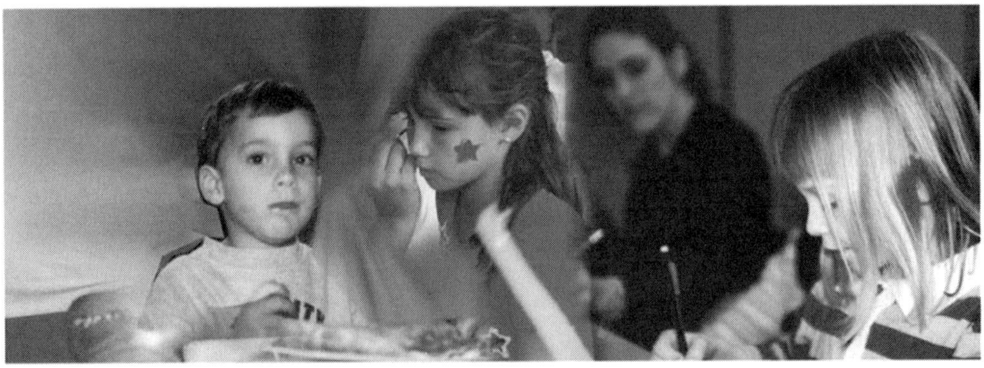

Part V

Other Editions in the **Healthy Dining** Book Series

Questionnaire

Book Order Form with Discount

Healthy Dining in Los Angeles

Participating Restaurants:

Acapulco
Allegria
Anastasia's Asylum
Baja Fresh
Beau Rivage
Bluewater Grill
Bombay Café
Border Grill
Bristol's Café at Bristol Farms
Buon Gusto
Buona Vita
Ca'Brea
Ca' del Sole
Cafe Luna
Café Pinot
Café Santorini
California Wok
Carmine's
Chang's
Charo Chicken
Chaya Brasserie
Chaya Venice
Chili My Soul
Chin Chin
China Grill
Coco's Bakery Restaurant
Crocodile Café
Crustacean
El Pollo Loco
El Torito
Empress Harbor Seafood
Gaetano's Restaurant
Havana Mania
Hotel Bel Air
il Forno
il Moro
Jack Sprat's Grill
Jamba Juice
Junior's Restaurant & Deli
Khoury's Restaurant
Kincaid's Bay House
King's Fish House
Koo Koo Roo
La Salsa
Lisa's Bon Appétit
Malvasia
McCormick & Schmick's
Mi Piace
Ocean Avenue Seafood
Old Spaghetti Factory
One Pico
Palomino
Pane e Vino
Patina
Pick Up Stix
Pinot Bistro
Pinot Hollywood
PJ's Thai Restaurant
Pradeep's
Prego Ristorante
Real Food Daily
Riviera Mexican Grill
Rock'N Fish
Rosti
Ruby's Diner
Sammy's Woodfired Pizza
Santa Monica Seafood
Sharky's
Shenandoah Café
Sisley Italian Kitchen
Skew's Fresh & Fire Grilled
Souplantation
Spaghettini
The Spot Natural Food Restaurant
Susan's Healthy Gourmet
Twin Palms
Wahoo's Fish Taco
Wasabi Japanese Restaurant
Whole Foods Market
Zax

To order any of the **Healthy Dining** editions, see pages 191-192 or call 1-800-DINE (3463)

Healthy Dining in San Diego

Participating Restaurants:

Andre's Cuban Restaurant
Anthony's Fish Grotto Restaurants
Baja Fresh
Bandar Fine Persian Cuisine
The Beach House
Bob's on the Bay
Boll Weevil
The Brigantine
Café India
Café Pacifica
Casa de Bandini
Casa de Pico
Casa Guadalajara
Celadon Fine Thai Cuisine
Chili's Grill & Bar
Chin's Szechwan Cuisine
Cilantro Live!
Cuvee Wine Country Cuisine
Daily's Restaurant
Dave & Buster's
El Callejon
El Indio Mexican Restaurant
El Pollo Loco
El Torito Restaurants
Firenze Trattoria
The Fish Market
The Fish Merchant
The Flame Broiler
The French Gourmet
Fresh Seafood Restaurant
G5–Georges on Fifth
Galoka Vegetarian Fine Dining
Harry's Bar & American Grill
Il Fornaio
India Palace
Jack in the Box
Jamba Juice
Jay's Gourmet
Jimbo's…Naturally!
Karihan Filipino Food
Kensington Grill
Ki's Restaurant & Juice Bar
Koo Koo Roo
La Salsa
Leucadia Pizzeria
Lino's Italian Restaurant
Los Cabos Mexican Mesquite Grill
Meritage Restaurant & Bar
Milton's Restaurant & Bakery
The Mission
Mr. Charlie's Fortune Cookie
Mucho Gusto Express Mexican Grill
Nicolosi's Italian Restaurant
Nine-Ten at the Grande Colonial Hotel
The Old Spaghetti Factory
On Tap Bistro & Brewery
Pacific Coast Grill
Pat & Oscar's
Pick Up Stix
Pizza Nova
Prego Ristorante
Quails Inn
Rainwater's On Kettner
Rancho el Nopal
Ranchos Cocina Mexican & Vegetarian Rest.
Red Oak Steakhouse
Roppongi Restaurant
Round Table Pizza
Ruby's Diner
St. Germain's Café
Sammy's Woodfired Pizza
SandCrab Café
Sbicca
Sizzler
Solana Beach Fish House
Souplantation
Spices Thai Café
Star of India
Stir Fresh Mongolian Grill
Subway
Susan's Healthy Gourmet
Tio Leo's
Tony Roma's
Top of the Cove
Trattoria La Strada
Trellises at the Town & Country Hotel
Tutto Mare
Villa Manila
Wahoo's Fish Taco
Whole Foods Market
Zio Fine Italian Restaurant

To order any of the **Healthy Dining** editions, see pages 191-192 or call 1-800-DINE (3463)

Say "Thank You" to Restaurant Management

Restaurants that honor your special requests and take active steps to serve healthier meals need to hear from you, the consumer. Write a note of thanks on the restaurant's customer comment card. Or...you can photocopy the next page and clip these Thank You notes to give to restaurant managers. Use your **Healthy Dining** book to select which restaurants to visit, order menu items featured in the book, and tell management whenever possible that you appreciate the restaurant's participation in **Healthy Dining**, that you use the book and recommend it to your friends and family.

You can also give these notes to restaurants that are not in the **Healthy Dining** book. Tell management about the program and encourage them to get involved. Call the **Healthy Dining** office with any names of potential restaurants for future publications.

Restaurants listen to you, the "Healthy Diner." Together, we can lead the way to a healthier community.

✂ Clip Here

Dear Restaurant Owner/Manager:

THANK YOU…for serving such satisfying food that is lower in calories, fat, cholesterol, and sodium – and dishes that include fruits and vegetables. The top killers of Americans – heart disease, cancer, stroke and diabetes – are closely linked with diet. Your "healthy" leadership is helping to improve – even save – lives in Southern California!

To learn more about **Healthy Dining**, call 1-800-953-DINE

Dear Restaurant Owner/Manager:

THANK YOU…for serving such satisfying food that is lower in calories, fat, cholesterol, and sodium – and dishes that include fruits and vegetables. The top killers of Americans – heart disease, cancer, stroke and diabetes – are closely linked with diet. Your "healthy" leadership is helping to improve – even save – lives in Southern California!

To learn more about **Healthy Dining**, call 1-800-953-DINE

Dear Restaurant Owner/Manager:

THANK YOU…for serving such satisfying food that is lower in calories, fat, cholesterol, and sodium – and dishes that include fruits and vegetables. The top killers of Americans – heart disease, cancer, stroke and diabetes – are closely linked with diet. Your "healthy" leadership is helping to improve – even save – lives in Southern California!

To learn more about **Healthy Dining**, call 1-800-953-DINE

Dear Restaurant Owner/Manager:

THANK YOU…for serving such satisfying food that is lower in calories, fat, cholesterol, and sodium – and dishes that include fruits and vegetables. The top killers of Americans – heart disease, cancer, stroke and diabetes – are closely linked with diet. Your "healthy" leadership is helping to improve – even save – lives in Southern California!

To learn more about **Healthy Dining**, call 1-800-953-DINE

Dear Restaurant Owner/Manager:

THANK YOU…for serving such satisfying food that is lower in calories, fat, cholesterol, and sodium – and dishes that include fruits and vegetables. The top killers of Americans – heart disease, cancer, stroke and diabetes – are closely linked with diet. Your "healthy" leadership is helping to improve – even save – lives in Southern California!

To learn more about **Healthy Dining**, call 1-800-953-DINE

Dear Restaurant Owner/Manager:

THANK YOU…for serving such satisfying food that is lower in calories, fat, cholesterol, and sodium – and dishes that include fruits and vegetables. The top killers of Americans – heart disease, cancer, stroke and diabetes – are closely linked with diet. Your "healthy" leadership is helping to improve – even save – lives in Southern California!

To learn more about **Healthy Dining**, call 1-800-953-DINE

$5.00 OFF

your next purchase of **Healthy Dining**

We want to know more about you and your thoughts about **Healthy Dining**. So we'll give you $5.00 off your next copy of **Healthy Dining** if you'll return this questionnaire (information is confidential). To thank you, we will contact you when new editions are published and offer $5.00 off the retail price. You may also order now at the discount price (see reverse side).

1. How did you learn about **Healthy Dining in Orange County**?

____ Newspaper ____ Family or friend ____ Dietitian
____ Radio ____ Restaurant ____ Personal Trainer/Fitness Ctr.
____ Television ____ Health Organization ____ Special Event __________
____ Internet ____ Physician ____ Workplace
____ Store __________ ____ Other ______________________

2. Are you on any of these special diets?

____ Weight loss ____ Low-cholesterol ____ Diabetic ____ General health-conscious
____ Low-fat ____ Low-sodium ____ Vegetarian ____ Other ______________

3. Please list your favorite restaurants from this book:

4. What other restaurants would you like to see in the next edition?

5. Please list your favorite recipes from the book:

6. On average, how many times per month do you dine out? _____ Do you use the coupons? _____

7. Is this book primarily used by: ___ female ___ male ___ both ____ how many?

8. What is the age of the primary user of this book?

____ Under 30 ____ 30 to 45 ____ 45 to 60 ____ over 60

9. What other food or health-related publications or websites do you read? (*Health Magazine, Berkeley Wellness, Nutrition Action Healthletter, Eating Well, Cooking Light*, WebMD.com, cyberdiet.com, etc.)

10. If you would like information about fund-raising, seminars, or wholesale prices for **Healthy Dining**, please provide your phone number (_____)______________ and e-mail ____________________

We'd like to keep in touch! Please visit us at **www.healthy-dining.com** to get more information and sign up for your **FREE e-newsletter** and other offers.

Other Comments?

Please complete name and address on reverse side, fold and mail. Photocopy acceptable. OC5

Fold on lines with address on outside.

Name: ______________________

Address:_____________________

____

Stamp

Healthy Dining
8305 Vickers Street, Suite 106
San Diego, CA 92111

Special $5.00 OFF **Healthy Dining** books.

Order as many as you want at the special discount! It's our thank-you for answering our questionnaire. You will also receive the $5.00 discount on future editions. Orders normally processed within 1 week.

Quantity			Price
_____	**Healthy Dining in Orange County**	$19.95 - $5.00 discount = $14.95	_________
_____	**Healthy Dining in San Diego**	$19.95 - $5.00 discount = $14.95	_________
_____	**Healthy Dining in Los Angeles**	$19.95 - $5.00 discount = $14.95	_________

Call (800) 953-3463 for more information. Wholesale rates also available.

Subtotal _________

Tax (7¾% in Orange County) _________

Postage ($1.84 for 1st book + 24¢ each for additional books) _________

____ Check enclosed Total _________

____ VISA/Mastercard # ______________________________ exp._______ Signature_______________

Phone (_____) __________________ e-mail ______________________________________

Please fill out questionnaire on reverse and your name & address above. If sending check, make to **Healthy Dining** and fasten your check securely to this sheet or use a separate envelope. Thanks.

Part VI

Coupons

See pages 191-192 for special offer on additional Healthy Dining books!

Coupon — *Healthy Dining in Orange County* — Coupon

Free Entrée

with purchase of one entrée of equal or greater value.
Maximum value $8.00. Only one coupon per table. Not valid with any other offer.

Angie's

Cuisine Italiano
14425 Newport Ave.
Tustin, CA 92780
(714) 832-3434

Coupon — *Healthy Dining in Orange County* — Coupon

Free

32 oz. Sports Cup

with a purchase of any entrée or food order!
A $1.99 value. One coupon per customer.
Cannot be combined with any other offer. No cash value.
Not valid if reproduced. Cashier code (media promo)

22 locations in Orange County. Visit www.bajafresh.com for a location near you.

Coupon — *Healthy Dining in Orange County* — Coupon

50% OFF

Second Entree

Buy one entrée, get 50% off a 2nd entrée of equal or lesser value.

Not valid with any other offer.

BeachFire

Bar & Grill
204 Avenida Del Mar Suite D
San Clemente, CA 92672
(949) 366-3232

Coupon — *Healthy Dining in Orange County* — Coupon

Free Meal

with purchase of one meal of equal or greater value.
Maximum $10.00
Not valid with any other offer.

Blackboard Bistro

1198 Pacific Coast Highway
Seal Beach, CA 90740
(562) 596-9556

Coupon — *Healthy Dining in Orange County* — Coupon

Free Cup of Chowder

with any purchase.

Not valid with any other offer.

Bluewater Grill

Newport Beach: 630 Lido Park Dr.
(949) 675-3474
Santa Ana: 1621 W. Sunflower Ave.
(714) 546-3474

Healthy Dining in Orange County

Healthy Dining in Orange County

Healthy Dining in Orange County

Healthy Dining in Orange County

Healthy Dining in Orange County

Coupon | *Healthy Dining in Orange County* | Coupon

$3.00 OFF

with minimum purchase of $15.00

Not valid with any other offer.

CAFÉ Chin Chin
ASIAN FAST CASUAL

Café Chin Chin

Lakewood Mall: Candlewood Restaurant Row (562) 616-7171
Tustin Market Place: 2945 El Camino Real (714) 689-3131

Coupon | *Healthy Dining in Orange County* | Coupon

Free Meal

with purchase of one meal of equal or greater value.

Not valid with any other offer.

EST. 1990 BAKERY - RESTAURANT - CATERING
The Cafe de France .com

Café de France

4213 Campus Dr., Irvine 92612
(949) 854-5002

Coupon | *Healthy Dining in Orange County* | Coupon

Free Meal

with purchase of one meal of equal or greater value.
Maximum $7.00

Not valid with any other offer.

CAFÉ HEIDELBERG

CAFÉ VIENNA

Café Heidelberg

1100 S. Coast Hwy. #116
Laguna Beach (949) 497-4594

Café Vienna

31542 S. Coast Hwy.
Laguna Beach (949) 499-3015

Coupon | *Healthy Dining in Orange County* | Coupon

15% OFF
Entire Meal

Alcoholic beverages excluded.
Up to 4 in party.
Not valid with any other offer.

CALIFORNIA WOK
Natural Chinese and Thai Cuisine

California Wok

4466 Cerritos Avenue
Los Alamitos, CA 90720
(714) 527-0226

Coupon | *Healthy Dining in Orange County* | Coupon

$2.00 OFF

any whole chicken with two sides of your choice!

Not valid with any other offer.

WE DELIVER!

CHARO CHICKEN
NATURALLY DELICIOUS

Charo Chicken

Locations: Costa Mesa, Dana Point, Foothill Ranch, Huntington Beach, Irvine, Lake Forest, Lakewood, Long Beach, Los Alamitos, Murrieta, Redondo Beach, San Clemente, Seal Beach & Tustin.

Healthy Dining in Orange County

Healthy Dining in Orange County

Healthy Dining in Orange County

Healthy Dining in Orange County

Healthy Dining in Orange County

Coupon — *Healthy Dining in Orange County* — Coupon

Free Meal

with purchase of one meal of equal or greater value.

Not valid with any other offer.

Chin's Chinese Kitchen

13771 Newport Ave., Tustin
(714) 838-0603

Coupon — *Healthy Dining in Orange County* — Coupon

Free Meal

with purchase of one meal of equal or greater value. Maximum $8.00.

Valid at Brea & Long Beach only.
Not valid with any other offer.

The Culinary Wrap

Brea: 2435 E. Imperial Hwy.,
(714) 672-9727
Cal State Long Beach: 6049 E. 7th St.
(562) 494-9727

Coupon — *Healthy Dining in Orange County* — Coupon

50% OFF

Second Entree

Buy 1 entrée, get 50% off a 2nd entrée of equal or lesser value.

Not valid with any other offer.

Diho Siam

Thai/Chinese Cuisine

Costa Mesa: 1835 Newport Blvd. (949) 645-3259
Lake Forest: 23600 Rockfield #2L (949) 859-4192
Mission Viejo: 27001 La Paz, Suite 100 (949) 597-1550
THAI DISHES: Fountain Valley: 10065 Garfield Ave. (714) 962-1312

Coupon — *Healthy Dining in Orange County* — Coupon

$1.00 OFF

Pollo Choice Skinless Breast Meal: Flame-grilled skinless chicken breast with fresh vegetables, garden salad and house sal

El Pollo Loco

Over 40 locations in Orange County.
Valid at participating locations.
Not valid with any other offer.
Expires 12/31/05.

Coupon — *Healthy Dining in Orange County* — Coupon

Free Meal

with purchase of one meal of equal or greater value.

Not valid with any other offer.

Ferdussi

Taste of Persia

3605 S. Bristol Street, Santa Ana
(714) 545-9096

Healthy Dining in Orange County

Healthy Dining in Orange County

Healthy Dining in Orange County

Healthy Dining in Orange County

Healthy Dining in Orange County

Coupon | *Healthy Dining in Orange County* | Coupon

Free Meal

with purchase of one meal of equal or greater value.

Maximum $10.00

Not valid with any other offer.

Finbars

Italian Kitchen

Costa Mesa: 901-C South Coast Dr.
(714) 641-3000
Seal Beach: 550 Pacific Coast Highway #111
(562) 430-4303

Coupon | *Healthy Dining in Orange County* | Coupon

20% OFF

Entire Meal

Alcoholic beverages excluded.
Up to 4 in party.
Not valid with any other offer.

Fitness Grill

Brea: 103-A W. Imperial Hwy.
(714) 672-0911

Fitness Pizza

Yorba Linda: 18246 Imperial Hwy.
(714) 993-5421

Coupon | *Healthy Dining in Orange County* | Coupon

20% OFF

Total bill.

Not valid with any other offer.

The Flame Broiler

Costa Mesa: 204 E. 17th St. #103 (949) 650-6939
Orange: 2316 W. Chapman Ave. (714) 938-1156
Fullerton: 1203 E. Chapman Ave. (714) 526-1128
Stanton: 12700 Beach Blvd. (714) 899-1863

Coupon | *Healthy Dining in Orange County* | Coupon

$3.00 OFF

any meal $8.00 or more.

Not valid with any other offer.
PLU 3583

Gelson's Markets

Irvine: 5521 Alton Parkway (949) 551-6093
Dana Point: 24 Monarch Bay Plaza (949) 488-8147
Newport Beach: 1660 San Miguel Dr. (949) 644-8660

Healthy Dining in Orange County | Coupon

Free Entrée

with purchase of one entrée of equal or greater value.

Not valid with any other offer.

Green Parrot Café

2035 North Main Street
Santa Ana, CA 92706
(714) 550-6040

Healthy Dining in Orange County

Healthy Dining in Orange County

Healthy Dining in Orange County

Healthy Dining in Orange County

Healthy Dining in Orange County

Coupon *Healthy Dining in Orange County* Coupon

Free Dinner

with purchase of one dinner of equal or greater value. Maximum $15.00

Valid after 5 pm. Not valid with any other offer.

The Health Emporium

Open 7 days/week 7 am to 10 pm
3347 Pacific Coast Highway
Corona del Mar (949) 673-2244

Coupon *Healthy Dining in Orange County* Coupon

10% OFF

your purchase of $25.00 or more.

PLU #5022 Disct. Amt. ______

Henry's Marketplace

Costa Mesa: 3030 Harbor Blvd.
Laguna Niguel: 27271 La Paz
Mission Viejo: 27765 Santa Margarita Pkwy.
Yorba Linda: 17482 Yorba Linda Blvd.
Call (619) 258-2900 for other locations.

Coupon *Healthy Dining in Orange County* Coupon

Free Entree

with purchase of one entrée of equal or greater value.

Maximum $8.00. Excludes Sunday Brunch. Not valid with any other offer

Ho Sum Bistro

3112 Newport Blvd
Newport Beach, CA 92663
(949) 675-0896

Coupon *Healthy Dining in Orange County* Coupon

Free Meal

with purchase of one meal of equal or greater value. Maximum $8.00

Good Sunday through Thursday. Not valid with any other offer.

il Farro

Caffé Trattoria

111 21st Place
Newport Beach, CA 92663
(949) 723-5711

Coupon *Healthy Dining in Orange County* Coupon

Buy 2 Smoothies and get

$1.00 OFF

No other discounts apply.
One coupon per customer.

Jamba Juice

Orange County locations in Anaheim, Brea, Costa Mesa, Fullerton, Huntington Beach, Irvine, Irvine Spectrum, Laguna Beach, Long Beach, Newport Beach, Orange, Seal Beach, Tustin & Westminster.
Call 1-888-JAMBA12 for the nearest location.

Healthy Dining in Orange County

Healthy Dining in Orange County

Healthy Dining in Orange County

Healthy Dining in Orange County

Healthy Dining in Orange County

Coupon *Healthy Dining in Orange County* Coupon

15% OFF

Entire Meal

Alcoholic beverages excluded.
Up to 4 in party.
Not valid with any other offer.

J T Schmid's

Brewhouse & Eatery

2610 E. Katella Ave.
Anaheim, CA 92806
(714) 634-9200

Coupon *Healthy Dining in Orange County* Coupon

Original Breast Combo for $5.99

Includes one chicken breast, two sides and a regular drink. Juicy and delicious! At less than 1½ g of fat per oz. for the breast portion, you can't beat it for tasteful, healthy dining. Not valid with any other offer.

Koo Koo Roo®

13792 Jamboree Road
Irvine, CA 92612
(714) 508-9900

Coupon *Healthy Dining in Orange County* Coupon

Free Dinner

with purchase of one dinner of equal or greater value. Maximum $10.00.

One coupon per table.
Not value Friday, Saturday, or holidays.
Not valid with any other offer.

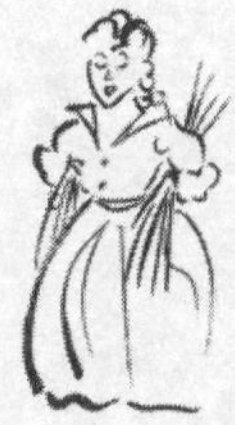

Luciana's Ristorante

24312 Del Prado (PCH)
Dana Point, CA 92629
(949) 661-6500

Coupon *Healthy Dining in Orange County* Coupon

Free Dinner

with purchase of one dinner of equal or greater value. Maximum $10.00.

Not valid with any other offer.

Luigi's D'Italia

801 S. State College, Anaheim
(714) 490-0990

Coupon *Healthy Dining in Orange County* Coupon

20% OFF

Entire Meal

Up to 4 in party.
Not valid with any other offer.

Marrakesh

Moroccan Authentic Cuisine

1976 Newport Blvd.
Costa Mesa, CA 92627
(949) 645-8384

Healthy Dining in Orange County

Healthy Dining in Orange County

Healthy Dining in Orange County

Healthy Dining in Orange County

Healthy Dining in Orange County

Coupon *Healthy Dining in Orange County* Coupon

Free Meal

with purchase of one meal of equal or greater value, any weekday.

Not valid with any other offer.

McCormick & Schmick's

2000 Main Street
Irvine, CA 92614
(949) 756-0505

Coupon *Healthy Dining in Orange County* Coupon

$10.00 Off

with purchase of $50.00 or more for web or phone orders.

Code: HL500

Not valid with any other offer.

Melissa's

World Variety Produce, Inc.
www.melissas.com
(800) 588-0151

Coupon *Healthy Dining in Orange County* Coupon

Free Entree

with purchase of one entrée of equal or greater value, up to $8.00 value.

Not valid with any other offer.

Mother's

Market & Kitchen

Costa Mesa: 225 E. 17th St. (949) 631-4741
Irvine: 2963 Michelson Dr. (949) 752-6667
Huntington Beach: 19770 Beach Blvd. (714) 963-6667
Laguna Woods: 24165 Paseo De Valencia (949) 768-6667

Coupon *Healthy Dining in Orange County* Coupon

$5.00 Off

Second Meal

Buy one meal, get $5.00 off the price of a second meal.

Not valid with any other offer.

Newport Beach Brewing Co.

2920 Newport Blvd.
Newport Beach, CA 92663
(949) 675-8449

Coupon *Healthy Dining in Orange County* Coupon

Free Italian Cream Soda

with purchase of an entree.

Not valid with any other offer.

The Old Spaghetti Factory

Newport Beach: 2110 Newport Blvd.
Fullerton: 110 East Santa Fe Ave.
Riverside: 3191 Mission Inn Ave.
Rancho Cucamonga: 11896 Foothill Blvd.

Healthy Dining in Orange County

Healthy Dining in Orange County

Healthy Dining in Orange County

Healthy Dining in Orange County

Healthy Dining in Orange County

Coupon *Healthy Dining in Orange County* Coupon

$10.00 OFF

with purchase of $40.00 or more.

Not valid with any other offer.

Pane e Vino

240 S. Brea Blvd.
Brea, CA 92821
(714) 256-7779

Coupon *Healthy Dining in Orange County* Coupon

Free Mandarin Garden Side Salad

with fat-free cilantro lime dressing with purchase of any entrée.

Not valid with any other offer.
Valid at participating locations only.

© Pick Up Stix 2004

Pick Up Stix

Please visit
www.pickupstix.com
for locations near you.

IT Code: HDining

Coupon *Healthy Dining in Orange County* Coupon

Free Meal

with purchase of one meal of equal or greater value. Maximum $8.00.

Not valid with any other offer.

Red Rock Chili Co.

Fashion Island, Atrium Court
401 Newport Center Dr. #A106
Newport Beach, CA 92660 (949) 760-0752

Coupon *Healthy Dining in Orange County* Coupon

$3.00 OFF **Extra Large Pizza**
$2.00 OFF **Large Pizza**
$1.00 OFF **Medium Pizza**

Dine-in, carry-out, or delivery. Limited delivery area & hours. Delivery fee may apply. One coupon per pizza. Not valid with any other offer, promotion or discount.

Round Table Pizza

Valid at participating locations in Costa Mesa, Dana Point, Fountain Valley, Huntington Beach, Irvine, Lakewood, Lake Forest, Long Beach, Mission Viejo, Newport Beach & San Clemente.

Coupon *Healthy Dining in Orange County* Coupon

Free Healthy Dining Entrée

with purchase of any other entrée of equal or greater value.

Not valid with any other offer.

Sammy's

18315 Brookhurst Street
Fountain Valley, CA 92708
(714) 593-5800

Healthy Dining in Orange County

Healthy Dining in Orange County

Healthy Dining in Orange County

Healthy Dining in Orange County

Healthy Dining in Orange County

Coupon
#606000

Healthy Dining in Orange County

Coupon
#606000

10% OFF

2 Adult dinners

Valid with coupon only. Not valid with any other offer/discount. Valid for up to 2 adult meals. Beverages, cookies and kids' meals not included. Expires 12/31/05.

Souplantation.

Souplantation locations:

Brea, Costa Mesa, Fountain Valley, Foothill Ranch/Lake Forest, Fullerton, Garden Grove, Irvine, Laguna Niguel, and Tustin.

Coupon

Healthy Dining in Orange County

Coupon

Free Dinner

with your first purchase of $30 or more.

Not valid with any other offer.

SUSAN'S Healthy Gourmet
fresh · delicious · delivered

Susan's Healthy Gourmet

fresh, delicious, delivered

1-888-EZ-MEALS (396-3257)
www.susanshealthygourmet.com

Coupon

Healthy Dining in Orange County

Coupon

Free Combo Meal

with purchase of one combo meal of equal or greater value.

Not valid with any other offer.

THE TACO Company
"REAL MEXICAN FOOD"

The Taco Company

1009 N. Tustin Ave.
Orange, CA
(714) 289-8006

Coupon

Healthy Dining in Orange County

Coupon

Free Meal

with purchase of one meal of equal or greater value. Maximum $8.00

Not valid with any other offer.

Thai Specialty 2
RESTAURANT

Thai Specialty 2

13572 Newport Ave.
Tustin, CA 92780
(714) 731-1711

Coupon

Healthy Dining in Orange County

Coupon

$5.00 OFF

with purchase of $15.00 or more.

Not valid with any other offer.

VIE DE FRANCE

Vie de France

3333 Bristol Ave.
#1420 South Coast Plaza
Costa Mesa, CA 92626
(714) 557-1734

Healthy Dining in Orange County

Healthy Dining in Orange County

Healthy Dining in Orange County

Healthy Dining in Orange County

Healthy Dining in Orange County

Coupon | *Healthy Dining in Orange County* | Coupon

$10.00 OFF

with purchase of
$40.00 or more.

Valid lunch or dinner, seven days.
Not valid with any other offer.

Walt's Wharf

201 Main Street
Seal Beach, CA 90740
(562) 598-4433

Coupon | *Healthy Dining in Orange County* | Coupon

$2.00 OFF

Any Pizza

For up to 4 members in party.
Not valid with any other offer.

Z Pizza

Orange County locations: Aliso Viejo, Belmont Shore, Corona Del Mar, Crystal Cove, Huntington Beach, Laguna Beach, Lake Forest, Newport Beach, San Clemente, Seal Beach, & South Coast Metro. For other locations, please visit www.zpizza.com.

Healthy Dining

See page 192 for special $5.00 discount on additional *Healthy Dining* books!

Healthy Dining in Orange County

Healthy Dining in Orange County

Healthy Dining in Orange County

Healthy Dining in Orange County

Healthy Dining in Orange County

Part VII

Indexes

Restaurant Menu Indexes

Cuisine 216
Location 218
Alphabetical 222

Other Indexes

Health Resource Guide 171
Recipe Index 116

Index by Cuisine

American, Family
The Back Bay Rowing & Running Club 49
Blackboard Bistro 53
Charo Chicken 59
The Gypsy Den 74
Pat & Oscar's 92
Red Rock Chili Co. 94
Ruby's Diner 97
Souplantation 100
Yard House 110

Bakery, Café
Café Heidelberg 57
Café Vienna 57
The Gypsy Den 74
Vie de France 106

California
BeachFire Bar & Grill 52
The Culinary Wrap 61
Fitness Grill 70
Fitness Pizza 70
Green Parrot Café 73
Ho Sum Bistro 76
J. T. Schmid's 78
Koo Koo Roo 80
Newport Beach Brewing Co. 88
Sammy's Woodfired Pizza 98
The Sundried Tomato 101
Z Pizza 111

Chinese
Café Chin Chin 55
California Wok 58
Chin's Chinese Kitchen 60
Diho Siam 63
Ho Sum Bistro 76
Pick Up Stix 93

Deli, Market
Gelson's Market 72
The Health Emporium 75
Henry's Marketplace 179
Mother's Market & Kitchen 87
Whole Foods Market 109

European
Café Heidelberg 57
Café Vienna 57

Fast Casual – see Quick Serve

French
Café de France 56
Pascal Epicerie & Wine 91
Pascal Restaurant 91
Vie de France 106

Greek
Daphne's Greek Café 62

Home Delivery, On-line
Melissa's/World Variety Produce, Inc. 181
Susan's Healthy Gourmet 102

Indian
Royal Khyber 96

Index by Cuisine, continued

Italian
Angie's Cuisine Italiano 48
Finbars Italian Kitchen 67
il Farro Caffe Trattoria 77
Luciana's Ristorante 82
Luigi's D'Italia 83
The Old Spaghetti Factory 89
Pane e Vino Trattoria 90

Juice Bar
Jamba Juice 79

Korean
The Flame Broiler 71

Mediterranean
Fitness Grill 70
Fitness Pizza 70

Mexican, Southwest
Acapulco 47
Baja Fresh Mexican Grill 50
El Pollo Loco 64
El Torito 65
La Salsa 81
Taco Bell 103
The Taco Company 104
Wahoo's Fish Taco 107

Moroccan
Marrakesh 84

Persian
Ferdussi Taste of Persia 66

Pizza
Fitness Grill 70
Fitness Pizza 70
Round Table Pizza 95
Sammy's Woodfired Pizza 98
Z Pizza 111

Quick Serve, Fast Casual
Baja Fresh Mexican Grill 50
Café Chin Chin 55
Charo Chicken 59
The Culinary Wrap 61
El Pollo Loco 64
The Flame Broiler 71
Jamba Juice 79
Koo Koo Roo 80
La Salsa 81
Pick Up Stix 93
Taco Bell 103
The Taco Company 104
Wahoo's Fish Taco 107

Seafood
The Beach House 51
Bluewater Grill 54
The Fish Market 68
The Fisherman's Restaurant 69
McCormick & Schmick's 85
McKenna's on the Bay 86
Santa Monica Seafood 99
Walt's Wharf 108

Thai
California Wok 58
Diho Siam 63
Thai Dishes 63
Thai Specialty 2 105

Vegetarian, Natural
The Gypsy Den 74
The Health Emporium 75
Henry's Marketplace 179
Melissa's/World Variety Produce, Inc. 181
Mother's Market & Kitchen 87
Whole Foods Market 109

Index by Location

Aliso Viejo – see Laguna Hills

Anaheim
El Pollo Loco 64
El Torito 65
J. T. Schmid's 78
Jamba Juice 79
Luigi's D'Italia 83
Susan's Healthy Gourmet 102
Taco Bell 103

Anaheim Hills
Baja Fresh Mexican Grill 50
Susan's Healthy Gourmet 102
Taco Bell 103

Brea
Baja Fresh Mexican Grill 50
The Culinary Wrap 61
Daphne's Greek Café 62
El Pollo Loco 64
Fitness Grill 70
Jamba Juice 79
Pane e Vino Trattoria 90
Pick Up Stix 93
Souplantation 100
Susan's Healthy Gourmet 102
Taco Bell 103

Buena Park, Cypress
Baja Fresh Mexican Grill 50
Charo Chicken 59
El Pollo Loco 64
El Torito 65
Pat & Oscar's 92
Susan's Healthy Gourmet 102
Taco Bell 103

Corona del Mar – see Newport Beach

Costa Mesa
Acapulco 47
The Back Bay Rowing & Running Club 49
Baja Fresh Mexican Grill 50
Charo Chicken 59
The Culinary Wrap 61
Daphne's Greek Café 62
Diho Siam 63
El Pollo Loco 64
The Flame Broiler 71
Finbars Italian Kitchen 67
The Gypsy Den 74
Henry's Marketplace 179
Jamba Juice 79
Marrakesh 84
Mother's Market & Kitchen 87
Pick Up Stix 93
Round Table Pizza 95
Ruby's Diner 97
Santa Monica Seafood 99
Souplantation 100
Susan's Healthy Gourmet 102
Taco Bell 103
Vie de France 106
Wahoo's Fish Taco 107
Yard House 110

Cypress – see Buena Park

Dana Point
The Beach House 51
Charo Chicken 59
El Pollo Loco 64
El Torito 65
Gelson's Market 72
Luciana's Ristorante 82
Pick Up Stix 93
Round Table Pizza 95
Ruby's Diner 97
Susan's Healthy Gourmet 102
Taco Bell 103

El Toro – see Lake Forest

Index by Location, continued

Foothill Ranch – see Lake Forest

Fountain Valley
Pick Up Stix 93
Round Table Pizza 95
Sammy's Woodfired Pizza 98
Souplantation 100
Susan's Healthy Gourmet 102
Taco Bell 103
Thai Dishes 63

Fullerton, Placentia
Daphne's Greek Café 62
El Pollo Loco 64
El Torito 65
The Flame Broiler 71
Jamba Juice 79
The Old Spaghetti Factory 89
Pick Up Stix 93
Ruby's Diner 97
Souplantation 100
Susan's Healthy Gourmet 102
Taco Bell 103
Wahoo's Fish Taco 107

Garden Grove, Stanton, Westminster
Acapulco 47
El Pollo Loco 64
El Torito 65
The Flame Broiler 71
Jamba Juice 79
Souplantation 100
Susan's Healthy Gourmet 102
Taco Bell 103

Huntington Beach
Baja Fresh Mexican Grill 50
Charo Chicken 59
El Pollo Loco 64
Jamba Juice 79
Mother's Market & Kitchen 87
Pick Up Stix 93
Round Table Pizza 95
Ruby's Diner 97
Susan's Healthy Gourmet 102
Taco Bell 103
Wahoo's Fish Taco 107
Z Pizza 111

Irvine
Baja Fresh Mexican Grill 50
Café de France 56
Charo Chicken 59
Daphne's Greek Café 62
El Pollo Loco 64
El Torito 65
The Fish Market 68
Gelson's Market 72
Jamba Juice 79
Koo Koo Roo 80
La Salsa 81
McCormick & Schmick's 85
Mother's Market & Kitchen 87
Pat & Oscar's 92
Pick Up Stix 93
Round Table Pizza 95
Ruby's Diner 97
Souplantation 100
Susan's Healthy Gourmet 102
Taco Bell 103
Wahoo's Fish Taco 107
Yard House 110

La Habra, La Mirada
Baja Fresh Mexican Grill 50
Daphne's Greek Café 62
El Pollo Loco 64
Susan's Healthy Gourmet 102
Taco Bell 103

Laguna Beach
The Beach House 51
Café Heidelberg 57
Café Vienna 57
Jamba Juice 79
Ruby's Diner 97
The Sundried Tomato 101
Susan's Healthy Gourmet 102
Taco Bell 103
Wahoo's Fish Taco 107
Z Pizza 111

Index by Location, continued

Laguna Hills, Laguna Woods, Aliso Viejo
Baja Fresh Mexican Grill 50
Daphne's Greek Café 62
El Pollo Loco 64
El Torito 65
La Salsa 81
Mother's Market & Kitchen 87
Ruby's Diner 97
Susan's Healthy Gourmet 102
Wahoo's Fish Taco 107
Z Pizza 111

Laguna Niguel
Acapulco 47
Baja Fresh Mexican Grill 50
El Pollo Loco 64
Henry's Marketplace 179
Pick Up Stix 93
Souplantation 100
Susan's Healthy Gourmet 102
Taco Bell 103

Laguna Woods – see Laguna Hills

Lake Forest, El Toro, Foothill Ranch
Baja Fresh Mexican Grill 50
Charo Chicken 59
Daphne's Greek Café 62
Diho Siam 63
El Pollo Loco 64
Pat & Oscar's 92
Pick Up Stix 93
Round Table Pizza 95
Souplantation 100
Susan's Healthy Gourmet 102
Taco Bell 103
Wahoo's Fish Taco 107
Z Pizza 111

Long Beach, Lakewood
Acapulco 47
Café Chin Chin 55
Charo Chicken 59
The Culinary Wrap 61
Daphne's Greek Café 62
El Pollo Loco 64
Jamba Juice 79
McKenna's on the Bay 86
Round Table Pizza 95
Susan's Healthy Gourmet 102
Taco Bell 103
Z Pizza 111

Los Alamitos – see Seal Beach

Mission Viejo
Baja Fresh Mexican Grill 50
El Pollo Loco 64
Diho Siam 63
Henry's Marketplace 179
Pick Up Stix 93
Round Table Pizza 95
Ruby's Diner 97
Susan's Healthy Gourmet 102
Taco Bell 103

Newport Beach, Balboa, Corona del Mar
Baja Fresh Mexican Grill 50
Bluewater Grill 54
Daphne's Greek Café 62
El Pollo Loco 64
Gelson's Market 72
The Health Emporium 75
Ho Sum Bistro 76
il Farro Caffe Trattoria 77
Jamba Juice 79
La Salsa 81
Newport Beach Brewing Co. 88
The Old Spaghetti Factory 89
Pascal Epicerie & Wine 91
Pascal Restaurant 91
Pick Up Stix 93
Red Rock Chili Co. 94
Round Table Pizza 95
Ruby's Diner 97
Susan's Healthy Gourmet 102
Taco Bell 103
Wahoo's Fish Taco 107
Z Pizza 111

Orange
Acapulco 47
El Pollo Loco 64
El Torito 65
The Flame Broiler 71
Jamba Juice 79
Pat & Oscar's 92
Santa Monica Seafood 99
Susan's Healthy Gourmet 102
Taco Bell 103
The Taco Company 104

Index by Location, continued

Placentia – see Yorba Linda

Rancho Santa Margarita
Baja Fresh Mexican Grill 50
Daphne's Greek Café 62
El Pollo Loco 64
Pick Up Stix 93
Ruby's Diner 97
Susan's Healthy Gourmet 102
Taco Bell 103

San Clemente
Baja Fresh Mexican Grill 50
BeachFire Bar & Grill 52
Charo Chicken 59
Daphne's Greek Café 62
El Pollo Loco 64
The Fisherman's Restaurant 69
Pick Up Stix 93
Round Table Pizza 95
Susan's Healthy Gourmet 102
Taco Bell 103
Wahoo's Fish Taco 107
Z Pizza 111

San Juan Capistrano
El Pollo Loco 64
Ruby's Diner 97
The Sundried Tomato 101
Susan's Healthy Gourmet 102
Taco Bell 103

Santa Ana
Acapulco 47
Baja Fresh Mexican Grill 50
Bluewater Grill 54
Daphne's Greek Café 62
El Pollo Loco 64
Ferdussi Taste of Persia 66
Green Parrot Café 73
The Gypsy Den 74
Pick Up Stix 93
Royal Khyber 96
Susan's Healthy Gourmet 102
Taco Bell 103
Z Pizza 111

Seal Beach, Los Alamitos
Baja Fresh Mexican Grill 50
Blackboard Bistro 53
California Wok 58
Charo Chicken 59
Daphne's Greek Café 62
El Pollo Loco 64
Finbars Italian Kitchen 67
Jamba Juice 79
Pick Up Stix 93
Ruby's Diner 97
Susan's Healthy Gourmet 102
Taco Bell 103
Walt's Wharf 108
Z Pizza 111

Stanton – see Garden Grove

Tustin
Angie's Cuisine Italiano 48
Café Chin Chin 55
Charo Chicken 59
Chin's Chinese Kitchen 60
Daphne's Greek Café 62
El Pollo Loco 64
El Torito 65
Jamba Juice 79
La Salsa 81
Pick Up Stix 93
Ruby's Diner 97
Souplantation 100
Susan's Healthy Gourmet 102
Taco Bell 103
Thai Specialty 2 105
Wahoo's Fish Taco 107
Whole Foods Market 109

Westminster – see Garden Grove

Yorba Linda, Placentia
El Pollo Loco 64
El Torito 65
Fitness Pizza 70
Henry's Marketplace 179
Pick Up Stix 93
Ruby's Diner 97
Susan's Healthy Gourmet 102
Taco Bell 103
Wahoo's Fish Taco 107

Alphabetical Index

Acapulco 47
Angie's Cuisine Italiano 48
The Back Bay Rowing & Running Club 49
Baja Fresh Mexican Grill 50
The Beach House 51
BeachFire Bar & Grill 52
Blackboard Bistro 53
Bluewater Grill 54
Café Chin Chin 55
Café de France 56
Café Heidelberg 57
Café Vienna 57
California Wok 58
Charo Chicken 59
Chin's Chinese Kitchen 60
The Culinary Wrap 61
Daphne's Greek Café 62
Diho Siam 63
El Pollo Loco 64
El Torito 65
Ferdussi Taste of Persia 66
Finbars Italian Kitchen 67
The Fish Market 68
The Fisherman's Restaurant 69
Fitness Grill 70
Fitness Pizza 70
The Flame Broiler 71
Gelson's Market 72
Green Parrot Café 73
The Gypsy Den 74
The Health Emporium 75
Henry's Marketplace 179
Ho Sum Bistro 76
il Farro Caffe Trattoria 77
J.T. Schmid's 78
Jamba Juice 79
Koo Koo Roo 80
La Salsa 81
Luciana's Ristorante 82
Luigi's D'Italia 83
Marrakesh 84
McCormick & Schmick's 85
McKenna's on the Bay 86
Melissa's/World Variety Produce, Inc. 181
Mother's Market & Kitchen 87
Newport Beach Brewing Co. 88
The Old Spaghetti Factory 89
Pane e Vino Trattoria 90
Pascal Epicerie & Wine 91
Pascal Restaurant 91
Pat & Oscar's 92
Pick Up Stix 93
Red Rock Chili Co. 94
Round Table Pizza 95
Royal Khyber 96
Ruby's Diner 97
Sammy's Woodfired Pizza 98
Santa Monica Seafood 99
Souplantation 100
The Sundried Tomato 101
Susan's Healthy Gourmet 102
Taco Bell 103
The Taco Company 104
Thai Dishes 63
Thai Specialty 2 105
Vie de France 106
Wahoo's Fish Taco 107
Walt's Wharf 108
Whole Foods Market 109
Yard House 110
Z Pizza 111